Geriatric

PHARMACOTHERAPY

A GUIDE FOR THE HELPING PROFESSIONAL

Notices

Geriatric
PHARMACOTHERAPY
A GUIDE FOR THE HELPING PROFESSIONAL

CYNTHIA G. OLSEN

WILLIAM N. TINDALL

MARK E. CLASEN

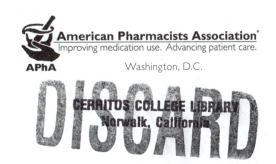

American Pharmacists Association®
Improving medication use. Advancing patient care.
APhA

Washington, D.C.

Managing Editor: L. Luan Corrigan
Acquiring Editor: Sandra J. Cannon
Indexer: Lillian R. Rodberg
Book Design and Layout: Roy A. Barnhill
Cover Design: Scott Neitzke

© 2007 by the American Pharmacists Association
APhA was founded in 1852 as the American Pharmaceutical Association.

Published by the American Pharmacists Association
1100 15th Street, NW, Suite 400
Washington, DC 20005-1707
www.aphanet.org

To comment on this book via e-mail, send your message to the publisher at aphabooks@aphanet.org.

Library of Congress Cataloging-in-Publication Data

Geriatric pharmacotherapy : a guide for the helping professional /
  [edited by] Cynthia G. Olsen, William N. Tindall, Mark E. Clasen.
    p. ; cm.
    Includes bibliographical references and index.
    ISBN-13: 978-1-58212-072-0
    ISBN-10: 1-58212-072-2
    1. Geriatric pharmacology. 2. Older people--Drug use.
  I. Olsen, Cynthia G. II. Tindall, William N. III. Clasen, Mark E.
  IV. American Pharmacists Association.
    [DNLM: 1. Drug Therapy--methods. 2. Aged.   WT 166 G3694
  2007]
    RC953.7.G469 2007
    615.5'80846--dc22   2006026846

How to Order This Book
Online: www.pharmacist.com
By phone: 800-878-0729
VISA®, MasterCard®, and American Express® cards accepted

*Dedicated to the memory of Alan C. McKelvey (1958–2006),
a very special pharmacist who was a blessing to so many**

---

* Alan C. McKelvey authored Chapter 12, "Natural Medicines Used by the Elderly:
A Common Sense Dose of Reality."

Contents

7 Issues in Geriatric Dermatology   137

ALICE A. HOUSE

8 Dealing with the Dread of Dementia and Alzheimer's Disease   163

KATHY KEMLE AND JONIE FAWLEY

9 Diagnosis and Treatment of Depression in the Geriatric Population   177

DIPESH PATEL AND JOHN M. BOLTRI

Foreword

If only old age did not come with its burden of chronic diseases and vexing symptoms. If only old age did not require medicines to prevent, treat, and control those diseases and symptoms. If only old age did not alter our physiology so that both the dynamics and kinetics of medications are changed. If only the health professionals who prescribe, dispense, administer, and observe the effects of medicine knew all they needed to know to prescribe optimally and to manage therapeutics optimally; then and only then, would we be able to help with avoiding preventable and terrible side effects that often harm elderly patients.

What the typical health professional does not know about the special nature of medication use in the elderly could fill a book; fortunately, what we do know can fill several. Such was not the case a generation ago when the best we could say were generalizations such as, "Start low and go slow," or "Avoid polypharmacy." Such admonitions meant well but provided scant guidance to a clinician. Beginning with pioneering research in the 1980s (largely supported by The John A. Hartford Foundation), we began to learn about how age-related physiological changes alter the effects of medications and which types of medications most commonly used cause side effects in the elderly. We learned more about the mechanisms of medication toxicity and that information led pharmaceutical companies to develop safer medications and determine the safest dosages for the elderly. At the beginning of the 1980s, a very small cadre of academics could claim to be expert in the area of geriatric pharmacotherapy, especially after several fellowships were established (primarily by the pharmaceutical industry) to ensure that the

United States would have the experts it needed to provide leading research in the field. Today, that expertise benefits the entire world with knowledge in the use of medications in the elderly. Research on drug use in the elderly is a robust activity today as drug developers, academic institutions, and public agencies pay special attention to the effects of the aging process on the use of drugs. Leaders in the field of geriatric pharmacology lecture frequently and, fortunately, write books. Books—whether printed or distributed in electronic format—remain the most efficient way to distribute this collective knowledge to the broadest public in a way that can change prescribing and drug therapy management behavior. I for one am indebted to the authors of this volume for sharing their knowledge; in turn and in fair recompense, I urge all helping professionals to commit to applying this shared knowledge at every opportunity.

What then is the content of the collective knowledge on how to optimize the use of medications in the elderly? That content is not restricted to the traditional parameters of pharmacology. It includes information on epidemiology, access to care, and communication. Lack of sufficient knowledge in any one area becomes the weakest link, undermining the strength of the chain.

In this book, my colleagues provide an overview of these topics. Together, the chapters in this book provide the underpinning for a process. That process has three critical components:

- First, a health practitioner must have adequate knowledge about any drug being considered for the elderly. He or she must understand the pharmacology of the chosen medication and the medications not chosen. It is through such a comparison that a clinician can determine if there has been optimal prescribing.
- Second, the health practitioner must know the patient and be able to answer questions such as: What co-morbid conditions might alter the choice of medications? What personality or familial factors might make it difficult for the patient to follow recommendations? Are there circumstances that might impede the patient's filling the prescription in the first place or adhering to instructions?
- Third, because elderly people differ one from another more substantially than any other cohort, the health practitioner must remain vigilant and work as an advocate on behalf of his/her geriatric population. Experience gained with dozens of older patients on any medication can be turned upside down when, in another, the response is markedly different. Thus, helping health professionals must always

remain vigilant and suspicious, and must continuously monitor drug therapy with a bent toward a willingness to change drugs and directions for their use at any time. Finally, because clinicians are often quite paternalistic and too often are eager to prescribe, dispense, or administer drugs, they are often reluctant to adjust or discontinue a medication and can contribute to a patient's nonadherent behavior.

Medications provide the most powerful and useful interventions for the care of older people. We have developed medications to help many older people prevent, control, and cure disease and troubling symptoms. But, primo no nocere: The changes of aging and the enormous formulary of available drugs complicate the choices of medications used in the elderly. There is no such thing as prescribing without risk. But, working together as a team, helping health professionals can do far more than what they are currently doing to maximize effects and minimize side effects. This book, *Geriatric Pharmacotherapy, A Guide for the Helping Professional,* provides a starting point for those who want to reconnect with why they became health professionals and hopefully can serve to further empower them to redouble their commitment to the goal of helping the elderly get the best use of their medicines.

Mark H. Beers, MD
Editor-in-Chief, The Merck Manuals

Preface

This book was written as a guide for health professionals who want to provide help for the elderly who too often are forgotten or go unseen by their younger health professionals and caregivers. Although the poem that follows was written to nurses, its poignant message applies to all health professionals. It was written by an elderly woman after she was admitted to a geriatric ward of a small hospital near Dundee, Scotland. This simple but elegant poem encourages us all to look at the aging as hungry for a much different kind of care from taking one more pill. This is the lament of an elderly woman in a nursing home.

What do you see, nurses?
What do you see?
What are you thinking,
When you're looking at me?

A crabby old woman,
Not very wise,
Uncertain of habit,
With faraway eyes.

Who dribbles her food,
And makes no reply,
When you say in a loud voice,
"I do wish you'd try!"

Who seems not to notice,
The things that you do,
And forever is losing
A stocking or shoe.

Who, resisting or not,
Lets you do as you will,
With bathing and feeding,
The long day to fill.

Is that what you're thinking?
Is that what you see?
Then open your eyes, nurse,
You're not looking at me.

I'll tell you who I am,
As I sit here so still,
As I do at your bidding,
As I eat at your will.

I'm a small child of ten,
With a father and mother,
Brothers and sisters,
Who love one another.

A young girl of sixteen,
With wings on her feet,
Dreaming that soon now,
A lover she'll meet.

A bride soon at twenty,
My heart gives a leap,
As I make the vows
That I promised to keep.

At twenty-five now
I have young of my own,
Who need me to guide them
In a secure happy home.

A women of thirty
My young now grow fast
Bound to each other
With ties that should last.

At forty my young sons
Are grown and now gone,
But my man is besides me
To make sure I don't mourn.

At fifty once more,
Babies play round my knee,
Again we know children
My loved one and me.

Dark days are upon me
My husband is dead,
I look at the future,
I shudder with dread.

For my young are all rearing
Young of their own,
And I think of the years
And the love I have known.

For I am now an old woman
And nature is cruel,
'tis jest to make old age
Look like a fool.

The body it crumbles,
Grace and vigor depart,
There now is a stone
Where I once had a heart.

But inside this carcass
A young girl still dwells,
And now and again
My battered heart swells

As I remember the joys
As I remember the pain,
And I am loving and living
Life all over again.

Contributing Authors

Robert J. Belloto, PhD, RPh, CGP, FASCP, is a Fellow of the American Society of Consultant Pharmacists and a Certified Geriatric Pharmacist consulting for Continuum Care Pharmacy in Middletown, Ohio. Dr. Belloto received his pharmacy training at The Ohio State University College of Pharmacy, where he also received the MS and PhD degrees in the areas of pharmaceutics, pharmaceutical chemistry, and pharmacokinetics. He has completed certification programs in anticoagulation therapy and lipid management and is also a staff pharmacist at Good Samaritan Hospital in Dayton, Ohio. Dr. Belloto has more than 11 years of experience serving as a consultant pharmacist for numerous nursing home facilities. His work as an expert in pharmacokinetics has allowed him to present expert testimony in court cases. He also serves as an editorial adviser to *Annals of Pharmacotherapy.*

John M. Boltri, MD, is Professor of Family Medicine at Mercer University School of Medicine. He graduated from The Ohio State University School of Medicine and completed his residency training in Family Medicine at Akron City Hospital. He completed his fellowship training at the McLennan County Research and Education Foundation Faculty Development Center of Texas. He currently serves as Vice Chair for Faculty Development in the Department of Family Medicine and Associate Director of the Family Medicine Residency Program at the Medical Center of Central Georgia.

Mark E. Clasen, MD, PhD, is currently Professor and Chair of the Department of Family Medicine at Wright State University Boonshoft School of Medicine in Dayton, Ohio. He is also Vice President of Wright State Physicians, Inc., and the Medical Director of the Kettering College of Medical Arts. Dr. Clasen is listed in *Best Doctors in America* and has been principal investigator on numerous grants and contracts based on his interest in cardiovascular risk reduction and geriatrics. He serves as an adviser to a special program, Frail and Elderly People of Dayton, as well as Associate Medical Director of Hospice of Dayton. He is board certified in geriatrics. A proud native of Minnesota, he earned his MD and PhD from the University of Mississippi.

Y. Monique Davis-Smith, MD, is an Assistant Professor of Family Medicine at Mercer University School of Medicine. She graduated from Wayne State University School of Medicine and completed her residency training in Family Medicine at Southwest Georgia Residency, Phoebe Putney Memorial Hospital. Currently, Dr. Davis-Smith serves as Associate Director of the Family Medicine Residency Program at the Medical Center of Central Georgia and is a member of the Research Division of the Family Medicine Department.

Jonie Fawley, PA-C, is a Physician Assistant who has served on the staff of the Yellow Springs Family Medicine Clinic in Yellow Springs, Ohio. She has served there since graduating in 2001 from the Kettering College of Medical Arts. She provides geriatric medical services to three nursing homes (Friends Care Nursing Home, Hospitality House, and Greene Oaks Nursing Home). Her undergraduate degree, a BS Ed, was earned in 1986 at The Ohio State University. She is also an adjunct faculty member of the Wright State University Department of Family Medicine, where she provides primary care instruction for undergraduate medical students. She is highly recognized for her elder care programs and especially for bringing to the area's elderly the yellow labrador "therapy dog" called Zolti.

Kristina L. Griffiths, PharmD, is a graduate of the Doctor of Pharmacy Program at Ohio Northern University in Ada, Ohio. She has several years of experience in community pharmacy and is now completing a pharmacy residency program. She has completed a clerkship in geriatric pharmacy at the Yellow Springs Family Health Center of Wright State University.

Paul J. Hershberger, PhD, is Professor of Family Medicine at Wright State University. He is a PhD psychologist and sees patients through the Good Samaritan Family Medicine Center of Wright State University and the Veterans Administration Hospital in Dayton, Ohio. A native of Ohio, he has also served as a Methodist pastor.

Alice A. House, MD, FAAFP, CMD, is a Fellow of the American Academy of Family Physicians, an Assistant Professor of Family Medicine at Mercer University School of Medicine, the Medical Director of a nursing home, and a Certified Medical Director with the American Medical Directors Association. Dr. House received her medical training at Mercer University School of Medicine and completed a Family Medicine residency at the Medical Center of Central Georgia.

Kathy Kemle, PA-C, is an Assistant Professor in the Division of Geriatrics within the Department of Family Medicine at Mercer University School of Medicine and the Medical Center of Central Georgia. She completed her physician assistant studies at the University of Texas Southwestern Medical School in Dallas, Texas, and her master's degree in clinical gerontology at the University of Texas Medical Branch in Galveston, Texas.

Karen Kovach, PhD, is Assistant Professor in the Department of Family Medicine and Director of the Biomedical Ethics Program at Mercer University School of Medicine. She received her doctorate in moral philosophy from the Graduate School of the City University of New York and fellowship training in bioethics at the Mount Sinai School of Medicine in New York City.

Alan C. McKelvey, RPh, is the pharmacist-in-charge of the Fred A. White Outpatient Pharmacy on the campus of Wright State University. He has been in charge of this pharmacy since 1982. In addition, he continues to work two weekends per month in a community pharmacy. As a community pharmacist, he publishes a newsletter featuring his passionate writing efforts to bring to the public accurate and helpful information on nonprescription and natural medicines. Pharmacist McKelvey is a graduate of the Ohio Northern University Raabe College of Pharmacy in Ada, Ohio. He is a certified smoking cessation program facilitator for the American Lung Association and is certified as a diabetes educator for Walgreens.

Cynthia G. Olsen, MD, is a 1985 graduate of Wright State University's School of Medicine and currently serves as Professor and Executive Vice Chair of the Department of Family Medicine. Dr. Olsen is also the Medical Director of Yellow Springs Family Health Center and two care facilities for the elderly, Friends Care Center in Yellow Springs and Hospitality Homes in Xenia, Ohio. In addition to her Board Certification in Family Practice, Dr. Olsen is a Certified Medical Director and holds a Certificate of Added Qualifications in Geriatric Medicine, an area in which she is well known and to which she is strongly committed, resulting in her often being sought out for her expertise. Other areas of clinical expertise for Dr. Olsen are the medical care of adults with mental retardation/developmental disabilities and the primary care of women. Dr. Olsen holds membership in the American Association of Family Practice, the American Medical Society, the American Geriatrics Society, the Academy of Family Practice, the Society of Teachers in Family Medicine, and the American Medical Directors Association.

Dipesh Patel, MD, is Assistant Professor of Family Medicine at Mercer University School of Medicine. He received his medical school training at B. J. Medical College, New Civil Hospital School of Medicine, and his family medicine residency training at the Medical Center of Central Georgia. He subsequently completed a Fellowship in Geriatrics at Emory University School of Medicine. Dr. Patel is currently involved in the development of a geriatric medicine fellowship program at Mercer University School of Medicine.

William N. Tindall, RPh, PhD, is Professor of Family Medicine at the Wright State University Boonshoft School of Medicine in Dayton, Ohio, where he teaches pharmacology to physician assistants and oversees the Alliance for Research in Community Health. Prior to joining Wright State University's medical school in 2002, he served for 18 years in the Washington, D.C., area as an association executive for two pharmacy associations and one physicians' association. He earned his BS in Pharmacy from the University of Saskatchewan, his MS from Long Island University, and his PhD from the University of Pittsburgh. He has served on the faculty of Creighton University, the University of Rhode Island, and Ferris State College. He is author or coauthor of six books and has published extensively in matters affecting pharmacy practice.

Philip S. Whitecar, MD, is Associate Professor in the Department of Family Medicine at Wright State University School of Medicine, Dayton, Ohio. He also serves as Associate Program Director for the Dayton Community Family Practice Residency Program and Director of Family Medicine Education at Kettering (Ohio) Medical Center. Dr. Whitecar received his medical degree from the University of Illinois College of Medicine, Urbana-Champaign, and completed a family practice residency at the University of Missouri–Columbia School of Medicine. He practices medicine at the Indian Ripple Family Medicine Center in Kettering, Ohio, and is recognized for his expertise in treating chronic pain.

1

Medication Needs of the Ambulatory Elderly

WILLIAM N. TINDALL AND MARK E. CLASEN

It is not enough for a great nation merely to have added new years to life—our objective must also be to add life to those years.

—**John F. Kennedy**

OVERVIEW

Aging is a process that is hard to stop. While modern medicines may help stretch the process, such medications must be administered appropriately by professionals who understand the unique needs of the elderly. This chapter presents a practical overview of why the elderly need sound medication management and why health professionals must be consistently and constantly aware of the diseases and physiological changes that occur in the elderly and that alter drug effects. The elderly are in special need of management because medications often are overutilized and/or inappropriately prescribed for this vulnerable group. In addition, a high rate of adverse drug reactions (ADRs) occurs in this susceptible population. Medication management interventions are required to address issues surrounding drug interactions that may cause or increase mental confusion, sedation, and urinary retention, to evaluate medication usage, and to monitor effectiveness and side effects.

However, initially health professionals must consider polypharmacy as a plausible cause of any new symptom. Many opportunities exist for health professionals to assist the elderly with their medication needs when helpful relationships are developed with such patients.

Mary Todd is normally a cheerful 82-year-old. She is witty and articulate and describes herself as "being nothing more than middle-aged but with a touch of arthritis in one hip." She walks with a cane, and her manner of dress causes most people to assess her as lower class or poor. One day, looking unusually disheveled, she goes into a pharmacy and stops by the pain control center. As she tries hard to read the fine print on a bottle of Advil®, the pharmacist notices her, walks up behind her, and says in a gruff and loud voice, "What's the matter; can't you read the label?" Startled, Mary grimaces, turns, and says, "What in heck are you shouting at me for? You darn fool; you scared me half to death. I should whack you with my cane. I am here because I've used up the last of that arthritis drug that was just pulled off the market, and now I need something to replace it. My hip is killing me. How do I know I can trust your advice?"

- What is going on here?
- What is it about Mary that the pharmacist should have assessed before approaching her?
- How could the pharmacist have approached Mary in a manner that indicates he has a good understanding of her needs?

UNDERSTANDING MEDICATION NEEDS DUE TO AGING

Once a person matures, the body begins its long slow process through a series of either very noticeable changes or very subtle changes. Hopefully, the longer these changes take place over time, the better it is. Thus, aging is an inevitable event and is deemed "a progressive degeneration of biological function that is universal among all living organisms." Some scientists believe it is caused by the manifestations of a preprogrammed internal clock that determines life span. Others believe aging stems from a slow, progressive accumulation of metabolic damage, and still others believe aging is caused by the generation of free oxygen radicals, which, once inside cells, accelerate the aging process.

Whatever the premise, theory, or evidence about aging, it is commonly accepted among researchers and clinicians that aging is a multifaceted process within which the inherited aspects of one's life account for 35% of its variance, while 65% is accounted for by enhanced metabolic capacity and an increased ability to respond to stress.[1] What would be more helpful is for health professionals to consider two general categories of aging: healthy older adults (successful aging) or the frail elderly (less successful aging). Health professionals can help the elderly in both of these categories maximize their independence; research shows that many elderly persons, even if in a state of dependency, find satisfaction and meaning, including moments of vivid alertness, through intimacy with family members and spiritual revival.[2]

However the aging process occurs, it affects everyone and does so in such a way as to elicit changes in sensory functions, intellectual ability, and memory and changes that limit activity and/or affect overall health. Or as it is often said, aging brings changes that reduce one's quality of life. Thus, if aging is the sum total of all physiological changes that occur with the passage of time, it presents opportunities for physicians, pharmacists, nurses, and other health care professionals to work together to improve the health-related quality of life for the elderly.

In many elderly persons, the manifestations of aging have become intertwined and so complex that they are difficult to manage, especially by any one health professional working alone. Thus, a "team" approach is fast becoming a necessity for improving health among the elderly. In 1956, Dr. Louis Lasagna summarized the then state of knowledge of how drug effects are modified by aging and concluded that, "What is obviously required is a good deal more work and a good deal less talk."[3]

During the five decades since Dr. Lasagna's comment, a good deal more work has been done and much of it supports the necessity of having multidisciplinary teams tackle this issue. Today, it is commonplace to see teams of health professionals, such as physicians, pharmacists, nurses, physiotherapists, and others develop and deliver programs for the elderly. Their work results in improved mobility, improved mental health status, reduced incidence of depression, and better management of medication therapy so that the elderly can function more independently. Those who take the time to better understand the elderly and their needs know that this group presents complexities. Such complexities mean that the elderly should not be given pill upon pill as the only means of returning to good health. In fact, taking too many drugs is often the culprit behind a declining quality of life for many elderly patients. Thus, it behooves those entrusted with care of the elderly to answer questions such as:

- How does aging affect elderly patients and how they function?
- How do physiological changes affect drug dosing?
- How do drug-related problems occur when health system elements fail the elderly?
- How do the elderly lose out on access to care and insurance programs and fall victim to health disparities because of stereotyping and other noncaring attitudes?

C. Everett Koop, MD, former U.S. Surgeon General, once wrote, "All the demographic, social, political, and biomedical indicators tell us the single most significant change in the character of American society is the growth of that segment of our population that is over the age of 65."[4] Twenty years after he made that remark, the United States had 35 million people or 13% of its population classified as "over 65 years of age." That number continues to grow and today that age group consumes nearly one-third of all prescriptions and 40% of nonprescription remedies.[5] From a demographic point of view, those who are between the ages of 65 and 74 are significantly different from those who are more than 85 years of age. This is true also when comparing those who live in nursing homes and other care facilities to those living in their own homes or with families. In fact, only about 10% of the elderly live in institutions, which means 90% are residing in communities throughout the nation, suggesting that health care professionals have many opportunities to help them.

The latest U.S. census predicts that the percentage of the U.S. population over 65 will grow by 1%–3% per year. If this occurs, by 2030, one in five persons in this country will be over 65. In addition, the "over 85" population is expected to grow so that by 2050 nearly 850,000 persons in the United States will be more than 100 years of age.[6] The social composition of American seniors is also expected to shift by 2050. White elders will decline to become two-thirds of the total elderly, down from 85% in 2000, and at the same time Hispanic and African-American elders will grow in numbers and percentages. The main reason the number of elderly is increasing in the United States is because life expectancy has increased from less than 50 years at the beginning of the 20th century to more than 76 years at the beginning of the 21st century, causing the number of elderly to double since 1960.[7] Because life expectancy is increasing, health professionals can anticipate that their daily activities will include interactions and interventions with more persons who have geriatric concerns brought about by chronic conditions such as cardiovascular disease and diabetes.[8]

Finally, although many elderly couples live in communities and enjoy their independence, it is likely that, as they age, one of them will end up living alone. This scenario should cause caregiving professionals to ask, "How do we balance our services, our programs, and our collaborating so that we work together to help the elderly continue to live independently?"

WHAT KEEPS THE ELDERLY FROM LIVING INDEPENDENTLY?

Eventually many elderly succumb to one or more chronic conditions impairing their ability to live independently, which may eventually drive them from their community homes. The list of chronic conditions that limit or impair the elderly has changed very little over the past two decades; the most common of these chronic conditions are shown in Table 1.[9]

It is these chronic conditions, with their ability to impair, that make the elderly America's biggest consumers of health resources, medical interventions, and medication, both prescription and nonprescription. But the prevalence of these chronic conditions has caused many health professionals to rethink their clinical skills and services and develop new ones to help stem the flood of elderly into the health care system and better manage chronic issues. In the past few decades especially, health professionals have made great strides on behalf of the elderly by intervening in the treatment of heart disease, cancer, chronic obstructive pulmonary disease (COPD), influenza, kidney disease, falls, dementia, and Alzheimer's disease. Yet the fact remains that the elderly, who constitute 13% of the U.S. population, still account for 34% of prescription expenditures,[10] even though many are poor and many have no prescription benefits, either public or private.

HOW AGING INFLUENCES THE NEED FOR CARE

Illnesses among the elderly are typically chronic and usually occur against a backdrop of underlying medical problems and aging changes. For example, those over 75 tend to present with greater numbers of chronic illnesses, which in turn may result in their falling victim to the ravages of polypharmacy. Health care professionals who care for those over 75 must be especially vigilant in looking for increased ADRs, drug–drug interactions, drug–disease interactions, and untoward side effects.

Table 1 Chronic conditions that impair the elderly[a]

Chronic Conditions	Percent of Elderly Population
Arthritis	45
Hypertension	34
Loss of hearing	28
Cardiovascular disease	25
Cataracts	16
Mobility impairment	15
Sinusitis	11
Diabetes	9
Tinnitus	8
Vision impairment	8

[a] Authors' unpublished data.

Aging influences the elderly person's need for care because it affects the senses, cognition and memory, behavior related to disease, and physiology.

Altered Senses

It is not uncommon as someone becomes "older" to notice, but often to deny, some loss of sensory functioning. This is because the loss is often so slow that it is not immediately recognized or, because of health beliefs, the loss is simply accepted or the individual adapts. Because nerves and neurons do not divide and turn over as other body cells do, neurons are as old as the person in whose body they reside. As a consequence, it is quite normal for senses to diminish in function as a person ages. The physician, pharmacist, nurse, or other caregiver must adjust their services to meet the needs of someone whose sight, hearing, smell, taste, and touch have altered over time. Wise health professionals also know these losses in sensory perception among the elderly may also be due to lifestyle habits. For example, alcohol use, tobacco use, and food preference can change a person's senses over time. Additionally, as people age, they may not be able to perceive colors correctly nor are they able to adapt to changes in light as younger people do.[11] Thus, even when an elderly person has no acute or chronic diseases, it is still possible for loss of hearing, vision, taste, touch, or smell to be mistaken for a disease process when, in fact, the issue is normal aging.

Sensory loss is often frustrating to the elderly, especially among those who have worked hard to maintain their independence or those who have tried to compensate for any sensory loss by adapting or by ignoring it. The health professional who understands that sensory changes are normal will find that new and novel ways to help the elderly maintain independence are appreciated. Because the elderly frequently must deal with loss of the accommodation reflex, opacities of the lens due to cataracts, loss of visual acuity and peripheral vision, and shifts in color perception, they need help to distinguish their medications; the pharmacist should consider use of large print on labels, different size prescription containers, and brightly colored auxiliary labels. Research studies show that the elderly prefer block lettering on pastel paper over block lettering on white paper, and many health professionals now provide labels and patient education materials using pastels.[12]

Diminished hearing is another sensory loss due to aging; however, when it does occur, it is usually loss of higher frequency sounds.[13] Thus, many health professionals have learned there is no reason to stereotype the elderly by shouting or by talking loudly to them; rather, it is more effective to just speak a little slowly and in near normal tones. Finally, because of possible sensory loss in elderly patients, health professionals find counseling is more effective if the counseling area is well lit, has nonglare surfaces, and is free from ambient or background noises.

Altered Cognition and Memory

Those who stereotype the elderly often paint them as being forgetful and unable to recall simple instructions. Research related to the elderly's ability to think, reason, and solve problems shows their life experiences give them an edge when such characteristics are measured against patients who are much younger.[14] To the physician, pharmacist, or health professional trying to teach the elderly, this means the elderly can be taught new habits, but they will assimilate new information using coping skills, problem-solving skills, attitudes, and values acquired in the earlier part of their lives. Thus, when an elderly person and a much younger person try to talk with each other, it often ends in frustration for both, as neither one knows how the other is thinking or engaging in problem-solving. Even when loss of any one of the senses is great, health professionals should keep in mind that the elderly do keep their capacity for intelligent reasoning, as only small numbers of them are cognitively impaired by such things as dementia, Alzheimer's, or the ravages of atherosclerosis.

Those who live to be elderly have had to make many "adjustments" during their lifetime. These adjustments have most often been made to compensate for uncomfortable emotional events, such as changes in economic status, loss of friends and family, unfulfilled leisure time, and a narrowing of interests. Younger persons should always remember that their elders have something they do not have: a perspective on life tempered by experience. The younger health professional should also remember that life adjustments are stressful for any person, but especially so among the elderly, for these adjustments and attendant coping are often the root cause of much clinical depression or other mood disorders.

The elderly do not usually treat people any differently in their older years than they did during their younger years. Thus, the sweet old man who values honesty and integrity was once a sweet young man with these same values. Another truism about the elderly is that many never see themselves as old and will often label themselves as "middle-aged." These are the elderly who typically look forward to each day, because they see it as a time for a new adventure, an opportunity for helping others, or a day in pursuit of hobbies, intellectual exercises with others of similar values and interests, or just being with family members and friends who appreciate them.

One research project involved a study to quantify how a senior's ability to take oral prescription medication safely correlated with age, sex, socioeconomic status, education, cognitive impairment, depression, and self-management. When a team of physicians, nurses, and pharmacists worked together, the ability of the elderly to take oral medications safely was most influenced by cognitive function and economic status.[15]

Altered Behavior Due to Disease

Uncomplicated aging is a rare thing and is a wonderful gift that few experience. Yet, when asked, the elderly tend to perceive themselves as healthier than they really are,[16] with the result that many elderly avoid asking for help, seeking routine medical care, or complying with medication regimens. While most chronic diseases affect the elderly in a physiological way, many of those diseases also alter behavior in a way that affects how health professionals and others provide care. For example, diseases such as stroke, Alzheimer's, and cancer can result in a pharmacist, physician, nurse, or caregiver developing a closer relationship with the elderly patient than he or she has with family and friends. This offers the health professional an opportunity to build an honest, open, and trusting relationship with someone who needs and is likely to appreciate this special effort.

Altered Physiology

While all organs age, the elderly are especially prone to aging effects on the kidneys. Because of high blood flow into and out of the kidneys and because of how the kidneys excrete and metabolize drugs, this organ is especially prone to injury by medications. In the elderly, renal function can also be reduced by age and comorbidities, helping to induce a high incidence of ADRs. All health professionals need to pay particular attention to any elderly patient taking nonsteroidal anti-inflammatories, angiotensin-converting enzyme (ACE) inhibitors, antibiotics, and immunosuppressives.[17]

Because of all the alterations that can take place in an aging body, when starting any drug therapy in older individuals, prescribers are admonished to "start low and go slow."[18] The related concept of "therapeutic burden" is a means to better understand the effects and disposition of drugs in the elderly; all concurrent medications and their doses are scrutinized and rationally evaluated to make sure they are working to improve quality-of-life once they are "on-board."[19]

BUILDING CARING RELATIONSHIPS WITH THE ELDERLY

When a helping relationship exists between an elderly person and a caring professional, the health professional is faced with the challenge of how best to build and use that relationship so health needs are appropriately met. Health professionals serving the needs of the elderly frequently may play several roles, including biological, psychological, and social ones:

- **Biological role:** Involves helping the elderly deal with the symptoms and outcomes of their disease(s), such as aphasia and paralysis due to stroke, pain due to cancer, or memory loss due to Alzheimer's.
- **Psychological role:** Involves helping the elderly live with their need to maintain self-esteem, pride, and self-worth while reducing feelings of helplessness and hopelessness.
- **Social role:** Involves helping the elderly patient learn to trust those in the health care system and to enjoy relationships with people in whom they have confidence and who will address their health, medication, and medical care needs in a manner that keeps them independent and living in the community.

To be able to provide health services to the elderly in a comprehensive biological–psychological–social manner requires a specially trained and committed individual. A better alternative would be a well-trained cadre of people who want to work together building honest, open, and trusting (H.O.T.) relationships with the elderly. However, not all caregivers are so equipped professionally and not all relevant health professionals are talking with each other on a level that would result in coordinated, comprehensive care to be delivered on an optimal level. Good and helping relationships with the elderly can be achieved and they begin with a health professional who is able to:

- Avoid stereotyping the elderly.
- See the elderly as needing the very best in services.
- See the relationship as an opportunity to help someone focus on the positive aspects of being any age.
- Commit to the elderly in the same manner they would prefer, should the age difference be reversed.

In essence, building caring relationships with the elderly is all about providing them age-appropriate care and seeing them as valuable members of society able to make their own independent decisions.

INAPPROPRIATE MEDICATION USE IN THE ELDERLY

One report noted that 28% of all hospital admissions involved the elderly and were due to nonadherence to medication regimens or an ADR.[20] In addition, a landmark study in 1996 calculated that drug-related events in ambulatory care resulted in 6.5 admissions/100 people to a hospital, of which 13% proved fatal. Also in that year, 23% of the deaths among 198,000 people involved drug-related problems. The annual cost of all this was $76.6 billion.[21] Thus, to protect the elderly, it is essential that they receive appropriate treatment rather than falling victim to problems resulting from polypharmacy.[21,22]

Another study using data from 1995–2000 found that inappropriate prescribing for ambulatory care visits to a physician had an incidence rate of 7.8%. Of the ADRs resulting from this inappropriate prescribing, 27.6% could have been prevented, and among the most serious life-threatening ADRs, 42.2% were determined to be preventable.[23] The most common medication categories associated with these preventable ADRs included:

- Cardiovascular agents (24.5%)
- Diuretics (22.1%)
- Nonopioid analgesics (15.4%)
- Hypoglycemic agents (10.9%)
- Anticoagulants (10.2%)

How did these errors occur? Errors that occurred during the prescribing stage (i.e., use of the wrong dose, the wrong drug, or the wrong therapeutic category; insufficient patient education; and use of interacting drugs) accounted for 58.4% of preventable ADRs.[24] However, patients were also found to be at fault with errors in compliance (i.e., taking the wrong dose, continuing to take medicines despite instructions to discontinue them, refusing to take necessary medicines, continuing to take a medicine despite the appearance of adverse effects, and taking another person's medications) that accounted for another 21.1% of these preventable ADRs in older outpatients.

Frustration and concern continue to increase over the growing number of geriatric patients who suffer complex drug–drug and drug–disease interactions that may severely compromise their mental health. According to Dianne Tobias, PharmD, past-president of the American Society of Consultant Pharmacists, the percentage of patients in U.S. nursing facilities who are receiving nine or more routine medications a day—the currently accepted definition of polypharmacy—rose from 17% in 1997 to nearly 27% in May 2000.[25] The slippery slope known as polypharmacy begins when Drug A causes an ADR that is interpreted as a new medical condition. Drug B is then prescribed to treat the "new" condition. Drug B causes an ADR or interaction, which is then interpreted as a new condition, and subsequently Drug C is prescribed; the end point could be a patient taking upward of a dozen drugs. While age-related changes in the elderly can and do impact the efficacy of medicines, they are still an important part of treating the illnesses of the elderly. But when the elderly, their illnesses, and their medications come together, it sometimes leads to physical, mental, and nervous system side effects, such as reduced mental functioning, sleep disturbances, and falls leading to hip fractures.[26] Furthermore, comorbidities and polypharmacy complicate things, especially when polypharmacy medications include drugs deemed "inappropriate for the elderly."[27]

In 1991, physician Mark Beers and a group of physicians and pharmacologists with expertise in geriatric medicine and medications identified 20 medications that should generally be avoided in the frail elderly. Since then, studies using the Beers' criteria indicate that between 14% and 40% of the frail elderly are given at least one medication deemed inappropriate. The inappropriate drugs most often given are long-acting benzodiazepines, dipyridamole, propoxyphene, and amitriptyline.[28] Later, Beers began a review of his list in order to apply it to all persons over 65 years of age, and he grouped these medications according to: (1) medications inappropriate due to the person's disease and (2) medications inappropriate due to relative ineffectiveness, ADRs, and existence of safer or more effective alternatives.

Later, this list became the focus of several research studies and led to the discovery that the largest group of inappropriate medications given to those over 65 included the psychotropics. One out of every four to six patients in ambulatory settings is given a psychotropic agent inappropriately. Most of these drugs were long-acting benzodiazepines, amitriptyline, and doxepin.[29] These agents are considered inappropriate for use in the elderly because they induce a high rate of anticholinergic effects that range from sedation to delirium to urinary retention.

Drug-induced delirium is common and is associated with anticholinergic activity caused by tricyclic antidepressants, neuroleptics, benzodiazepines, and, to a lesser extent, sedatives; it is also associated with dopamine-activating drugs, antiepileptics, histamine H_2-receptor blockers, digitalis, and analgesics.[30] The use of alternative medicines such as SSRIs would be of greater help to the elderly because these medications do not induce anticholinergic effects and because they can be used safely at doses one-third to one-half of those used in younger persons.[31] Other studies using the Beers' criteria have shown inappropriate use of long-acting benzodiazepines to be a large contributing factor to falls and hip fractures among the elderly.[32]

In 2003, growing interest in the Beers' criteria caused the related list of medications to become the focus of a report by the U.S. Government Accounting Office (now the Government Accountability Office) (GAO). That GAO report lists several behaviors that contribute to inappropriate medication use in the elderly population. When it came to the elderly, chief among those behaviors were:

- Physician-prescribing practices were based on outdated information.
- Pharmacists were not conducting appropriate reviews and monitoring drug use.
- Health professionals and their patients were not communicating with each other.

Despite the updates of the Beers' list in 1997[28] and in 2003[33] the list's validity and its merits are still being scrutinized. While some experts consider the list reasonable, many others report that many elderly patients are able to tolerate drugs described as inappropriate and do so with no untoward problems.[34] Where does this leave the Beers' list? Recently, the Centers for

Medicare and Medicaid Services adopted the Beers' list as a measuring tool for quality care indicators in nursing homes in its draft revisions on unnecessary drugs and pharmacy services. These are now in its reference *Guidance to Surveyors of Long Term Care Facilities.*[35]

Although the incidence and prevalence of serious ADRs, polypharmacy, and inappropriate prescribing vary from study to study (i.e., study design and other study-related factors can affect the results), those incidence and prevalence numbers have not ranged widely during the past 40 years. Continuing professional education programs and other educational pursuits have raised awareness, but the incidence of drug-induced mortality and morbidity remain high to the point that nearly every health professional knows of at least one incident. At the moment, it would appear that the best way for health professionals to reduce the effects of ADRs is to assemble current information on the patient's medications and needs, and then work with other professionals to rationally minimize the number of medications without compromising therapeutic goals.[36]

Interest in ADRs involving the elderly has never been higher, and the research community that reviews published literature on ADRs has become quite sophisticated. Such reviewers sometimes downgrade the literature on ADRs by saying that prospective data are missing, ADRs are poorly described, and analytical methods are questionable.[37] While all this leads to imprecise and generalized outcomes based on data that are statistically in question, it does not in any way diminish the fact that the existence of ADRs is clinically significant. Nonetheless, one recent study of elderly persons enrolled in HMOs indicated that more than 28% received at least one of 33 medications deemed potentially inappropriate for their age group, and 5% received one of 11 drugs categorized as totally inappropriate for use in older patients.[22]

Inappropriate medication use among the elderly in ambulatory care, home health care, and long-term care settings continues to be pervasive throughout the United States despite decades of research. This situation is complicated by the fact that today's medicines are often delivered as home intravenous therapy in multiple drug regimens that treat multiple chronic diseases; also, a growing group of ambulatory patients are presenting with high degrees of complexity and acuity. While longevity is increasing, the elderly still are at increased risk for drug-related problems.[38] Obviously, much work still needs to be done if health professionals are going to help the elderly obtain better health care outcomes through better management of their medication therapy needs. Pharmacists especially need to be recruited to assist with:

- Promoting safer prescribing practices.
- Making sure elderly patients understand their medication regimen before they leave a pharmacy.
- Providing in-service programs for nursing home residents and staff as well as local community centers.
- Reviewing medication regimens of the elderly using the power of their computers to check for potential drug interactions and ADRs.
- Supplying the elderly with appropriate age-related containers, labels, and compliance aids.
- Serving on drug formulary and auditing committees.
- Helping the elderly dispose of unwanted, outdated, and unusable medications.
- Conducting in-store "brown bag" or medication review programs.

KEY POINTS

- On average, those over 65 years of age are taking twice as many medications as those under 65.
- The elderly have more chronic diseases, and the aging process increases the complexities of their diseases.
- Because of the number of drugs taken and the complexity of the diseases, the elderly are susceptible to many more ADRs.
- Medication needs of the elderly are influenced by:
  - inappropriate prescribing based on outdated information,
  - insufficient drug utilization reviews and monitoring of both prescription and nonprescription medications, and
  - lack of collaboration among health professionals, their elderly patients, and families.
- The elderly need medication management; all health professionals must become more observant and aware of such patients.
- Health professionals, especially pharmacists, must help avoid the use of unnecessary medications in the elderly, particularly antidepressants and antianxiety agents.

REFERENCES

1. Bearon LB. Successful aging: what does the good life look like? Concepts in Gerontology, The Forum for Family and Consumer Issues, North Carolina State University 1(3), Raleigh, NC; Summer 1996.
2. Rovira II, Finkel T. Mechanics of aging. *Geriatr Times*. 2002(July/Aug):19.
3. Lasagna L. Drug effects as modified by aging. *Res Publ Assoc Res Nerv Ment Dis.* 1956;35:83–9.

4. Koop CE. Clinical perspectives on geriatric drug use. In: Moore SR, Teal TW. *Geriatric Drug Use*. New York: Pergamon Press; 1985:3.

5. National Institutes of Health. *Action Plan for Aging Research: Strategic Plan for Fiscal Years 2001–2005*. Bethesda: U.S. Department of Health and Human Services, National Institutes of Health, National Institute on Aging; May 2001: NIH Publication 01–4951.

6. American Geriatric Society Foundation: http://www.healthinaging.org/agingintheknow/chapters_ch_trial.asp?ch=2 (accessed June 20, 2006).

7. Gist YJ, Hetzel LI. We the People: Aging in the United States, Census 2000 Special Reports. U.S. Department of Commerce, U.S. Census Bureau; December 2004. Washington, DC: http://www.census.gov/prod/2004pub/censr-19.pdf (accessed June 20, 2006).

8. Schwarze M. Selecting therapy for elderly at risk for coronary heart disease or stroke. *Clin Geriatr*. 2000;8(10):24–33.

9. Grossberg GT, Grossberg JA. Epidemiology of psychotherapeutic drug use in older adults. *Clin Geriatr Med*. 1998;14(1):1–5.

10. Chrischilles EA, Foley DJ, Wallace RB, et al. Use of medications by persons 65 and over: data from established populations for epidemiologic studies of the elderly. *J Gerontol*. 1992;47:M137–44.

11. Larsen P. Assessment and management of sensory loss in elderly patients. *AORN J*. 1997 Feb; 65:432–7.

12. Tindall WN. Physical, emotional, and attitudinal influences on effective communication with the elderly. In: *Pharmacy Practice for the Geriatric Patient*. Alexandria, VA: American Association of Colleges of Pharmacy; 1985.

13. Ebaugh FC. *Management of Common Problems in Geriatric Medicine*. Menlo Park, CA: Addison Wesley; 1980:24–7.

14. Holyoak KJ, Morrison RG. *The Cambridge Handbook of Reasoning and Thinking*. New York: Cambridge University Press; 2005.

15. Raehl CL, Bond CA, Woods T, et al. Individualized drug assessment use in the elderly. *Pharmacotherapy*. 2002;22:1239–48.

16. American Medical Association Council on Scientific Affairs, Report 5, Improving the Quality of Geriatric Pharmacotherapy: http://ama-assoc.org/pub/article/print/2036-7955.html (accessed June 20, 2006).

17. Bennett WM. Drug related renal dysfunction in the elderly. *Geriatr Nephrol Urol*. 1999;9(1):21–5.

18. Rochon P, Anderson GM, Tu JV, et al. Age- and gender-related use of low-dose drug therapy. *J Am Geriatr Soc*. 1999;47(8):954–9.

19. Abernathy DR. Aging effects on drug disposition. *Geriatr Nephrol Urol*. 1999;9(1):15–9.

20. American Medical Directors Association. White Paper on Quality Pharmaceutical Care in Long Term Care, proceedings of a Symposium on Quality in Pharmaceutical Care. Montreal, Quebec; November 1998.

21. Field TS, Gilman BH, Subramanian S, et al. The costs associated with adverse drug events among older adults in the ambulatory setting. *Med Care*. 2005;43(12):1171–6.

22. Goulding MR. Inappropriate medication prescribing for elderly ambulatory care patients. *Arch Intern Med*. 2004;164:305–12.

23. Gurwitz JH, Field TS, Harrold LR, et al. Incidence and preventability of adverse drug events among older persons in the ambulatory setting. *JAMA*. 2003;289:1107–16.

24. Moore AR, O'Keefe ST. Drug-induced cognitive impairment in the elderly. *Drugs Aging*. 1991 Jul;15(1):15–28.

25. Chutka DS, Evans JM, Fleming KC, et al. Symposium on geriatrics—part 1: drug prescribing for the elderly. *Mayo Clin Proc*. 2003;70(7):694–702.

26. Ray WA, Griffin MR, Schaffner W, et al. Psychotropic drug use and the risk of hip fracture. *N Engl J Med*. 1987;316:363–9.

27. Aparasu RR, Mort JR. Inappropriate prescribing for the elderly. *Ann Pharmacother*. 2000;34:338–46.

28. Beers MH. Explicit criteria for determining potentially inappropriate medication use in the elderly: an update. *Arch Intern Med*. 1997;157:1531–6.

29. Aparasu RR, Mort JR, Sitzman S. Psychotropic prescribing for the elderly in office-based practice. *Clin Ther*. 1998;20(3):603–16.

30. Karlsson I. Drugs that induce delirium. *Dement Geriatr Cogn Disord*. 1999;10(5): 412–5.

31. Salzman C. Practical considerations for the treatment of depression in elderly and very elderly long-term care patients. *J Clin Psychiatry*. 1999;60(Suppl 20):30–3.

32. Burke WJ, Folks DG, McNeilly DP. Effective use of anxiolytics in older adults. *Clin Geriatr Med*. 1998;14(1):47–65.

33. Fick DM, Cooper JW, Wade WE, et al. Updating the Beers criteria for potentially inappropriate medication use in older adults: results of a U.S. consensus panel of experts. *Arch Intern Med*. 2003;163:2716–24.

34. Pasquale DA, Nace DA, Lindblad CI, et al. Update on drug-related problems in the elderly. *Am J Geriatr Pharm*. 2005;3(1):50–1.

35. Centers for Medicare and Medicaid Services Revised Guidance to Surveyors of Long Term Care Facilities: http://www.ascp.com/public/ga/nfsurvey/changes04/stateOps. pdf (accessed June 20, 2006).

36. Azad N, Tierney M, Victor G, et al. Adverse drug events in the elderly population admitted to a tertiary care hospital. *Healthcare Manage*. 2002;47(5):295–305.

37. Atkin PA, Veitch PC, Veitch EM, et al. The epidemiology of serious adverse drug reactions among the elderly. *Drugs Aging*. 1999;14:141–52.

38. Simon SR, Chan KA, Soumerai SB, et al. Potentially inappropriate medications used by elderly persons in the U.S. health maintenance organizations. *J Am Geriatr Soc*. 2005;53:227–32.

2

Enhancing Medication Adherence: An Opportunity to Improve Drug Therapy in the Elderly

PAUL J. HERSHBERGER AND WILLIAM N. TINDALL

The most helpful thing I have ever done with noncompliant patients has been to ask them questions.

—**Fred Kleinsinger, MD (2003)**

OVERVIEW

This chapter examines the ongoing problem of nonadherence; many patients simply do not adhere to their prescribed medication regimens, especially the elderly. A new perspective is offered on this costly medical problem and contributing factors are outlined. Furthermore, health system barriers that prevent medication adherence are described and recommendations are offered for improving adherence. The scientific and clinical literature on this complex topic is extensive and confounding. The multifaceted elements of adherence/nonadherence prohibit an exhaustive review in a single chapter. Therefore, this chapter emphasizes only the most important features of nonadherence relevant to clinical practice. Behavioral theories that contribute to understanding and managing medication adherence are discussed briefly. The chapter concludes with several recommendations for health care professionals that can serve as management strategies to enhance medication adherence in the elderly.

Gloria Gladdings, PharmD, a recent pharmacy school graduate, practices in a clinic of 50 physicians. The 600-sq.-ft. pharmacy fills 150 prescriptions each day, most of them for elderly patients who come into the clinic to see one of the family medicine physicians who specializes in geriatric care. Over the last few weeks, Gloria has struck up a friendship with Mrs. Joyce Lord, who seems to be a regular at the clinic. During their first encounter, Mrs. Lord had admonished Gloria for calling her by her first name. Gloria simply took this as a sign that her own generation was a little less formal than that of Mrs. Lord, who was now 81 years old. On a recent visit, Mrs. Lord approached Gloria and said, "I am here to refill my prescriptions but I decided against taking that lisinopril drug 3 weeks ago because I learned from an Internet search that I should not take this pill at the same time I am taking my water pill. In fact, I am not sure I should be on the water pill either as I have had no swelling in my ankles for months now. What do you think?"

Gloria was dumbfounded; she thought the elderly worshipped their doctors and would never stray from their instructions. She thought the only reason the elderly missed taking their pills was because of declining memory, that is, they simply forgot to take them. Or they found the complexity of their medication regimen too difficult to keep straight, again because of declining cognitive skills.

- Is noncompliance in older persons a problem?
- Is it often intentional, as with Mrs. Lord?
- What other reasons might cause nonadherence to a medication regimen in the elderly?
- What can pharmacists and prescribing physicians do to minimize the problems caused by nonadherence?
- How frustrating has it been for you as a professional to find that patients do not always follow what you consider to be perfectly good and helpful advice?
- Do you know what causes patients to put themselves at risk by not taking medicines as prescribed?
- Do you have a plan to identify, intervene, monitor, and modify your patient's nonadherent behavior?

NONADHERENCE: A COSTLY AND UBIQUITOUS PROBLEM

Nonadherence is ubiquitous in health care. The term, however, is too broadly defined. For instance, everyone can identify some type of health care recommendation or treatment to which her or his adherence is either incomplete or nonexistent (e.g., flossing teeth, avoiding sun exposure, following dietary or physical activity recommendations). Although taking medications is only one aspect of health care, nonadherence to medications is a pervasive and costly problem, especially when today's array of medications could be so helpful to the elderly if only the elderly would adhere to a medication regimen. What, then, predisposes the elderly to medication misadventures when age per se is **not** a precipitating factor?[1]

The most common estimate of medication nonadherence in the general population is 50%, and a range of 26% to 60% for elderly patients has been reported.[2–4] In the professional literature, nonadherence rates in clinical trials are reported to range from 22% to 57%.[5] Given such great variability about nonadherence in the clinical literature, it is reasonable to assume that about 50% of older adults with chronic illnesses are medication nonadherent in some fashion.[6] Thus, because the problem is so prevalent, anything pharmacists, physicians, and other health professionals can do to enhance medication adherence represents the best opportunity to increase and optimize the effectiveness of pharmacotherapy among the elderly.

TERMINOLOGY OF MEDICATION NONADHERENCE

The most common term used by health professionals to define the situation in which patients do not follow a prescribed treatment regimen is **noncompliance**. Because this term implies disobedience to an authority and because it also has a pejorative connotation when used to describe a patient, the term **nonadherence** has become increasingly accepted as a more appropriate term when speaking in health care circles about patients who do not take their medicines as prescribed. Nonadherence suggests that a patient is in control of the nonadherent behavior and is in control as the decision-maker who freely chooses whether or not to follow a prescribed regimen of medication.

More recently, the term concordance has been promoted, especially by the British, as a term that more fully depicts the idea that there exists a provider–patient relationship marked by shared decision-making and consultation.[7,8] While the term concordance is consistent with a type of professional relationship most conducive to helping a patient follow through on a medication regimen, this chapter uses the more commonly accepted term of nonadherence when referring to behavior of the elderly in which a medication regimen is not completely followed.

Medication adherence ranges from 0% to more than 100% (i.e., it will be more than 100% if a patient takes more medication than prescribed) among various groups as reported in many types of literature by different researchers. The real issue is just what is nonadherence and how did the researcher define it. For example, is a patient nonadherent if she takes the prescribed amount of medication but takes it at inappropriate times or under inappropriate circumstances (e.g., with or without food)? It is not uncommon to have a physician write a prescription stating that the patient should take the medication once a day in the morning, but for various reasons the patient willingly and regularly takes it once a day with his noon meal or just before bedtime. Indeed, some types of partial nonadherence may have few, if any, adverse consequences, whereas complete nonadherence typically comes at a high cost and also without any health benefit, unless there has been a mistake on the part of the writing physician or dispensing pharmacist. Therefore, one challenge when discussing nonadherence is identifying what does or does not constitute nonadherence. For purposes of this chapter, the term nonadherence is used to refer to any use or nonuse of a prescribed medication that is inconsistent with the intent of the prescription.

COSTS OF MEDICATION NONADHERENCE

The most important cost associated with medication nonadherence is the cost of dealing with poor health outcomes and with the reduction in quality of life that occurs in the older patient for whom the medication was prescribed. That cost is difficult to quantify, but nonetheless it is enormous. For example, hypertension, which is generally controllable, remains uncontrolled in nearly three-quarters of those in whom it is diagnosed, and a major reason for uncontrolled hypertension is medication nonadherence.[8]

Four factors contribute to medication nonadherence: polypharmacy, cognitive issues, adverse drug reactions, and cost of the medication.[9] While money matters are identifiable and arguably an issue in nonadherence, the additional money spent by patients, employers, and society on medications that are not properly taken represents a waste of health care resources and results in increased health care expenditures. In the late 1980s, medication nonadherence in the elderly was determined to cost the U.S. economy $8.5 billion annually,[10] a figure that by the early 1990s had grown to be $100 billion.[11] What assumptions were made to come up with each figure and which figure is more accurate does not matter. What does matter is that medication non-adherence costs a sizable sum. It leads to increased utilization of other health care resources when nonadherence exacerbates existing health care problems or causes the development of new problems. Looking at this another way, approximately one-quarter of the hospitalizations of persons over 75 years of age may be related to some type of medication nonadherence, leading to unnecessary and costly prescribing of additional medications, diagnostic studies, and referrals for specialty evaluation and care.[12]

FACTORS CONTRIBUTING TO NONADHERENCE

The health care literature is replete with studies designed to identify factors that contribute to medication nonadherence; many of them specifically look at older patients. One underlying goal of these studies has been to identify ways in which medication nonadherence can be predicted. Indeed, there are factors that increase the likelihood that medication nonadherence will occur, although it has also been found that it is very difficult to predict which individual patient will be nonadherent and with which particular medication. Thus, studies and reviews attempting to describe the nonadherent patient have largely failed.[13] However, it is possible to categorize contributing factors to nonadherence into four groups:

- Those that pertain to the patient.
- Those that pertain to the medication.
- Those that pertain to relationships with health care providers.
- Those that pertain to weaknesses in the health care system.

Patient Factors

Demographic variables such as marital status, income level, age, gender, and educational level typically are not reliably related to adherence.[5] For any given patient, however, such a demographic variable can be a contributing factor—for example, when a recently widowed patient loses the support system that resulted from his reliance on having his spouse manage his medications. Personality variables are not predictive of medication nonadherence,[14,15] but the cognitive functioning of an older adult is clearly relevant to medication adherence. Thus, to assist the elderly, the helping professional should determine if the patient has the requisite ability to understand what his/her medical condition is and if the patient has the ability to understand the need for the prescribed medication.

In addition, the health professional should ascertain if the patient is able to remember any complexities in the medication regimen. Physicians often administer a mini-mental status questionnaire to their older patients, and they have found that those scoring less than 24 are 2.5 times more likely to be nonadherent with medication than those with scores over 24.[16]

Impairments in vision, hearing, ambulation, or other functional abilities can also impede adherence. Such impairment can exacerbate existing cognitive difficulties. The presence of psychiatric disorders may affect medication adherence, for example, when depression induces a lack of motivation or interest in following a medication regimen. Another example is when extreme anxiety about side effects induces annoyance or fear about taking a drug. A common example is the angiotensin-converting enzyme (ACE) inhibitors, which induce a dry hacking cough in 10%–30% of those who take one. Psychotic illnesses, such as paranoid ideation or delusional beliefs, may impair or distort a person's understanding of his/her condition and the role of the prescribed medications.

Illiteracy in general, or medical illiteracy in particular, contributes to medication nonadherence. The literature promotes corrective interventions that rely on providing written information when conducting drug therapy management or simply counseling a patient. However, this strategy may be applied incorrectly if the health professional assumes he or she has patients who are all literate.

A serious and important patient element in nonadherence is the patient's health beliefs about his/her illness or the prescribed medications. Health beliefs are important to consider when asking the elderly why they are not adherent to their medication regimen. Finally, not all the blame for poor medication adherence can be placed on the shoulders of patients. A considerable body of literature suggests that nonadherence is a function of the following elements:[17-19]

- A medication regimen that is too complex.
- A failure on the part of the health professional to explain the benefits of a medication as well as its side effects.
- A failure to adjust a medication regimen in consideration of a patient's life-style.
- A failure to consider the impact of the costs of a medication.
- A failure between the health professional and the patient to develop a good therapeutic or helping relationship.

A therapeutic or helping relationship between patients and health professionals is important in this age of computers, especially now that patients have access to resources that can make them as literate about their diseases as their health professional. Without an open, honest, and trusting relationship, many patients may disagree about a medication or treatment; any element of mistrust can cloud the necessity and appropriateness of a particular medication. Furthermore, the health professional should also remember that a patient's attitude toward the value of certain medications or the patient's cultural background and beliefs may be strong influencers over the extent to which a patient will accept and use a prescribed medication.[20] Finally, it is quite common to find that generational differences, such as the life experiences and values that differ between an elderly patient and a younger professional, will also impede open communication and/or trust.

Medication Factors

The complexity of a drug regimen appears to be one of the most important and controllable factors in medication nonadherence in older adults, although studies have yielded inconsistent results.[21] As the number of medications and their differing dosing intervals increases, one can expect the likelihood of some or complete nonadherence to increase also, simply because the demands on the older patient are greater.

The side effects of medications also impact nonadherence. Obviously, nonadherence tends to increase with more troublesome side effects, especially when the medication is used to treat an asymptomatic condition such as hypertension.[21]

Health Care Provider Factors

The quality of the relationship between the patient and the physician, as well as the relationship between the patient and other members of the health care team, is the responsibility of the involved health care professionals. A well-intentioned and capable older adult may be nonadherent with a medication regimen solely because communication was not clear, patient understanding was not assessed, or conflicting information was given to the patient by one or more professionals. Health care professionals may fail to anticipate and discuss potential barriers to adherence, or they may fail to help the patient overcome such barriers (e.g., failing to prescribe a less costly medication when possible). Providers are profound facilitators of nonadherence when they do not speak clearly (because of pace, volume, or an accent), write clearly, or are inattentive to overt and covert indicators of patient misunderstanding.

Health Care System Factors

Many factors related to the health care environment constitute potential barriers to medication adherence, and among these are medication costs. Older adults, especially, often decide not to fill a prescription because of cost; this is called intentional nonadherence.[22] In these days of managed care and prescription benefit programs, the prohibitive expenditure is often not the cost of a medication but rather the cost of multiple copays. Even when the patient has insurance that takes care of the bulk of medication costs, the tiered and cumbersome pharmacy benefit packages (i.e., obtaining prior authorization, forced mail delivery, forced generic substitution) can be factors in patient nonadherence.

Another health system contributor to medication nonadherence is inadequate communication between the professionals on the patient's health care team. Although this may not be a direct factor, it is clearly an important reason why some older adults face the ravages of polypharmacy or unnecessary drug interactions.

Finally, the manner in which medications are packaged may also be a factor in nonadherence behavior for the older adult. For example, many elderly find that screw-top containers, child-resistant closures on prescription vials, and blister or foil packs are too difficult to open.[3]

BEHAVIORAL THEORIES THAT EXPLAIN MEDICATION NONADHERENCE

Several behavioral theories have been used to frame and better understand why patient health beliefs and expectations affect medication adherence. One is the **theory of reasoned action**, which states that individuals decide their intentions in advance of voluntary actions and that these intentions predict what people will do.[23] A second is the **health belief theory**, which is a model that suggests patients behave in response to their perceptions of the following four key dimensions:[24]

- Perceived susceptibility to an illness or problem.
- Perceived seriousness of the threat or problem.

- Perceived benefits of the proposed treatment or action.
- Perceived barriers to taking action.

Finally, a third explanation is found in the **transtheoretical model of change** that is used to explain the stages of thinking a person goes through before deciding on a course of health behavior.

The health belief model and the theory of reasoned action are based on an underlying premise that an individual's behavior is founded on the strengths of that person's belief that he/she has the skill or ability to execute a behavior that is required to accomplish a task.[25] For example, a woman's belief in her own self-efficacy is the basis for her taking a medication three times a day. Adherence to that medication regimen is found in that person's belief that she can indeed establish a routine whereby she will remember to take the medication as prescribed. A related concept is outcome efficacy, which refers to the belief that if the target behavior is accomplished, then a desired outcome will occur. Thus, if an elderly man truly believes that joint stiffness will be reduced (an outcome) if he takes the medication three times a day, then he is adherent to this regimen because of his belief that it will work (a reasoned action).

These theories suggest that patients are most likely to exhibit adherent behavior when there is highly perceived seriousness for a health threat (if I smoke I will get lung cancer like the rest of my family), when there is a highly perceived susceptibility to the threat (all my sisters and my mom had breast cancer; I'm likely to have it too, so I better do something now to avoid it), when there is high response–efficacy (if I get a PSA test every 6 months, I'm sure I can avoid prostate cancer), and when there is intention to perform the behavior (if I start exercising and eating right I can avoid diabetes).[26] Unfortunately, these theories have not yielded significant advances in the development of broad-based interventions to enhance adherence. They can, however, guide one's approach to an individual patient.

Another explanation for medication nonadherence is the transtheoretical model of change, also known as the stages-of-change model. This theory postulates that persons go through a series of stages when committing to a behavioral change. While it has been widely applied to explain and examine health behavior such as deciding to quit smoking, medication adherence also has been studied using this model.[27,28] The five stages in the transtheoretical model of change are:

- **Precontemplation:** the individual is not yet giving any consideration to the change.
- **Contemplation:** the individual is thinking about making the change.
- **Preparation:** the individual is actually making plans to implement the change.
- **Action:** the individual makes the change.
- **Maintenance:** the individual monitors and sustains the change.

This model provides any health practitioner with a framework for understanding the perspective of an older patient for whom a new prescription is written. To begin, the health professional determines which stage the patient is in relative to the new prescription. Then the health professional helps the patient to complete the stages of change until the patient tries and then accepts the new behavior (i.e., the new prescription). Ideally, sufficient interpersonal communication and educational interventions have occurred so that the patient appreciates the need for medication adherence and is moving forward through the stages to become someone willing to do what is necessary to implement the medication regimen. However, there may be cases in which the patient does not appreciate the severity of the condition or the necessity of taking medication so that, with respect to taking a new medication, the patient remains "stuck" in the precontemplation or contemplation stage. To reduce medication nonadherence, it is important to identify the stage a patient is in. Such identification guides the type of education and communication needed in any particular situation.

Health professionals must strive for high-quality interpersonal communication with patients and an accurate understanding of the patient's lifestyle, life setting, and health beliefs or perspectives. Patient-centered interviewing is a model for interaction with patients in which the emphasis is clearly on the patient, rather than on the provider, disease, or treatment.[29] Guides for learning patient-centered interviewing are readily available[30] and data support how it improves medication adherence as a result of enhancing communication between patient and provider.[31] Patient-centered interviewing can take more of a health professional's time, but it does work to avoid many problems that can result when clear and quality-focused communication between health professional and patient does not exist. Being involved in patient-centered interviewing also helps reduce malpractice suits and the number of patients switching pharmacies; it also generates better health outcomes, providing benefits to all when everyone addresses nonadherence through better interpersonal communication.[32]

STRATEGIES FOR ENHANCING MEDICATION ADHERENCE

Because medication nonadherence is so prevalent, it obviously is a problem that reduces the effectiveness of drug therapy in the elderly. Thus, it is not a great leap to state that effective interventions to enhance medication adherence are the best means to improve drug therapy. Some medication management therapy strategies should be built into every patient encounter by every member of the health care team, especially those encounters with elderly patients. However, because the problem of medication nonadherence is so complex, generalities and general strategies have not proved to be widely effective.[33,34] Pharmacists and health professionals must remember that researchers define and measure adherence rates differently. However, no matter what they use to define and measure adherence, rates are well below 100% and, for long-term therapies, are more like 50%.[35] Thus, it behooves every health care professional to work with each patient on an individual basis in order to maximize medication adherence.

General Strategies for Enhancing Medication Adherence

The following guidelines and strategies have been routinely used with older patients in the interest of improving medication adherence:

- Use the least number of medications possible and use the simplest dosing schedule possible for each medication.
- Have each member of the health care team assume responsibility for enhancing patient adherence. Beyond the physician and nurse, it is appropriate for the receptionist to ask a patient upon checkout whether there are any questions about medications that haven't been answered (and ensures that an available health care professional sees the patient to address the concern). To ensure accurate understanding, pharmacists are well advised to ask patients to repeat the dosing instructions after the prescription has been filled.
- Remember that education about medication regimens is important and necessary but frequently is insufficient to change behavior.
- Keep in mind that each patient's situation is unique and further individualization of adherence-enhancing strategies may be necessary, as nonadherence should be anticipated. Ensure that there is open and clear communication, which involves ongoing assessment of the extent to which the patient understands the treatment plan and its rationale. It has been suggested that if there is any common thread in the research examining the effectiveness of adherence-enhancing

interventions, frequent interaction with patients is beneficial. The need for open and clear communication extends to the patient's other providers as well. The involvement of family members is often useful and is especially important in cases where the older adult may not be capable of understanding or retaining information.

Individualized Strategies for Enhancing Medication Adherence

Individualizing medication adherence strategies must be done in the context of a professional relationship established between the elderly patient and his/her pharmacist or health care professional. The professional who has utilized interviewing strategies that are truly patient-focused and has accurate knowledge of that patient's needs, beliefs, desires, and motivations is the best person in the best position to best help that patient achieve the best medication adherence.

The process of individualizing adherence management strategies involves four steps that have been proven to work. These four steps are based on a model that first appeared in the mid-1990s, and this method was later taught to more than 120,000 pharmacists and others.[36] The first word in these four steps forms the acronym RIMM, which stands for:

1. **R**ecognize the barriers to adherence for the patient.
2. **I**ndividualize a plan with the patient to address the barriers.
3. **M**onitor adherence.
4. **M**odify the plan as necessary.

In step 1, a pharmacist or any health professional must **recognize** that there are barriers to adherence and some are on the part of the patient. While some adherence barriers may be obvious based upon one's knowledge about a given patient (e.g., cost, memory problems, physical disability), the wise and caring professional will ask important questions of each elderly patient. To help identify the potential for medication nonadherence, the health professional should ask the patient questions such as: "What difficulties have you had in the past with taking your medications?" and "What concerns do you have about taking this particular medication?"

In step 2, the caring professional must **individualize** a plan to create better adherence and do this with the patient as a full partner. This helps to address the barriers and the patient's best means for overcoming them. Because numerous factors may affect adherence, the helping professional must look for multidimensional means to overcome the barriers. For example, an elderly and arthritic patient might request that the pharmacist use an easier-to-open container rather than one with mandated childproof caps, or the pharmacist might suggest some type of cue to remind the patient to take the medication. Examples of such cues might be the time at which an elderly patient feeds her beloved cat or the time at which an elderly patient brushes his teeth.

Sometimes the intervening pharmacist can get approval for a once-a-day sustained-release medication, knowing that such a dosing regimen can be matched to a patient's agreed upon routine. Other cueing aids may be to have the elderly patient follow a simple diary in which he/she writes down the time each medication is taken.

If resources allow, many helping professionals arrange for themselves or other caregivers to make an occasional phone call to the patient or to stop by and review the medication adherence plan with the patient. While pharmacists have refill records to determine the frequency and quantity of medications dispensed, such records may not address all adherence problems. The process of individualizing a plan can help build a relationship with an elderly patient, a benefit that is in itself adherence-enhancing and also creates a long-term benefit.

The third step in a medication adherence program is to **monitor** medication adherence. Medication adherence can be monitored or measured in various ways, including self-reports, diaries, pill counts, refill intervals, direct observation, and even undertaking laboratory analyses. Unfortunately, none of these is without problems. Newer electronic monitoring systems can be more accurate, but they are quite costly. Nonetheless, one or more methods should be utilized to gain some knowledge of adherence patterns, and with that knowledge the pharmacist should be able to conduct extended discussions of adherence behavior with the patient.

Occasionally, a patient may become defensive about being "watched" via monitoring. The caregiver should indicate that many patients on the same medication have difficulty following this regimen and that monitoring a patient's behavior prevents many problems from developing. Thus, medication monitoring is a professional responsibility and an important task in the ongoing process to identify barriers to adherence and to address the factors that improve it.[22]

The final step in this medication adherence model is to **modify** the plan as necessary. Using the information gained from the monitoring system, along with additional patient-centered interviewing to get the patient's perspective of their experience with the medication regimen, the pharmacist, physician, or others should be able to negotiate necessary modifications. While modifications based on factors such as side effects routinely occur, there may be less obvious changes that would help the patient and prevent him/her just stopping the drug. A good example would be a patient with hypertension who is started on a beta-blocker such as metoprolol following a mild heart attack. Many patients actually feel worse for 6 months because of this drug and may stop taking it after a few weeks, not realizing that the slowing of their heart by the drug is of great benefit in preventing a second heart attack or stroke. To help these people remain adherent, it may be possible to add a second drug at one-half the usual dose for both drugs and obtain a synergistic effect that keeps blood pressure down and does so without troublesome side effects.

Finally, no matter what is being done, medication nonadherence in general and in older patients in particular is a health care problem that has been widely studied. Although efforts to come up with strategies to readily identify which patients are most likely to be nonadherent as well as endeavors to develop panacean interventions that will make huge reductions in the problem have largely been futile,[37,38] nevertheless health professionals should keep trying to make a difference in the lives of those in their care.

KEY POINTS

- Nonadherence in older patients remains a daunting, costly, and complex problem, but it provides opportunities for health professionals to enhance the effectiveness of pharmacotherapy.
- Nonadherence can be related to the patient, the medication, relationships with other health care providers, and weaknesses inherent in the health care system.
- Application of behavioral models such as the theory of reasoned action, the health belief theory, and the transtheoretical model of change can be helpful.
- Improvements in adherence can:
  - lower overall health care costs,
  - decrease the risk of hospitalization,
  - reduce the incidence of drug reactions and interactions,

- lessen the problem of drug errors and misuse, and
- enhance health.
- Health professionals should assume that nonadherence is a potential problem for every patient, not only the elderly.
- Adherence rates among the elderly can be improved if health professionals:
  - take the time to help the patient better understand the medication,
  - facilitate their motivational factors to take it,
  - remove the hindering barriers by learning what unique experiences and challenges each patient faces, and
  - address the issues with strategies designed to remove medication-taking variation.
- Any health professional who wants to improve the medication therapy outcomes of an elderly patient will have to engage in more than a one-time encounter.
- As a health professional, you cannot expect patients to change their behavior because you say so.

REFERENCES

1. Gurwitz JH, Avorn J. The ambiguous relationship between aging and adverse drug reactions. *Ann Intern Med*. 1991;114(11):956–66.
2. MacLaughlin EJ, Raehl CL, Treadway AK, et al. Assessing medication adherence in the elderly: which tools to use in clinical practice? *Drugs Aging*. 2005;22:231–55.
3. McGraw C, Drennan V. Older people and medication management: from compliance to concordance. *Rev Clin Gerontol*. 2004;14:145–53.
4. Balkrishnan R. Predictors of medication adherence in the elderly. *Clin Ther*. 1998;20: 764–71.
5. Osterberg L, Blaschke T. Adherence to medication. *N Engl J Med*. 2005;353:487–97.
6. Murray MD, Morrow DG, Weiner M, et al. A conceptual framework to study medication adherence in older adults. *Am J Geriatr Pharmacother*. 2004;2:36–43.
7. Jackevicius CA, Mamdani M, Tu JV. Adherence with statin therapy in elderly patients with and without acute coronary syndrome. *JAMA*. 2002; 288:495–7.
8. Neutel JM, Smith DHG. Improving patient compliance: a major goal in the management of hypertension. *J Clin Hypertens*. 2003;5:127–32.
9. Ascione F. Medication compliance in the elderly. *Generations*. 1984;18(Summer): 28–33.
10. Kusserow RP. *Medication Regimens: Causes of Non-compliance*. Washington, DC: Office of the Inspector General, U.S. Department of Health and Human Services; 1990: Report #WOE1-04-89–8912.
11. Johnson MJ, Williams M, Marshall ES. Adherent and nonadherent medication-taking in elderly hypertensive patients. *Clin Nurs Res*. 1999;8:318–35.
12. Chan M, Nicklason F, Vial JH. Adverse drug events as a cause of hospital admission in the elderly. *Intern Med J*. 2001;31:199–205.

13. Vik SA, Maxwell CJ, Hogan DB. Measurement, correlates, and health outcomes of medication adherence among seniors. *Ann Pharmacother.* 2004;38:303–12.

14. Dunbar-Jacob J, Burke LE, Puczynski S. Clinical assessment and management of adherence to medical regimens. In: Nicassio PM, Smith TW, eds. *Managing Chronic Illness: A Biopsychosocial Perspective.* Washington, DC: American Psychological Association; 1995:313–49.

15. Meichenbaum D, Turk DC. *Facilitating Treatment Adherence: A Practitioner's Guidebook.* New York: Plenum Press; 1987.

16. Gray S, Mahoney J, Blough D. Medication adherence in elderly patients receiving home health services following hospital discharge. *Ann Pharmacother.* 2001;35:539–45.

17. Elliott WJ, Moddy R, Toto R, et al. Hypertension in patients with diabetes: overcoming barriers to effective control. *Postgrad Med.* 2000;107:29–32, 35–6, 38.

18. Black HR. Will better-tolerated antihypertensive agents improve blood pressure control? JNC VI revisited. *Am J Hypertens.* 1999;12:225S–30S.

19. Ickovics JR, Mead CJ. Adherence to HAART among patients with HIV. *HIC Care.* 2002;14:309–18.

20. Horne R, Weinman J. Patients' beliefs about prescribed medicines and their role in adherence to treatment in chronic physical illness. *J Psychosom Res.* 1999;47: 555–67.

21. Cramer JA. Enhancing patient compliance in the elderly. Role of packaging aids and monitoring. *Drugs Aging.* 1998;12(1):7–15.

22. Mojtabai R, Olfson M. Medication costs, adherence, and health outcomes among Medicare beneficiaries. *Health Aff.* 2003;22:220–9.

23. Ajzen I, Fishbein M. *Understanding Attitudes and Predicting Social Behavior.* Englewood Cliffs, NJ: Prentice Hall; 1980.

24. Rosenstock IM, Strecher VJ, Becker MH. Social learning theory and the Health Belief Model. *Health Educ Q.* 1988;15:175–83.

25. Bandura A. *Self-Efficacy: The Exercise of Control.* New York: Freeman; 1997.

26. Damrosch S. Facilitating adherence to preventive and treatment regimens. In: Wedding D, ed. *Behavior and Medicine.* 2nd ed. St. Louis: Mosby; 1995:379–88.

27. DiClemente CC, Ferentz K, Velasquez MM. Health behavior change and the problem of "noncompliance." In: Hass LJ, ed. *Handbook of Primary Care Psychology.* New York: Oxford University Press; 2004:157–72.

28. Willey C, Redding C, Stafford J, et al. Stages of change for adherence with medication regimens for chronic disease: development and validation of a measure. *Clin Ther.* 2000;22:858–71.

29. Platt FW, Gaspar DL, Coulehan JL, et al. "Tell me about yourself": the patient-centered interview. *Ann Intern Med.* 2001;134:1079–85.

30. Smith RC, Marshall-Dorsey AA, Osborn GG, et al. Evidence-based guidelines for teaching patient-centered interviewing. *Patient Educ Couns.* 2000;39:27–36.

31. Rosal MC, Ebbeling CB, Lofgren I, et al. Facilitating dietary change: the patient-centered counseling model. *J Am Diet Assoc.* 2001;101:332–41.

32. Beck RS, Daughtridge R, Sloane PD. Physician–patient communication in the primary care office: a systematic review. *J Am Board Fam Pract.* 2002;15:25–38.

33. Haynes RB, Yao X, Degani A, et al. Interventions to enhance medication adherence. *Cochrane Database Syst Rev.* 2005 Oct. 19:CD000011.

34. McDonald HP, Garg AX, Haynes RB. Interventions to enhance patient adherence to medication prescriptions: a scientific review. *JAMA.* 2002;288:2868–79.

35. *Crossing the Quality Chasm: A New Health System for the 21st Century.* Washington, DC: Institute of Medicine; 2001.
36. Pharmacist–patient consultation program, unit 3, counseling to enhance patient compliance. New York: Pfizer Inc; 1995.
37. Peterson AM, Takiya L, Finley R. Meta-analysis of trials of interventions to improve medication adherence. *Am J Health System Pharm.* 2003;60:657–65.
38. Van Eijken M, Tsang S, Wensing M, et al. Interventions to improve medication compliance in older patients living in the community: a systematic review of the literature. *Drugs Aging.* 2003;20:229–40.

3

Altered Pharmacokinetics in an Aging Population: A Silent Epidemic

ROBERT J. BELLOTO

Stora was a victim of a silent epidemic that afflicts millions of seniors. Everyone knows the benefits of pharmaceutical drugs. But many of those same medications are inappropriate for seniors or can be deadly if taken improperly or in combination with incompatible remedies.

—Howard Gleckman in *BusinessWeek*

OVERVIEW

This chapter describes those factors that affect responses to a drug by the aging human body and how those responses result in an altered ability of the elderly to absorb, distribute, metabolize, and excrete medications. The clinical impact of common variations in drug response is described, leading to a better appreciation of such things as how a decrease in hepatic metabolism in the elderly can cause the half-life of a drug to be lengthened. Frailty itself is a risk factor for the elderly when it comes to dosing and choice of medication. Finally, how renal excretion of a drug is influenced by aging is discussed, with the conclusion that many drugs need to be carefully titrated and then monitored when given to the elderly.

Patient Al Jolson is a widowed 87-year-old. He is 5'8" (173 cm) and weighs 78 kg. Mr. Jolson is also a nursing home resident who was admitted during the current month due to worsening dementia. Regulations stipulate that a medication review be performed monthly.[1] The admitting diagnoses include several chronic diseases, most having 20 years or more duration: dementia—Alzheimer's type, hypertension, gout, hypercholesterolemia, and benign prostatic hyperplasia (BPH).

A blood analysis run as follow-up to Mr. Jolson's nursing home admission disclosed the abnormal values listed in Table 1. His current medications and administration regimens are listed in Table 2.

- What do you think Mr. Jolson's drug-related problems are?
- What drug-related problems do you think he has because of age-related changes in physiology?
- What does his blood chemistry tell you?
- What changes to his current medications would you recommend?
- How would you know if Mr. Jolson's quality of life improved because of what you recommended?

Mr. Jolson's decreased total protein and albumin levels have likely resulted from his worsening dementia and an inability to feed himself properly. Given his renal function,[2] the hypouricemia is most likely the result of an excessive dose of allopurinol. His creatinine clearance, estimated using the Cockcroft–Gault method, is 39 mL/minute. The recommended dosage for allopurinol based upon his renal function is 150 mg/day.

A recommendation, written by a pharmacist, to reduce the dose of allopurinol to one-half tablet daily was accepted by the patient's physician. Repeat blood chemistries showed improvements in total protein and albumin and a uric acid level in the normal range. Serum creatinine was essentially unchanged at 1.2 mg/dL. The patient did not experience a gout attack as a result of the change in drug therapy.

This case illustrates one of the most common scenarios encountered in the care of the elderly: a patient given the standard dose of a drug has diminished ability to eliminate the drug renally because of declining renal function induced by normal aging. Knowing the metabolic fate of a drug given to an elderly person is helpful in determining appropriate doses and in understanding drug interactions and why side effects often occur with increased prevalence in the elderly.

Table 1 Blood chemistry for Mr. Al Jolson

Chemistry	Value (Normal Range)
Total protein	5.5 (6.0–8.0 g/dL)
Albumin	3.0 (3.5–5.0 g/dL)
Uric acid	1.4 (3.5–7.2 mg/dL)
Creatinine	1.3 (0.5–1.2 mg/dL)

Table 2 Current medication list for Mr. Al Jolson

Drug	Dose	Frequency
Allopurinol	300 mg	daily
Triamterene/hydrochlorothiazide	37.5 mg/25 mg	daily
Tamsulosin	0.4 mg	daily
Finasteride	5 mg	daily
Pravastatin	40 mg	daily
Atenolol	50 mg	daily
Galantamine	4 mg	twice daily

CHANGES IN PHARMACOKINETIC PROCESSES IN THE AGING BODY

Pharmacokinetics is the study of the rate processes of absorption, distribution, metabolism, and excretion of chemicals, along with their pharmacologic, therapeutic, or toxic response in humans and animals.[3] Pharmacokinetic knowledge supplies the clinician with a scientific basis for determining a drug's appropriate dose and how that dose should be adjusted because of physiological changes, such as those due to aging.

Physiologic- and disease-related changes in organ and enzyme systems can and do alter the pharmacokinetics of drug products in the elderly. Renal drug elimination typically declines with age, along with the fall in creatinine clearance, and is the most common effect seen in the elderly. Many metabolized drugs show a decreased rate of elimination in the elderly, particularly those eliminated by the cytochrome P-450 enzyme system. Transdermal absorption of drugs is also altered in the elderly, when compared to younger individuals, and this is due to changes in skin integrity and altered muscle and fat changes.

Both water-soluble and fat-soluble drugs distribute differently in the elderly, thereby altering a drug's volume of distribution (Vd). Although these changes are not as pronounced as renal alterations in elimination of a drug, knowledge of these alterations in drug disposition is helpful in understanding dosage recommendations and adjusting doses.

There are many texts on pharmacokinetics.[4-6] The goal of this chapter is to clarify and use practical examples to explain why drug dosages often need to be reduced in the elderly. A second goal is to help a clinician do at least some of the dosage adjustments without expert help.

DRUG ABSORPTION AS A COMPLEX PROCESS

Drug absorption is a more complex process than is usually appreciated by health professionals, although most drug absorption occurs due to a simple concentration gradient, which results in a first-order process. This process can be explained by the following equation:

$$\frac{dA}{dt} = -k_a A$$

where A is the amount of drug remaining, k_a is a first-order absorption rate constant (since the exponent on A is unity), and dA/dt represents the instantaneous rate of absorption. However, things are not always so simple.

A favorite example used to explain the drug absorption process is vitamin C; its pharmacokinetics have been thoroughly investigated.[7] Ascorbic acid is actively absorbed; that is, a carrier enzyme that apparently becomes saturated limits the absorption and the fraction of the dose absorbed decreases with increasing dose. The average plasma level reaches a plateau at a dose of approximately 250 mg/day and changes little with doses up to 2500 mg/day. The overall pharmacokinetic model of ascorbic acid is complex and contains a fair number of carrier-mediated processes.

The second major model of absorption as an active process is the **Michaelis–Menten model of enzyme kinetics**.

In general, since absorption is primarily a passive process, aging does not alter the rate or extent of drug absorption (termed bioavailability) except in a few cases.[8] Ciprofloxacin, a fluoroquinolone antibiotic, has an increased extent of absorption (72% versus 58% of a 250-mg dose) in the elderly, although this characteristic is not shared with the other available fluoroquinolones.[9] The reason for the increased absorption seen in the elderly is not understood at present, and the primary reason for dosage reduction in the elderly is their declining renal function.

Another class of drugs in which the extent of absorption is increased in the elderly is the narcotic analgesics. The extent of morphine absorption increases from 36% to approximately 46% for both a solution and a sustained-release preparation.[8] The extent of nalbuphine absorption almost quadruples in elderly patients compared to a population of younger patients serving as controls. Again, various researchers have not been able to satisfactorily explain these changes.

When addressing drug absorption, there is no single rule that can be universally applied. For example, indomethacin has a reduced, rather than an increased, extent of absorption in the elderly; however, whether or not this applies to other nonsteroidal anti-inflammatory drugs has apparently been little studied.[8]

Bioavailability may also be affected by intestinal cytochrome P-450 activity and by P-glycoprotein, which is an efflux transporter, although again, these processes do not appear to be altered to any great extent due to aging. In summary, aging can and does affect drug bioavailability but only in a few cases that are not well understood or explained. For the most part, aging has little effect on the rate and extent of drug absorption.

DRUG DISTRIBUTION AND PROTEIN BINDING

Drugs bind to albumin and $alpha_1$-acid glycoprotein, and this binding is a function of both the levels of the drug and the levels of the protein.[10] Albumin levels generally decrease with age, while $alpha_1$-acid glycoprotein levels are unaltered. Changes in the protein binding of drugs is generally not age-related but rather is pathological, since drug disposition is altered more by disease states such as congestive heart failure and decreased renal function. The most common effect that the author has encountered in the elderly is increased free levels of phenytoin due to decreases in plasma albumin levels.

The apparent volume of distribution of a drug is related to the clearance and half-life according to:

$$Cl = \frac{\ln 2}{t_{1/2}} \times Vd$$

and thus changes in either the volume of distribution or the half-life can alter drug clearance. It is important to appreciate that clearance is the fundamental parameter that will aid one in fully understanding drug disposition, although it is abused quite often in the published literature. Furthermore, like the apparent volume of distribution, clearance can be based on blood, plasma, or serum, depending on how the drug is assayed. Care must also be taken in the interpretation of clearance or volumes calculated using nonspecific assays, that is, assays that measure the drug and a metabolite rather than just the drug itself. Notice also that the volume of distribution is an apparent volume. It is termed apparent because it does not refer to any physiological volume. In general, only a small fraction of the drug is in the blood; most of it is distributed to the tissues.

The apparent volume of distribution for diazepam increases with age, but the clearance remains constant across different ages, being offset by an increase in the half-life.[11] This volume of distribution change is most likely due to changes in the lean body mass or the ratio of fat to muscle in the individual, since the total clearance of diazepam did not change, as evidenced by an increase in the half-life. Another drug that behaves similarly is lidocaine.

Drugs that are somewhat hydrophilic have a smaller volume of distribution, which in turn results in higher drug levels in the elderly, assuming negligible tissue binding. Drugs in this category are the aminoglycosides, cimetidine, ethanol, and theophylline.[12]

DRUG METABOLISM

Aging is also associated with a smaller liver and a decrease in liver blood flow. However, caution should be exercised in interpreting studies that compare young and elderly patients since, by default, the elderly group is a more censored sample than the younger groups; that is, the experimental results may differ if the same sample of subjects was followed longitudinally for 40 years. Although it has generally been agreed that a larger person has a larger liver and can therefore metabolize more of a certain drug, not all experiments have been consistent with this assumption. In fact, the reasons why drug metabolism may be reduced with advancing age have not been clearly and unequivocally explained.[8] It has been demonstrated that cytochrome activity does not decrease with advancing age, thus removing one possible explanation. Probably the most promising explanation is a restriction of oxygen supply, specifically hepatocyte hypoxia, as the liver ages. The physiological changes involve pseudocapillarization of the sinusoidal endo-thelium of the liver.[13]

One example that has been cited is that of warfarin requirements decreasing with increasing age. However, an earlier study failed to find any reduction in clearance, and once again it is unclear what the cause or causes of the decreased dosage requirements were.

Regardless of the mechanism(s) by which these small reductions in hepatic metabolism take place, few, if any, are clinically significant. That is because these differences are usually dwarfed by renal clearance reductions. Thus the need to reduce the dose or change to another drug is usually caused by declines in renal function with age rather than by hepatic metabolism per se.

First-pass metabolism of drugs has been shown to differ due to age accord-ing to the route of administration for drugs with a high extraction ratio given intravenously, such as lidocaine, labetalol, and verapamil. But when these same drugs were administered orally, reductions in clearance were not evident.[8] Although this evidence is consistent with the hepatocyte hypoxia hypothesis, the clinical relevance is questionable.

DRUG EXCRETION

The most important reason for adjusting the dose of an elderly individual is the age-related decline in renal function. Drug excretion has been exten-sively studied, thus providing the most evidence explaining these changes. Interestingly, one of these changes, specifically a thickening of the intrare-nal vascular intima, is similar to that of the thickening that occurs in the endothelium of the liver. Studies have shown a progressive decline in renal function as measured by a decrease in the creatinine clearance, which is often used as a measure of the glomerular filtration rate (GFR). Thus, both a reduction in the number of glomeruli and a decrease in the function-ing ability of each glomeruli account for some of these changes. However, these changes were not absolute; the Baltimore Longitudinal Study of Aging reported that approximately one-third of the individuals monitored showed no decline in renal function whatsoever.[8]

Since many drugs are cleared by the kidneys, there is naturally a correlation between the glomerular filtration rate and the renal clearance of the drug. For drugs that are mainly eliminated via the kidneys, there exists a high correlation between the measured GFR and the clearance of the drug. It is important to remember that urinary excretion of a drug can involve either glomerular filtration, active tubular secretion, or passive tubular resorption,[4] or it can involve all three. For a drug that is neither secreted nor resorbed, there will be a strong correlation between GFR and clearance of the drug.

Recently, there has been a rekindling of the debate over which equation to use when a clinician wants to estimate the GFR in patients. This debate has raged since the 1970s and will most likely continue another 35 years. The two main competitors for estimating GFR are the **Cockcroft–Gault formula**[14] and the somewhat newer **MDRD (Modification of Diet in Renal Disease) formula**.[15]

Before choosing which formula to use, a clinician needs to first consider accuracy versus precision. Whether the MDRD formula is more accurate is questionable, although it is more precise. However, this extra precision does not necessarily entail a meaningful reduction in the variability and the predictions made. Furthermore, most, if not all, drug dosing is based on the Cockcroft–Gault formula; thus, there is still good reason to continue to use it. Another factor to consider is that these differences are mostly moot by the time a dose is rounded up to a practical figure on which to base the administration of a manufactured dosage to a patient.

However, if a good estimate of GFR in a patient is needed, it is best measured in that patient rather than using only one of the above-mentioned methods.

The Cockcroft–Gault formula is:

$$Cl_{cr} = \frac{(140 - age) \times weight~(kg)}{72 \times S_{cr}}$$

where age is given in years and serum creatinine, S_{cr}, is given in milligrams per deciliter. For females, multiply by 0.85. One of the MDRD formulas is:

$$GFR = 170 \times (S_{cr})^{-0.999} \times (age)^{-0.176} \times (SUN)^{-0.170} \times (ALB)^{0.318}$$

where age is in years, SUN is the serum urea nitrogen in milligrams per deciliter, and ALB is the serum albumin concentration in grams per deciliter. For females, multiply by 0.762, and for blacks, multiply by 1.18. Obviously, the Cockcroft–Gault formula is easier to use, but the use of both equations will be demonstrated.

Table 3 Recommended doses of vancomycin in patients with impaired renal function

Creatinine Clearance (mL/minute)	Dose (mg/24 hr)
100	1545
90	1390
80	1235
70	1080
60	925
50	770
40	620
30	465
20	310
10	155

As an example of looking for a difference between applying the Cockcroft–Gault formula or the MDRD formula, consider the following. An 85-year-old male Caucasian patient with a serum creatinine of 1 mg/dL, an albumin concentration of 4.2 mg/dL, and a serum urea nitrogen of 15 mg/dL is in need of a drug. This patient weighs 84 kg; the Cl_{cr} is needed in order to give a dose of vancomycin for an anaerobic infection. Use of the Cockcroft–Gault formula gives an estimated Cl_{cr} = 64.2 mL/minute, and use of the MDRD formula gives a GFR = 77.5 mL/minute.

Recommended dosages for vancomycin are given in Table 3. The Cockcroft–Gault value of 64.2 mL/minute results in a 990-mg dose, and the MDRD formula results in a dosage of 1196 mg. The dose administered would generally be rounded out, and since vancomycin is available in 1000-mg dosages, 1000 mg once every 24 hours is not an unreasonable recommendation, regardless of how the GFR was estimated. Blood levels can then be checked accordingly or if the patient experiences flushing (the so-called Red Man syndrome); if necessary, the dose could be reduced to 500 mg every 12 hours.

Any comprehensive listing of drugs that should be administered in reduced dosages to elderly patients would be quite large. Many patient care systems routinely provide clinicians with a list of patients and the drugs they take that require dosage reduction or monitoring of levels.[16] Clearly, any drug that depends upon renal elimination is a candidate, such as the aminoglycosides, digoxin, and even H_2-blockers. An extensive list of drugs whose dosage should be reduced in the elderly with suspected renal insufficiency is available.[17] Certain drugs should generally be avoided in the elderly; lists of these drugs are given elsewhere.[18]

Switching from the Cockcroft–Gault formula to the MDRD formulas is not without a certain risk. Since these formulas give slightly different estimates, the true test would be comparing the number of adverse drug reactions (ADRs) attributed to the different dosing schemes when in actual use.

KEY POINTS

- Drug disposition can be exceedingly complex; physiologic- and disease-related changes in organ and enzyme systems can and do alter pharmacokinetics in the elderly.
- Renal insufficiency is a serious matter related to drug disposition.
- Glomerular filtration rate is calculated using the Cockcroft–Gault formula and the newer Modification of Diet in Renal Disease formula.
- "Start low and go slow" applies.
- An attempt should be made to identify the cause of an ADR.
- In the elderly, certain drugs should generally be avoided. Lists of these drugs are available. Beers' list includes long-acting benzodiazepines such as diazepam, flurazepam, and chlordiazepoxide, which have possibly prolonged half-lives.
- In the elderly, taking into account variables other than renal function often requires a hit or miss approach since accurate prediction methods for dosing are not available.
- Constant vigilance on the part of all health professionals is likely the best way to serve the vulnerable elderly who are often overmedicated.

REFERENCES

1. Kidder SW. DUR by pharmacists. Lessons learned for MTMS. *Consult Pharm.* 2005; 20:1056–8, 1060–2.
2. Perez-Ruiz F, Hernando I, Villar I, et al. Correction of allopurinol dosing should be based on clearance of creatinine, but not plasma creatinine levels: another insight to allopurinol-related toxicity. *J Clin Rheumatol.* 2005;11(3):129–33.
3. Pharmacokinetics and biopharmaceutics: a definition of terms. *J Pharmacokinet Biopharm.* 1973;1:3–4.
4. Notari RE. *Biopharmaceutics and Clinical Pharmacokinetics: An Introduction.* 4th ed. New York: Marcel Dekker; 1987.
5. Shargel L, Wu-Pong S, Yu ABC. *Applied Biopharmaceutics and Pharmacokinetics.* 5th ed. New York: McGraw-Hill; 2005.

6. Gabrielsson J, Weiner D. *Pharmacokinetic and Pharmacodynamic Data Analysis: Concepts and Applications.* 3rd ed. Stockholm, Sweden: Swedish Pharmaceutical Press; 2000.

7. Graumlich JF, Ludden TM, Conry-Cantilena C, et al. Pharmacokinetic model of ascorbic acid in healthy male volunteers during depletion and repletion. *Pharm Res.* 1997;14:1133–9.

8. Cusack BJ. Pharmacokinetics in older persons. *Am J Geriatr Pharmacother.* 2004;2: 274–302.

9. Stahlmann R, Lode H. Fluoroquinolones in the elderly: safety considerations. *Drugs Aging.* 2003;20(4):289–302.

10. Grandison MK, Boudinot FD. Age-related changes in protein binding of drugs: implications for therapy. *Clin Pharmacokinet.* 2000;38:271–90.

11. Klotz U, Avant GR, Hoyumpa A, et al. The effects of age and liver disease on the disposition and elimination of diazepam in adult man. *J Clin Invest.* 1975;55:347–59.

12. Mangoni AA, Jackson SHD. Age-related changes in pharmacokinetics and pharmacodynamics: basic principles and practical applications. *Br J Clin Pharmacol.* 2004; 57(1):5–14.

13. Mclean AJ, Cogger VC, Chong GC, et al. Age-related pseudocapillarization of the human liver. *J Pathol.* 2003;200:112–7.

14. Cockcroft DW, Gault MH. Prediction of creatinine clearance from serum creatinine. *Nepron.* 1976;16:31–41.

15. Levey AS, Bosch JP, Lewis JB, et al. A more accurate method to estimate glomerular filtration rate from serum creatinine: a new prediction equation. *Ann Intern Med.* 1999;130:461–70.

16. Nash IS, Rojas M, Hebert P, et al. Reducing excessive medication administration in hospitalized adults with renal dysfunction. *Am J Med Qual.* 2005;20:64–9.

17. Brater DC. Drug dosing in renal failure. In: Brady HR, Wilcox CS, eds. *Therapy in Nephrology and Hypertension: A Companion to Brenner and Rector's the Kidney.* Philadelphia: WB Saunders; 1999:641–53.

18. Cusack B. Clinical pharmacology. In: Beers MH, Berkow R, eds. *The Merck Manual of Geriatrics.* Whitehouse Station: Merck Research Laboratories; 2000:54–74.

4

Pharmacotherapy Issues Related to Cardiovascular Disease and the Elderly

MARK E. CLASEN AND KRISTINA L. GRIFFITHS

Worry affects the circulation, the heart, the glands, the whole nervous system, and profoundly affects heart action.

—Dr. Charles H. Mayo

OVERVIEW

Cardiovascular disease (CVD) is the leading cause of morbidity and mortality in those 65 years of age and older. Elderly patients are often overlooked and preventative medicine is often underused due to a lack of research relative to the benefits of such therapy in the elderly. However, recent evidence suggests that CVD treatment and prevention are effective in the elderly and should be implemented when possible. Implementation must take into consideration the changes that take place in normal aging that may affect the pharmacology of medications. The elderly make up about 14% of the population, but the over 65 population consumes more than 30% of prescription drugs in the United States. It has been predicted by the U.S. Census Bureau that the geriatric population will more than double in the next 50 years due to the upcoming baby boomers and the increases in life expectancy. Therefore, the treatment of hypertension and hyperlipidemia along with lifestyle modifications and other preventative measures against stroke, peripheral vascular disease, and heart failure should be implemented to improve the health status and quality of life in the growing geriatric population.

Mrs. Rena Fernandez is a 78-year-old female of Hispanic origin. Seen wandering about the OTC display shelves in a pharmacy, she is approached by a clerk who asks, "Can I help you?" She responds, "I would like to see a lady pharmacist as I have a lady-like problem." The clerk goes to the dispensing area and asks Mary Sedral, PharmD, a recently graduated pharmacist, to come and help Mrs. Fernandez. The two women talk for a short time during which the elderly woman reveals that she is embarrassed to say that she has been having difficulty "moving her bowels" and could she be directed to a good laxative.

During further conversation, the pharmacist learns that Mrs. Fernandez has also been experiencing some facial redness, which is an annoyance because she says she is turning into a "Red Indian." The pharmacist then asks Mrs. Fernandez to wait a minute while she checks on her medication records. The records indicate that Mrs. Fernandez has been taking verapamil (Calan®) and she started this drug about 4 weeks ago. The pharmacist calls the prescribing physician and learns that Mrs. Fernandez is being treated for coronary heart disease, the beginnings of heart failure, and an irregular heartbeat, all of which were recently diagnosed.

- What do you think is going on here?
- What advice should Mrs. Fernandez receive?

Heart rate control by calcium antagonists is important for decreasing myocardial oxygen demand. Of all the calcium channel blockers available, verapamil has the most profound SA and AV nodal effects. But this class of drugs is associated with a variety of side effects, not all of which are found with use of each calcium channel blocker. Constipation is much more common with verapamil. Headache, facial flushing, hypotension, and bradycardia can occur with any of these medications.

HEART FAILURE

Heart failure is one of the more significant diseases affecting the elderly. It is estimated that more than 6 million Americans suffer from heart failure, and the morbidity, mortality, and health care expenditures because of it are significant: 84% of persons over the age of 65 die from this disease[1] and 400,000–700,000 new diagnoses are made each year. It used to be common to refer to heart failure as congestive heart failure (CHF), but that nomenclature is ceasing, since it is possible to have heart failure without congestion.

However, differences are observed when young and old hearts are compared, and these differences do not reflect an impairment of physiology and function. They simply represent changes due to advancing age, and there is no evidence that a normal aging heart cannot respond to stress by increasing its output. Cardiac output is determined by stroke volume times heart rate and, since the resting heart rate in the elderly changes very little (as is also the case in younger people), any change in cardiac output must occur through a change in stroke volume. Stroke volume in the elderly is affected by diastolic filling, ability of the ventricles to distend, the ability of the myocardium muscle to contract, and ventricular afterload.

Heart failure is best described as the failure to pump enough blood to adequately meet the oxygen or metabolic needs of body tissues. It is a highly lethal condition, with a 5-year mortality rate of about 50%.[2] Heart failure is not a traditional disease like asthma, for example, as it can be caused by several cardiac problems; however, once heart failure syndromes occur, they result in a specific pathological process independent of the cause. In older populations, the causes of heart failure are numerous, with the most common being coronary artery disease. Right- or left-sided symptoms center around whether or not there are differing etiologies. For example, 10 etiologies of left-sided failure include:

- Primary ischemic failure.
- Hypertension, which causes remodeling of the heart.
- Valvular regurgitation and other structural abnormalities such as hereditary congenital heart disease, one of which is valvular heart disease.
- Polyinfiltrates, such as viral and bacterial myocarditis.
- Toxins (cobalt, lead, alcohol) or toxic drugs such as disopyramide.
- Inflammation.
- Trauma, such as a gunshot wound.

Table 1   New York Heart Association Heart Failure Symptom Classification System

Class	Level of Impairment
I	No symptom limitation with ordinary physical activity
II	Ordinary physical activity somewhat limited by dyspnea (i.e., long distance walking, climbing two flights of stairs)
III	Exercise limited by dyspnea at mild work loads (i.e., short distance walking, climbing one flight of stairs)
IV	Dyspnea at rest or with very little exertion

- Constrictive etiologies, as exemplified by cardiac tamponade.
- Immunologic problems, exemplified by rheumatic heart disease.
- High output heart failure, such as that associated with systemic diseases (beriberi, anemia from any cause, and thyrotoxicosis).[3]

The New York Heart Association (NYHA) classification scheme is used to assess the severity of functional limitations and correlates fairly well with prognosis (Table 1).

Patients with heart failure syndrome should be regarded as having two pathologic processes occurring. The first is congestion, which manifests as an impairment of left ventricular function. The second pathology is myocardial failure, in which the myocardial tissue of the left ventricle ceases to function and induces pulmonary congestion, peripheral edema, hepatomegaly, fatigue, anorexia, and shortness of breath.[4]

As a decrease in cardiac function occurs, the heart relies on compensatory systems to maintain an adequate cardiac output. These systems are:

- Tachycardia and increased contractility of heart muscle as a result of sympathetic nervous system stimulation.
- Vasoconstriction.
- Ventricular hypertrophy and remodeling.
- A Frank–Starling response, whereby an increase in preload results in an increase in stroke volume.

The Frank–Starling response, or Law of the Heart, is named after two prominent 19th century physiologists who stated that, within physiological limits, the heart pumps all the blood that returns to it without undue damming of the blood in veins. Intrinsic regulatory mechanisms then permit adaption of the heart to rates of venous return that may vary from 2 L/minute at rest to 25 L/minute during exercise. Intrinsic regulation depends on the fact that stretching cardiac muscle results in a greater force of contraction. Thus, increased venous return stretches the heart and causes increased force of contraction (and a moderate increase in heart rate), resulting in a corresponding increase in cardiac output.[4] But when the heart is unable to meet the metabolic demands, the results are renal insufficiency, water retention, and elevated blood urea nitrogen (BUN) and creatinine, which then trigger the renin–angiotensin system, leading to the symptoms of heart failure and the rationale for drug interventions to correct the condition.

When an adult is at rest, cardiac output is approximately 5 L/minute. Under periods of exercise or other stresses, the average adult can pump 15 L/minute. Thus, the cardiac reserve is 300%, or three times the 5 liters at rest. The well-trained athlete running a marathon may be pumping 22 L/minute.

When heart failure occurs in the elderly, either there is not enough cardiac output or the heart is not pumping all the blood that comes to it. Either situation will lead to an increase in left atrial or right atrial blood pressure. If the left heart fails, there will be an increase in pulmonary artery pressure. If this pressure increases enough, pulmonary edema will result. If this pressure continues to increase, the right side of the heart will also fail. Thus, one common cause of right-sided heart failure is left-sided heart failure.

Symptoms of left-sided heart failure include paroxysmal nocturnal dyspnea, orthopnea, pulmonary edema, shortness of breath, and decreased exercise tolerance. If the right pump fails, there is decreased blood flow to the left side of the heart, resulting in decreased coronary artery perfusion, which then results in decreased myocardial perfusion. In this construct, right-sided heart failure can lead to left-sided heart failure. Symptoms of right-sided heart failure include jugular venous distension, hepatojugular reflux, and pedal edema.

If there is sudden damage to the left heart, as in an acute myocardial infarction, there is immediate decreased cardiac output. Within 30 seconds, the decreased output is followed by increased systemic venous pressure and a marked increase in norepinephrine in the circulation. This increase in norepinephrine stimulates receptors in the myocardium, causing a 100% increase of inotropic strength of the heart. There is then an increased venous pressure from 10 to 14 mm Hg, causing more venous return to the heart.

If there is less than normal cardiac output, a decrease in renal perfusion results, causing a marked increase in afferent arterial tone. This change activates the renin–angiotensin–aldosterone cascade, which causes:

- Markedly increased afferent arterial tone.
- Decreased peritubular capillary pressure.
- Markedly increased sodium and water retention.
- Increased antidiuretic hormone levels, causing fluid resorption.

The reason these changes occur is because the kidneys are responding per the Frank–Starling Law of the Heart. Here, the kidneys attempt to conserve fluid by not making urine and sending fluid back into the circulation and thus back to the heart. As it comes back into the heart, the heart pumps all of the fluid/blood that comes to it. In fact, the kidneys will not tolerate even the slightest decrease in perfusion from normal.

This increase in venous return to the heart causes the myocardium muscle fibers to stretch. The more the myocardium stretches, the stronger is the response of contraction. The increased contraction of the myocardium results in increased cardiac output, muscle hypertrophy, and a return of a normal cardiac output to satisfy the kidneys.

Systolic Heart Failure

The number one etiology of heart failure in the elderly is ischemic. Ischemic etiologies tend to cause systolic dysfunction heart failure. The patient's history is often one of an acute myocardial infarction or long-standing ischemia amplified with a history of angina. Physical examination of the patient with systolic dysfunction heart failure often reveals cardiac ataxia and a person without much vigor. Other features of this type of heart failure are cardiomegaly, an S3-gallup, a murmur of mitral regurgitation, or aortic insufficiency. A chest x-ray most likely will show the cardiomegaly and an echocardiogram will likely show dilated chambers with thin walls and floppy valves. Often, the left ventricular ejection fraction is less than 45%. The mechanism of this kind of heart failure is loss of or impaired muscle fibers, due to the so-called "remodeling of the heart."[5]

Diastolic Heart Failure

The number two etiology of heart failure among the elderly is diastolic heart failure. Often the patient's history includes long-standing hypertension. However, ischemia may also play a secondary role and, indeed, in many elders, diastolic and systolic heart failure coexist. The features of diastolic heart failure include:

- An S4-gallup.
- A systolic ejection murmur.
- A chest x-ray that might show normal heart size to slightly increased heart size.
- An echocardiogram that shows hyperdynamic, thick walls.
- A left ventricular ejection fraction often greater than 55%.

The mechanism here is fibrosis, altered collagen properties, and delayed cardiac relaxation.[6]

Pharmacotherapy Treatment of Heart Failure

Treatment of heart failure is usually dependent on its etiology. If looking at systolic dysfunction heart failure, most often due to ischemia, the following drugs are the most frequently used in the outpatient setting: digoxin (Lanoxin®), angiotensin-converting enzyme (ACE) inhibitors labeled for use in heart failure [e.g., enalapril (Vasotec®), captopril (Capoten®), fosinopril (Monopril®), lisinopril (Prinivil®), quinapril (Accupril®), and ramipril (Altace®)]; diuretics (hydrochlorothiazide, furosemide), nitrates, hydralazine (Zaroxolyn®); and beta-blockers that have reduced mortality in heart failure [e.g., bisoprolol (Zebeta®), carvedilol (Coreg®), and metoprolol (Toprol®)]. Sometimes, as this type of heart failure decompensates, the patient must come in for intravenous medications, including the sympathomimetics such as dobutamine (Dobutrex®) and dopamine (Inotropin®). Other drugs labeled only for use in heart failure include amrinone (Inocor®) and milrinone (Primacor®).

The treatment of heart failure, if it is primarily diastolic dysfunction heart failure, includes beta-blockers, ACE inhibitors, and certain calcium channel blockers. In chronic CHF conditions, aggressive tertiary prevention is very much in order. Aggressive pharmacologic management of hypertension, tobaccoism, hypercholesterolemia, diabetes, and obesity is an important therapeutic goal. In the treatment of this kind of heart failure, beta-blockers are an important addition in the outpatient setting in both systolic and diastolic dysfunction heart failure. Beta-blockers do prevent the down regulation of the beta 1 receptor. Keeping the beta 1 to beta 2 receptors intact is one strategy to prevent further remodeling of the heart. ACE inhibitors are almost always indicated in either type of heart failure, as is exercise and cardiac rehabilitation. Other factors in heart failure include anticoagulation, if indicated, and anti-inflammatory strategies.

Despite all of the literature that supports the use of ACE inhibitors, there is just as much literature supporting the fact that these agents are underused with heart failure. In fact, a significant number of patients who could benefit do not get ACE inhibitors and, of those who do get them, up to 50% are given doses **lower** than recommended.[7,8]

Part of the spectrum of ischemic heart disease also involves acute coronary syndromes. In the aftermath of these types of events, the following medications are often used: aspirin, beta-blockers, ACE inhibitors, statins, nitrates, and clopidogrel. The risk-to-benefit ratio of all these drugs and how they are used together or alone depends on the patient's particular situation. For hyperlipidemias, particularly LDL elevations, statins are often the drug of choice. For low HDL issues, niacin and fibrates are employed. As for hyper-triglyceridemia, sometimes two and three drug therapies are necessary. For antiplatelet action, clopidogrel and aspirin together or aspirin alone, according to some newer data, help with the anticoagulation issues or at least the antiplatelet aggregation issues that accompany these kinds of problems. If diabetes and hypertension are present, aggressive therapy for both comorbid conditions is indicated. Diabetes should be considered a coronary heart disease equivalent.

Dilemmas in Medicating the Geriatric Patient with Heart Failure
Polypharmacy

The geriatric dilemmas pertaining to prescribing for the elderly with heart failure involve the dynamic of polypharmacy versus improved outcome with targeted pharmaceuticals. There is no doubt that treating systolic hypertension with medications decreases the likelihood of a stroke. The suffering related to both coronary artery disease and stroke is mitigated by aggressive pharmacotherapy to reduce blood pressure. Likewise, if any coagulation is needed, particularly when there is atrial fibrillation, warfarin is most always indicated. Other issues of renal elimination and decreased portal blood flow frequently require clinicians to "start low and go slow" when adding medication. In terms of the number of drugs needed, if more than five drugs are prescribed for a heart failure patient, there is a 50–50 chance of a drug–drug interaction. Likewise, when a patient is taking more than five drugs, there are increased hospitalizations, compliance issues, and obvious economic issues.

Monotherapy

It is of note that monotherapy in the elderly:

- Rarely controls hypertension.
- Provides some optimal antithrombosis therapy.
- Rarely works for moderate-to-severe diabetes.
- Rarely works for severe dyslipidemia.

Monotherapy does work for isolated low-density lipoprotein (LDL) elevations.

Anticoagulation

Anticoagulation decreases the risks of sudden events; however, the INR for patients receiving warfarin has to be monitored carefully. Falls and traumatic injuries with warfarin therapy are very problematic. Other options such as aspirin and clopidogrel have an enhanced bleeding side effect. Low molecular weight heparin is another strategy that can be implemented for anticoagulation in older patients.

In summary, the goals of treating heart failure are:

- To prevent repeat acute coronary syndromes or other major ischemic events.
- To bring blood pressure down to 120/80.
- To target hemoglobin A1c at 6.
- To target lipids at LDL = < 60, high-density lipoproteins (HDL) = > 50, and triglycerides = < 159.
- To assess continually cardiovascular risks in heart failure patients by paying attention to the patient's medical history.

Assessing Risk Factors in the Medical History of the Patient and the Family

To be of greater assistance and to help an elderly patient with heart failure, all clinicians need to pay particular attention to the medical history of the patient and the family. Look for a history of hypertension, coronary artery disease, peripheral vascular disease, diabetes, stroke, chronic obstructive pulmonary disease (COPD), medication use, and nonprescription medication use. Risk factors in the medical history of the patient's family members should also be sought, including heart attacks, diabetes, heart failure, high cholesterol, hypertension, sudden death, and stroke. Risk factors in the patient's social history should also be assessed, including smoking, alcohol (either social or harmful), diet (helpful or harmful), occupational exposures, and drug usage. It is of note that drinking 1–2 oz of alcohol a day seems to have beneficial effects on cardiovascular disease and outcomes.

Risk factors from the physician's physical examination of the patient are also part of the clinical decision tree and include:

- Cardiac rhythm disturbances.
- Murmurs related to valvular heart disease.
- Bruits in the carotid, renal, or femoral arteries, which, of course, portend the coronary heart disease equivalent.
- Ankle-brachial index of > 0.9 (a rough indicator of arthrogenic load).

Pulse presence or absence helps determine whether peripheral vascular disease is present and, if so, whether it is a coronary heart disease equivalent. Waist circumference, skin texture, and quality of the lower extremities are again indicators to be assessed during physical examination.

Risk factors from the laboratory include fasting glucose, fractionated lipids, microalbumin, and a set of emerging markers. Risk assessments can be made using the global risk assessment from the Framingham study and evidence from EKGs, stress thalliums, echos, and cath labs.

Dealing with Comorbidities in the Elderly Heart Failure Patient

Hypertension

Interventions for hypertension involve weight loss and a target BP of 120/80.[9] Careful targeting in the elderly of blood pressure end points is highly advised. Beta-blockers should be part of the drug regimen in the postcoronary syndrome. ACE inhibitors are almost always indicated in both types of heart failure. Finally, diuretics are often indicated, particularly in systolic dysfunction congestive heart failure.

Diabetes

Diabetes should be considered a coronary heart disease equivalent. Exercise and weight loss are always a place to begin, but the main strategies to help the patient reach a hemoglobin A1c between 6 and 7 involve use of these four medication classes: (1) thiazolidinediones [troglitazone (Rezulin®)]; (2) sulfonylureas [glyburide (Micronase®)], glipizide (Glucotrol®), glimepiride (Amaryl®); (3) biguanides [metformin (Glucophage®)]; (4) alpha-glucosidase inhibitors [acarbose (Precose®)] plus insulin. In frail elderly patients, it is considered dangerous to control diabetes too tightly, particularly if the elderly are sedentary and unable to move to correct issues of hypoglycemia. Also, with diabetes in the elderly, the clinician must monitor all issues, including microalbuminuria. In cases of diabetic patients with heart failure, there is some rationale for an ACE inhibitor for blood pressure control; by keeping blood pressure lower, some of the nephropathy and protein loss associated with diabetic nephropathy are prevented.

Hyperlipidemia

A clinician's intervention relative to lipids, diet, and exercise is important. Set points include an LDL of less than 60, an HDL of greater than 50, and triglycerides less than 150. These are the goals when the patient has diabetes, hypertension, and hyperlipidemia.

Inflammation

When treating inflammation, aspirin continues to be the mainstay of anti-inflammatory medications for the elderly with heart failure. However, statins also exhibit some of the same qualities that aspirin does, particularly in the anti-inflammatory arena. Nonsteroidal anti-inflammatory drugs (NSAIDs) obviously are sometimes considered helpful in the elderly and may be protective with regard to Alzheimer's disease. However, NSAIDs do alter the enterons and prostaglandins and are well known to increase blood pressure, particularly in the elderly.

Thrombotic Risk

Finally, the use of aspirin reduces thrombotic risks whether or not clopidogrel is included. It probably would be wise to discontinue hormone replacement therapy, as estrogens are thrombogenic.

Sometimes, aspirin and clopidogrel are used together. One complication from this combination could be a surprise incidence of bleeding. Should deep vein thrombosis exist, warfarin or low molecular weight heparin might be indicated. For the patient in atrial fibrillation, strong evidence exists for the use of warfarin as a means to cut down on the incidence of stroke.

In summary, the issues attendant to the clinician's involvement with a heart failure patient are quite complex, and they involve issues of comprehensive screening for lipids, high blood pressure, and diabetes. Often, these comorbid conditions are so intermingled that they are part of the etiology of heart failure and present special and unique challenges to clinicians and caregivers.

HYPERTENSION

Hypertension in the Elderly

Hypertension is a modifiable risk factor in CVD and affects nearly 50 million people in the United States. More than two-thirds of the elderly population has hypertension; however, the geriatric population has the lowest rate of blood pressure control, and treatment is often underused because of a fear of harming elderly individuals. Additional care should be taken in the dosing of medications in the elderly; certain adjustments may be needed due to the changes that occur in aging, but overall, hypertension treatment in the elderly does not differ considerably from other individuals. Thus, the same general principles applied to younger patients should be applied to elderly hypertensive patients for adequate risk reduction for CVD.[10]

There is a progressive increase in blood pressure (BP) associated with aging. Several changes occur in the body that cause this increase. In general, an increase in peripheral vascular resistance occurs due to decreased vessel elasticity, increased aortic and large vessel wall thickness, and decreased vasodilatory responses to β-adrenergic receptors with preserved α-adrenergic vasoconstriction. Sodium retention and decreased plasma renin and aldosterone levels that occur with aging may also contribute to hypertension.[11]

Typically, both systolic and diastolic BP increase with age. Systolic blood pressure (SBP) usually rises until the age of 70 or 80. In contrast, diastolic blood pressure (DBP) increases until about age 50 or 60, and then tends to level off or decrease slightly. It is for this reason that isolated systolic hypertension (ISH) tends to occur more frequently in the elderly. Hypertension generally refers to a SBP ≥ 120 mm Hg and a DBP ≥ 80 mm Hg, whereas ISH refers to SBP ≥ 140 mm Hg and a DBP < 90 mm Hg. SBP is now believed to be a greater predictor of future cardiovascular events than DBP and is even believed to be an independent risk factor in itself in some instances.[12]

Why Treat Hypertension?

It has been demonstrated in many studies, including the Framingham study, that elevated BP increases the risk of all cardiovascular diseases, including CHF, peripheral vascular disease, left ventricular hypertrophy, and ischemic cardiopathy, that may result in a myocardial infarction. Chronic hypertension may also increase the incidence of strokes by leading to the narrowing of the lumen in multiple blood vessels, which then can affect cerebral blood flow. In addition, there is a correlation between mortality and hypertension, demonstrating hypertension as a major predictor of mortality. Lowering BP has been associated with a 35%–40% reduction in stroke, 20%–25% reduction in myocardial infarctions, and a decrease of more than 50% in heart failure incidence.[13] Therefore, it is imperative to treat hypertension, particularly in the geriatric population, which is at an increased risk for these cardiovascular diseases.

Diagnosis, Classification, and Cardiovascular Risk Factors

In an elderly hypertensive patient, a thorough diagnostic evaluation should be performed, including a history, physical exam, and laboratory evaluation using electrolyte measurements, creatinine levels, urinalysis, and electrocardiogram to assess any end organ damage or potential causes of hypertension. It is important to determine a patient's baseline BP. Diagnosis should be made using at least two accurate measurements of BP while the patient is seated comfortably in a chair for at least 5 minutes; measurements should take into account any alcohol, caffeine, or tobacco use, as well as anxiety. Occasionally, measurement of BP in the standing position may be indicated in those at risk for postural hypotension.

The JNC 7 Report on Prevention, Detection, Evaluation, and Treatment of High Blood Pressure[13] classifies hypertension in all individuals 18 years and older according to Table 2.

The JNC 7 goals of treatment include achieving a BP < 140/90 mm Hg to decrease the risk of CVD and stroke. In hypertensive patients with diabetes or chronic kidney disease, the BP goal is < 130/80 mm Hg; however, these goals are criticized as being somewhat strict in the elderly patient. Because the aging process involves increases in BP, it has been argued that elderly patients actually need a slightly higher BP to perfuse vital organs properly. In general, any 20-mm Hg decrease in BP decreases the risk of CVD. It is also important to lower BP slowly in geriatric patients with chronic hypertension, allowing their bodies to reset regulation to a more normal level, instead of the higher blood pressure to which their bodies had adapted.

Major cardiovascular risk factors include the following: hypertension, cigarette smoking, obesity (BMI ≥ 30), physical inactivity, dyslipidemia, diabetes mellitus, microalbuminuria or estimated GFR < 60 mL/minute, age (> 55 years for men, > 65 years for women), and family history of premature cardiovascular disease (men < 55 years or women < 65 years).[14]

Table 2   Classification and management of hypertension

BP Classification	Systolic BP, mm Hg	Diastolic BP, mm Hg	Lifestyle Modification	Initial Drug Therapy
Normal	< 120	< 80	Encourage	None
Prehypertension	120–139	80–89	Yes	None recommended.[a]
Stage 1 hypertension	140–159	90–99	Yes	Thiazide-type diuretics for most; may consider an ACE inhibitor, angiotensin-receptor blocker, beta-blocker, calcium channel blocker, or a combination.[a]
Stage 2 hypertension	≥ 160	≥ 100	Yes	Two-drug combination for most, usually a thiazide-type diuretic and an ACE inhibitor, angiotensin-receptor blocker, beta-blocker, or calcium channel blocker.

[a] Treat patients with medications appropriate for any compelling indications such as heart failure, postmyocardial infarction, diabetes, chronic kidney disease, peripheral vascular disease, or stroke prevention.

Benefits of Therapy

The first hypertension trial that demonstrated the efficacy of antihypertensives was the European Working Party on High Blood Pressure in the Elderly (EWPHE) trial. In the EWPHE trial, 840 hypertensive patients were assigned to diuretic therapy or placebo. Diuretic therapy was associated with a 27% reduction in cardiovascular mortality, a 60% reduction in fatal myocardial infarctions, a 52% decrease in stroke incidence, and a reduction in the incidence of heart failure.[15,16] In one of the next major trials, called the Swedish Trial in Old Patients with Hypertension (STOP-Hypertension), patients were given a diuretic, a beta-blocker, or a placebo. This trial revealed a 47% decrease in strokes, a 73% reduction in stroke mortality, and a 43% reduction in total mortality in the treatment groups.[17,18] Another major trial, called the Heart Outcomes Prevention Evaluation (HOPE), demonstrated a 22% decrease in risk of cardiovascular events with antihypertensive therapy.[19] Finally, the most recent trial, the Hypertension in the

Table 3   Lifestyle modifications for hypertension[a]

Modification	Recommendation	Approximate Systolic BP Reduction, Range
Weight reduction	Maintain normal body weight (BMI[b] 18–25).	5–20 mm Hg/ 10-kg weight loss
Adopt DASH[b] diet	Consume a diet rich in fruits, vegetables, and low-fat dairy products, with a reduced content of saturated and total fat.	8–14 mm Hg
Dietary sodium reduction	Reduce daily dietary sodium intake to no more than 100 mEq/L (2.4 g of sodium or 6 g of sodium chloride).	2–8 mm Hg
Physical activity	Engage in regular aerobic activity such as brisk walking at least 30 minutes/day most days of the week.	4–9 mm Hg
Moderation of alcohol consumption	Limit daily consumption of alcohol to no more than two drinks in men and no more than one drink in women and lighter weight persons.[c]	2–4 mm Hg

[a] Adapted from Reference 13.
[b] Abbreviations: BMI = body mass index, DASH = Dietary Approaches to Stop Hypertension.
[c] A drink refers to 1 oz or 30 mL of ethanol, 24 oz of beer, 10 oz of wine, or 3 oz of 80-proof whiskey.

Very Elderly Trial (HYVET), has indicated that a decrease in stroke incidence occurs when the very elderly (over 80) are treated for hypertension. The study began in 2001 in England. The HYVET study is an international randomized controlled trial designed to establish the balance of benefits and risks of antihypertensive therapy in persons 80 years of age or more; it is an ongoing study.[20]

Nonpharmacologic Treatment of Hypertension

Lifestyle modifications should be the initial treatment of any hypertensive patient, with or without drug therapy. Living a healthy life-style is a crucial part in the management of hypertension. Weight reduction, smoking cessation, sodium reduction, physical activity, moderation of alcohol consumption, and adoption of the Dietary Approaches to Stop Hypertension (DASH) diet are all lifestyle modifications that help decrease BP, enhance antihypertensive drug efficacy, and reduce cardiovascular risk. Table 3 summarizes important lifestyle changes to help manage hypertension.

Pharmacologic Treatment of Hypertension

The elderly are a segment of the U.S. population that has the highest prevalence of hypertension and accounts for a large proportion of persons seeking antihypertensive therapy.[21] The problem is that among the elderly hypertension is not only more prevalent, it is less well controlled and more severe, especially in elderly women.[22]

Thiazide-type Diuretics

Thiazide diuretics are the basis of hypertension therapy and should be considered first line or the drug of choice for hypertension. Several recent trials, including the Antihypertensive and Lipid-Lowering Treatment to Prevent Heart Attack Trial (ALLHAT), have proven that thiazide diuretics are superior to other agents in the reduction of stroke, cardiovascular events, and overall mortality.[23] In fact, the ALLHAT trial of 33,000 relatively high-risk patients who were treated over a 5-year period with chlorthalidone, a thiazide, amlodipine, or lisinopril found that those who received the thiazide experienced fewer overall cardiovascular events than those on other agents. There were no differences in end-point morbidity or mortality, however, just on selected outcomes. For example, those receiving the thiazides had a lower incidence of heart failure and stroke than the group randomized to lisinopril, especially so in African American populations.[24] The bottom line is that the ALLHAT results appear to have settled the debate about the benefits or risk of diuretics in the management of hypertension: for many years, physicians had argued that the metabolic issues surrounding diuretics might actually increase the risk for CVD.[25]

Thiazides work by inhibiting sodium and chloride reabsorption, promoting water loss, and reducing peripheral vascular resistance. They are effective in decreasing BP, are affordable, and enhance the hypertensive efficacy of multidrug regimens. Their major adverse effects include hyponatremia, hypokalemia, hyperuricemia, hypercalcemia, hyperglycemia, and possibly a rise in LDL cholesterol. Elderly patients may be more susceptible to the electrolyte disturbances of thiazides; metolazone is the only thiazide indicated in patients with renal insufficiency (CrCl < 30 mL/minute).

Despite hypertension treatment trials that demonstrate the benefit of diuretics and despite the repeated recommendations of the JNC for the use of diuretics as initial therapy, diuretic use decreased over the 20-year period of the 1980s and 1990s as newer drugs promised more exciting results.[26] With a decrease in the use of diuretics, an increased number of resistant hypertensives was anticipated. In several large clinics where resistant hypertension was defined as BP >160/100 mm Hg when patients received at least two or three medications, antihypertensive drug resistance disappeared in almost 50% of patients when the diuretic dosage was increased or diuretics were added to the treatment regimen. The bottom line is now quite a nondebate: diuretics are an important component of hypertension management. Unlike thiazides, loop diuretics and potassium-sparing diuretics are generally not recommended as monotherapy in hypertension. Although these agents can help reduce BP and have been shown to be safe in elderly individuals, they simply do not have the efficacy profiles demonstrated in other available agents.[27]

ACE Inhibitors

The recent trials describing benefits from treatment with ACE inhibitors or angiotensin-receptor blockers (ARBs) were not trials of monotherapy.[28-31] In most of these studies, more than 50%–60% of patients were receiving diuretics in addition to the study drugs. Improvement in outcomes, whether from heart or renal failure, usually resulted from the use of two or more medications with different mechanisms of action. There are clearly advantages to using more than one medication in the management of hypertension. Thus, when two or more agents are used, logically one of them should be a diuretic.

Generally, all ACE inhibitors and ARBs are similarly effective in treating hypertension, and their use is considered sage and well tolerated in the elderly. In many different comparative trials between ACE inhibitors and ARBs, there have been no significant differences in their antihypertensive activity. ACE inhibitors work by inhibiting the conversion of angiotensin I to the active hormone angiotensin II, which is a potent vasoconstrictor and stimulator of aldosterone secretion. ACE inhibitors also block the degradation of bradykinin, a potent vasodilator. It is by these mechanisms that they reduce peripheral vascular resistance and exert their antihypertensive effect. ARBs block the binding of angiotensin II to its receptor, working in a similar fashion as ACE inhibitors, except they have no effect on bradykinin. All ACE inhibitors except fosinopril and most ARBs except losartan and irbesartan are excreted primarily by the kidneys; therefore, lower initial doses are recommended in renal impairment (CrCl < 30 mL/minute). However, losartan and irbesartan are metabolized by the cytochrome P-450 system and thus should be monitored for drug interactions.

Common side effects of ACE inhibitors include hypotension, renal insufficiency, hyperkalemia, cough, and angioedema, whereas common side effects of ARBs include hyperkalemia, renal insufficiency, dizziness, diarrhea, fatigue, and, to a lesser degree, cough and angioedema. ACE- and ARB-induced renal insufficiency particularly occurs in those at increased risk, such as patients with hypotension, hyponatremia, severe heart failure, or renal artery stenosis or those receiving chronic NSAID therapy.

Beta-Blockers

The use of beta-blockers to reduce BP in elderly patients has proven to be safe, and all beta-blockers are equally effective; however, beta-blockers may differ pharmacologically and pharmacokinetically. Atenolol, metoprolol, bisoprolol, and acebutolol are selective beta-blockers working only on β_1-receptors in the heart. Labetalol and carvedilol have α_1-blocking properties and are nonselective beta-blockers, blocking both β_1- and β_2-receptors. These properties are important considerations when choosing a beta-blocker for an elderly patient. Adverse effects of beta-blockers include bradycardia, heart block, hypotension, fatigue, hyperglycemia, and hyperlipidemia. When used in combination with a diuretic, beta-blockers can be useful as initial therapy. Use caution when combining other agents, including digoxin and verapamil, with beta-blockers, since drug interactions can occur. Beta-blockers should be used with caution in some patient populations, such as those with pulmonary disorders (COPD or asthma) or conduction abnormalities.[32,33]

Calcium Channel Blockers

The two classes of calcium channel blockers are dihydropyridines and nondihydropyridines. The nondihydropyridines, such as verapamil and diltiazem, are negative inotropes and chromotropes (reduce contractility and heart rate). On the other hand, dihydropyridines such as nifedipine and nicardipine do not affect conduction through the AV node; however, these agents are negative inotropes as well, with the exception of amlodipine and felodipine. Despite their differences, all calcium channel blockers have similar antihypertensive effects. As part of the aging process, elderly patients' blood flow to the liver decreases, causing a decrease in the metabolism of agents by the liver. It is for this reason that geriatric patients may require lower initial doses of calcium channel blockers, which undergo extensive metabolism by the liver. The most common adverse effects of calcium channel blockers are constipation, particularly with verapamil; headache; tachycardia; dizziness; and flushing. Generally, calcium channel blockers are considered safe and well tolerated in the elderly, but the concomitant use of a calcium channel blocker with a beta-blocker should be avoided due to an increased risk of bradycardia.

Other Agents

Other agents for hypertension, including α_1-adrenergic blockers (doxazosin and terazosin), centrally and peripherally acting antiadrenergic agents (clonidine, methyldopa, reserpine), and direct vasodilators (hydralazine and minoxidil), can cause orthostatic hypotension and central nervous system side effects including sedation, dizziness, and confusion and should generally be avoided or used with extreme caution in the geriatric population. In situations where a patient has hypertension and benign prostatic hyperplasia (BPH), α_1-adrenergic blockers may be used to treat two conditions with one agent, and in these circumstances, use is warranted as long as caution and proper monitoring are utilized. If any one of these agents is initiated, start at low doses and titrate slowly, while monitoring for adverse effects.

HYPERLIPIDEMIA

Hyperlipidemia in the Elderly

Each year more than 1 million Americans have a heart attack, and nearly half of them do not survive. Close to 13 million Americans have coronary heart disease as a result of hyperlipidemia and atherosclerosis. In fact, hyperlipidemia is the most prevalent contributor to CVD risk, affecting almost one in two adults in the United States. The correlation between hyperlipidemia and CVD risk has been demonstrated in several clinical trials and has been illustrated in all age groups.

Drug therapy for hypercholesterolemia has remained controversial, mainly because of insufficient clinical trial evidence for improved survival. The Scandinavian Simvastatin Survival Study, or 4S trial, was designed to evaluate the effect of cholesterol lowering with simvastatin on mortality and morbidity in patients with coronary heart disease (CHD). The 4444 patients with angina pectoris or previous myocardial infarction and serum cholesterol of 5.5–8.0 mmol/L on a lipid-lowering diet were randomized to double-blind treatment with simvastatin or placebo. Over the 5.4-year median follow-up period, simvastatin produced mean changes in total cholesterol, LDL cholesterol, and HDL cholesterol of –25%, –35%, and +8%, respectively, with few adverse effects. According to the Scandinavian Simvastatin Survival Study (4S), CVD risk reduction occurs in those age groups < 65 as well as those > 65 in a similar fashion.[34]

Table 4 Positive and negative risk factors for hyperlipidemia[a]

Factors	Definition
Positive Risk Factor	
Cigarette smoking	Must be a current user
Hypertension	$\geq$ 140/90 or using antihypertensive medication
Low HDL	< 40 mg/dL
Family history of premature CHD	Males < 55 years old or females < 65 years old
Age	Males $\geq$ 45 years old or females $\geq$ 55 years old
Negative Risk Factor	
High HDL	$\geq$ 60 mg/dL

[a] Adapted from Reference 13 and from the Omnicare Formulary, Geriatric Care Guidelines, Omnicare, Inc., 2003.

Additionally, a retrospective analysis of the Long-Term Intervention with Pravastatin in Ischaemic Disease (LIPID) trial found that the benefit of treatment in patients 65–75 years old exceeded the benefit in younger adults.[35] Adequate treatment of hyperlipidemia can reduce the risk of total cardiac mortality by as much as 50% in the event of a myocardial infarction or stroke. Despite the benefits, many deaths occur each year, especially in the geriatric population, due to a failure to implement proper treatment. Thus, treatment of hyperlipidemia should be implemented in the geriatric population and should be no different from treatment used in the nonelderly.

Risk Factors and the Goals of Therapy

One of the most important elements when initiating treatment for hyperlipidemia is risk assessment. Risk assessment includes obtaining a fasting lipid panel and determining the number of risk factors a patient has in order to place the patient in an appropriate risk category for proper treatment. Risk factors for hyperlipidemia are cigarette smoking, hypertension, a low HDL level, age, and family history of premature CHD. Table 4 lists the positive and negative risk factors of hyperlipidemia.

After determining a patient's number of risk factors, the patient should be placed in the appropriate risk category to establish adequate goals and to decide when to start treatment. Table 5 breaks down risk categories, which correspond with the appropriate treatment goals. CHD risk equivalents include diabetes (type 1 or 2), peripheral artery disease, carotid artery disease, abdominal aortic aneurysm, and a 10-year Framingham risk >20%. Very high risk patients are those with established CHD who also have one

Table 5 Hyperlipidemia risk categories[a]

Risk Category	LDL Goal	Start TLC[b]	Start Drug Therapy
0 or 1 Risk factor	< 160 mg/dL	≥ 160 mg/dL	≥ 190 mg/dL
≥2 Risk factors	< 130 mg/dL	≥ 130 mg/dL	≥ 130–160 mg/dL
CHD or CHD equivalent	< 100 mg/dL	≥ 100 mg/dL	≥ 130 mg/dL
Very high risk CHD	< 70 mg/dL		

[a] Adapted from Reference 13.
[b] Therapeutic lifestyle recommendations.

of the following: major risk factors (diabetes), poorly controlled risk factors (smoking), multiple risk factors for metabolic syndrome (abdominal obesity, triglycerides >150, HDL < 40, etc.), or acute coronary syndrome.

Nonpharmacologic Therapy of Hyperlipidemia

Therapeutic lifestyle changes (TLC) have demonstrated beneficial effects in all age groups and should be recommended, either alone or in addition to pharmacologic therapy, in all patients who have hyperlipidemia. If implemented alone, the effectiveness of TLC should be assessed every 6 weeks; if not adequate after 3 months, pharmacologic therapy should be started. The basic lifestyle interventions include increased activity, decreased saturated fats, weight reduction, decreased cholesterol intake, smoking cessation, increased dietary fiber intake, and moderation of alcohol consumption. Specific recommendations are given in Table 6.

Pharmacologic Treatment of Hyperlipidemia

Statins

HMG-CoA reductase inhibitors are better known as statins. HMG-CoA reductase is the rate-limiting enzyme in cholesterol synthesis. It converts the HMG-CoA to mevalonic acid, the cholesterol precursor. By inhibiting this enzyme, these agents decrease cholesterol synthesis, which causes an increase in LDL receptor activity, and thus increases the clearance of LDL cholesterol. Statins also have been shown to decrease triglycerides and increase HDL, although the precise mechanism by which this occurs is unknown. In addition to their effects on cholesterol, statins have other beneficial effects, such as plaque stabilization and antiplatelet and antioxidant effects as well as anti-inflammatory effects.[36]

HMG-CoA reductase inhibitors are considered the drugs of first choice for cholesterol lowering, since, in addition to their many other beneficial

Table 6 Dietary recommendations[a]

Nutrient	Recommended Intake
Saturated fat	< 7% of total calories
Polyunsaturated fat	< 10% of total calories
Monounsaturated fat	< 20% of total calories
Total fat	25%–35% of total calories
Carbohydrates	50%–60% of total calories
Fiber	20–30 g/day
Protein	~15% of total calories
Cholesterol	< 200 mg/day
Total calories	Balance with total energy expenditure

[a] Adapted from Reference 13.

effects, they are the most effective for lowering LDL cholesterol. The safety and efficacy of all HMG-CoA reductase inhibitors have been firmly established in the elderly population through multiple clinical trials such as the Scandinavian Simvastatin Survival Study (4S), in which the results showed a 30% reduction in all-cause mortality and a 30%–40% reduction in major coronary events, with no significant difference between those over 65 years of age compared to those less than 65.

The results of 4S were supported by both the Prospective Study of Pravastatin in the Elderly at Risk (PROSPER)[37] trial and the Heart Protection Study (HPS).[38] PROSPER specifically examined the benefits of statins in the elderly population; the results of this large-scale international clinical trial confirmed for the first time that older persons (70–82 years of age) can reduce their risk of dying from CHD by almost a quarter and their risk of having a heart attack by almost a fifth through treatment with the cholesterol-lowering medication pravastatin. This large-scale trial studied 5804 men and women between 70 and 82 years of age. The participants were followed up for an average of 3.2 years. Half of the people in the study received the cholesterol-lowering medication pravastatin in addition to their regular treatments, and the other half were given a placebo. The results of PROSPER showed a 34% reduction in LDL cholesterol for statin-treated patients, with a 15% reduction of overall cardiac and cerebrovascular events.

The HPS analyzed the effect of statins on the prevention of cardiac events in several age groups (those < 65, 65–69, 70–74, and > 75). More than 20,000 persons participated in HPS and the study revealed similar results in both the elderly and the middle-aged, with a 25%–30% reduction in cardiac events.

Generally, statins are tolerated well in the geriatric population, with the most common adverse effects being gastrointestinal disturbances, myalgias, muscle weakness, headaches, and rash. A patient who does not tolerate one statin may tolerate another one better. Muscle aches and weakness can occur with or without a rise in the creatine phosphokinase level. Rhabdomyolysis and myoglobinemia can also occur, but they are rare. Creatine phosphokinase values should be measured at baseline and subsequently if the patient develops myalgia. Infrequent increases in hepatic transaminases can occur, but hepatitis is rare. Baseline liver function tests should be performed at initiation of therapy, then at 3 months, and, annually thereafter. Statins should be given at bedtime to coincide with optimal cholesterol biosynthesis in the body.

Drug interactions are a frequent occurrence with statins. All statins except pravastatin undergo extensive first-pass metabolism by the cytochrome P-450 system. Simvastatin and lovastatin are metabolized by CYP 3A4, and atorvastatin is partially metabolized by CYP 3A4 as well. Thus, CYP 3A4 inhibitors such as ketoconazole, itraconazole, erythromycin, clarithromycin, nefazodone, and grapefruit juice should be avoided. Fluvastatin and rosuvastatin may interact with drugs metabolized by CYP 2C9 such as tricyclic antidepressants, phenytoin, and warfarin. Cyclosporine increases the concentration of all statins and can increase the risk of rhabdomyolysis. Thus, cyclosporine should be avoided in the elderly taking a statin. The combination of gemfibrozil with a statin should also be avoided in the elderly, since gemfibrozil inhibits the metabolism of statins and can also increase the risk of rhabdomyolysis. Due to the plethora of drug interactions with statins, caution should be taken when coadministering other drugs with statins, particularly in the geriatric population.

Fibrates

Overall, fibrates are considered well tolerated and effective in the elderly. The precise mechanism of fibrates has not been established; however, the main effect is believed to be stimulation of lipoprotein lipase. Fibrates typically decrease triglycerides, increase HDL, and may lower or raise LDL. The most common adverse effect with fibrates is gastrointestinal discomfort, particularly with gemfibrozil. These agents may also increase the risk of rhabdomyolysis when combined with other agents known to cause myopathy, such as statins. Fenofibrate has been associated with increased serum creatinine and therefore should be avoided in severe renal impairment. Both gemfibrozil and fenofibrate have been associated with hepatotoxicity and are contraindicated in hepatic dysfunction. Fibrates may also increase the effects of anticoagulants and oral hypoglycemics. Gemfibrozil can be taken with or without food, but fenofibrate should be taken with food; if it is not, absorption can be decreased up to 35%.[39]

Niacin

In general, niacin decreases LDL levels by reducing hepatic very low density lipoprotein (VLDL) synthesis; triglyceride levels are also decreased by this action. Niacin also is the best agent available for increasing HDL, although the exact mechanism is unknown. Adverse effects can include increases in uric acid levels, precipitating gout, and increases in glucose levels, making it a relative contraindication in diabetics. In addition, niacin causes flushing and pruritus of the face and trunk, which may be severe. Flushing may be decreased by taking a 325-mg aspirin 30 minutes prior to taking the dose of niacin. Tolerance to the flushing generally develops when low doses are started initially and gradually titrated upward. Hepatotoxicity may occur in up to 50% of those using sustained-release niacin, but this effect is dose-related. Due to its poor tolerability, niacin use is limited. The best choice for use in the elderly is Niaspan® in daily doses up to 2 g, because it produces less flushing and hepatic toxicity.[40]

Cholesterol Absorption Inhibitors

Cholesterol absorption inhibitors like ezetimibe (Zetia®) inhibit the intestinal absorption of cholesterol by blocking its transport across the border of the small intestine. Used alone, Zetia has a moderate LDL-reducing effect, but taken in combination with a statin, the LDL-lowering effects of the two drugs are additive. Thus, a lower dose of a statin can be used in combination with Zetia to achieve the same reduction as a high-dose statin, with less risk of rhabdomyolysis. The most common adverse effects of these agents are flatulence and diarrhea. Pancreatitis, myalgia, and thrombocytopenia have been reported, but occurrence is rare.[41,42]

Bile Acid Sequestrants

Bile acid sequestrants bind bile acids in the intestinal lumen. The decrease in bile acids in the body increases the conversion of cholesterol to bile acids, upregulating the LDL receptors and decreasing LDL levels. Common adverse effects are gastrointestinal only, since these agents are not systemically absorbed. Such effects include constipation, heartburn, nausea, and bloating. Increasing fiber in the diet can help decrease constipation and bloating. Bile acids also have a tendency to bind up other drugs in the GI tract, decreasing the absorption and efficacy of these agents. Therefore, bile acid resins generally should not be used in the elderly population, since most elderly individuals take an average of four medications. Colesevelam is the only bile acid resin that can be used in the geriatric population, simply because it is much better tolerated and has fewer gastrointestinal side effects and drug interactions.[43]

KEY POINTS

- Enhancing patient outcomes among the elderly is arguably the most urgent priority in contemporary medical care.
- The elderly and society share an increasing burden of hospitalization and deaths due to cardiovascular disease and heart failure.
- Treatment is highly individualized.
- Cardiovascular disease and events are increasing in incidence, and they represent high levels of morbidity and mortality in the senior population.
- Large randomized clinical trials have provided strong evidence on which clinicians base their decisions and novel approaches.
- Atypical clinical presentations make diagnosing and treating cardiovascular issues a complex matter.
- The increasing prevalence of obesity, type 2 diabetes, and a host of psychologic–social–economic factors make lifestyle and pharmaceutical interventions necessary to improve quality of life.
- Aspirin and beta-blocker therapy have been shown to reduce overall mortality and morbidity.
- Lowering LDL cholesterol levels also results in a substantial reduction in CHD mortality and nonfatal myocardial infarctions in the elderly over 75 years of age.
- Systolic blood pressure elevation in the elderly should be aggressively treated using diuretics, beta-blockers, calcium channel blockers, and ACE inhibitors.

REFERENCES

1. Hanna TR, Wenger NK. Secondary prevention of heart disease in elderly patients. *Am Fam Physician.* 2005;71:2289–96.
2. Stevenson WG. Improving survival for patients with advanced heart failure: a study of 737 consecutive patients. *J Am Coll Cardiol.* 1995;26:1417–23.

3. Wynne J, Braunwald E. The cardiomyopathies and myocarditises. In: Braunwald E, ed. *Heart Disease: A Textbook of Cardiovascular Medicine.* Philadelphia: WB Saunders; 1997:1404–63.

4. Yakubov SJ, Bope ET. Cardiovascular disease in: Rakel RB. *Textbook of Family Practice.* 6th ed. Philadelphia: WB Saunders; 2002;776–8.

5. Katz AM. Ernest Henry Starling, his predecessors, and the "law of the heart." *Circulation.* 2002;106:2986–92.

6. Available at: http://www.emedicine.com/MED/topic3552.htm (accessed Mar. 31, 2006).

7. Stafford RS, Saglam D. National patterns of angiotensin-converting enzyme inhibitor use in congestive heart failure. *Arch Intern Med.* 1997;157:2460–4.

8. Roe CM, Motheral BR, Teitelbaum F, et al. Angiotensin-converting enzyme inhibitor compliance and dosing among patients with heart failure. *Am Heart J.* 1999;138:818–25.

9. Torosoff M, Philbin EF. Improving outcomes in diastolic heart failure, techniques to evaluate underlying causes and target therapy. *Postgrad Med.* 2003;113(3):67–74.

10. Moser M. Hypertension treatment and the prevention of coronary heart disease in the elderly. *Am Fam Physician.* 1999;59:1248–56.

11. Morimoto S, Uchida K, Miyamoto M, et al. Plasma aldosterone response to angiotensin II in sodium-restricted elderly subjects with essential hypertension. *J Am Geriatr Soc.* 1981;29(7):302–7.

12. Izzo JL, Levy D, Black HR. Clinical advisory statement. Importance of systolic blood pressure in older Americans. Coordinating Committee, National High Blood Pressure Education Program. Available at http://www.nhlbi.nih.gov/health/prof/heart/hbp/hbpstmt/index.htm (accessed Sept. 26, 2005).

13. Chobanian AV, Bakris GL, Black HR, et al. The seventh report of the Joint National Committee on Prevention, Detection, Evaluation, and Treatment of High Blood Pressure: the JNC 7 report. *JAMA.* 2003;289:2560–72.

14. Gaziano JM, Braunwald E. Atlas of cardiovascular risk factors. *Curr Medicine.* 2005.

15. O'Malley K, Cox JP, O'Brien E. Further learnings from the European Working Party on High Blood Pressure in the Elderly (EWPHE) study: focus on systolic hypertension. *Cardiovasc Drugs Ther.* 1991 Jan (4 Suppl 6): 1249–51.

16. Amery A, Birkenhager W, Brixko P, et al. Mortality and morbidity results from the European Working Party on High Blood Pressure in the Elderly. *Lancet.* 1985;1(8442):1349–54.

17. Dahlof B, Lindholm LH, Hansson L, et al. Morbidity and mortality in the Swedish Trial in Old Patients with Hypertension (STOP-Hypertension). *Lancet.* 1991;338:1281–5.

18. Staessen JA, Gasowski J, Wang JG, et al. Risks of untreated and treated isolated systolic hypertension in the elderly: meta analysis of outcome trials. *Lancet.* 2000;355:865–72.

19. Yusuf S, Sleight P, Pogue J, et al. Effects of an angiotensin-converting-enzyme inhibitor, ramipril, on cardiovascular events in high-risk patients. *N Engl J Med.* 2000;342(3):145–53.

20. Fields LE, Burt VL, Cutler JA, et al. The burden of adult hypertension in the United States 1999 to 2000: a rising tide of hypertension. *Hypertension.* 2004;44:398–404.

21. Lloyd-Jones DM, Evans JC, Levy D. Hypertension in adults across the age spectrum: current outcomes and control in the community. *JAMA* 2005;294:466–72.

22. Bulpitt C, Fletcher A, Beckett N, el al. Hypertension in the Very Elderly Trial (HYVET): protocol for the main trial. *Drugs Aging*. 2001;18(3):151–64.

23. Major cardiovascular events in hypertensive patients randomized to doxazosin vs. chlorthalidone: the Antihypertensive and Lipid-Lowering Treatment to Prevent Heart Attack Trial. Antihypertensive Therapy and Lipid Lowering Heart Attack Trial (ALLHAT) Collaborative Research Group. *JAMA*. 2000; 283:1967–75.

24. Cushman WC, Ford CE, Cutler JA, et al. Success and predictors of blood pressure control in diverse North American settings: the Antihypertensive and Lipid-Lowering Treatment to Prevent Heart Attack Trial (ALLHAT). *J Clin Hypertens*. 2002;4: 393–404.

25. Amer RP. The influence of non beta-blocking on the lipid profiles: are diuretics outclassed as initial therapy for hypertension? *Am Heart J*. 1987;114:998–1006.

26. Prevention of stroke by antihypertensive drug treatment in older persons with isolated systolic hypertension: final results of the Systolic Hypertension in the Elderly Program (SHEP). SHEP Cooperative Group. *JAMA*. 1991;265:3255–64.

27. Dahlof B, Devereux RB, Kjeldsen SE, et al. Cardiovascular morbidity and mortality in the Losartan Intervention for Endpoint Reduction in Hypertension study (LIFE): a randomized trial against atenolol. *Lancet*. 2002;359:995–1003.

28. Effects of ramipril on cardiovascular and microvascular outcomes in people with diabetes mellitus: results of the HOPE study and the MICRO HOPE substudy. Heart Outcome Prevention Evaluation (HOPE) Study Investigators. *Lancet*. 2000;355:253–9.

29. Lewis EJ, Hunsicker LG, Clarke WR, et al. Renoprotective effect of the angiotensin-receptor antagonist irbesartan in patients with nephropathy due to type 2 diabetes. *N Engl J Med*. 2001;345:851–60.

30. Agodoa L, Appel L, Bakris G, et al. Effect of ramipril vs. amlodipine on renal outcomes in hypertensive nephrosclerosis, a randomized controlled trial. African American Study of Kidney Disease and Hypertension Study Group (AASK). *JAMA*. 2001;285:2719–28.

31. Moser M. Diuretics revisited—again. *J Clin Hypertens*. 2001;3:136–8.

32. Roth B. Toxicity: beta blockers. In e-medicine at http://www.emedicine.com/emerg/topic59.htm (accessed Jan. 20, 2006).

33. Howard PA, Ellerbeck EF. Optimizing beta-blocker use after myocardial infarction. *Am Fam Physician*. 2000;62:1853-60, 1865–6.

34. Scandinavian simvastatin survival study (4S). Scandinavian Simvastatin Survival Study Group. Randomized trial of cholesterol lowering in 4444 patients with coronary heart disease. *Lancet*. 1994;344(8934):1383–9.

35. Prevention of cardiovascular events and death with pravastatin in patients with coronary heart disease and a broad range of initial cholesterol levels. The Long-Term Intervention with Pravastatin in Ischemic Disease (LIPID) Study Group. *N Engl J Med*. 1998;339:1349–57.

36. Sotiriou CG, Cheng JW. Beneficial effects of statins in coronary artery disease—beyond lowering cholesterol. *Ann Pharmacother*. 2000 Dec; 34:1432–9.

37. Shepherd J, Blauw GJ, Murphy MB, et al. On behalf of the PROSPER study group. Pravastatin in elderly individuals at risk of vascular disease (PROSPER): a randomized controlled trial. *Lancet*. 2002;360:1623–30.

38. Heart Protection Study Collaborative Group. MRC/BHF heart protection study of cholesterol lowering with simvastatin in 20,536 high-risk individuals: a randomized placebo-controlled trial. *Lancet*. 2002;360:7–22.

39. See Drugs.com accessed at http://www.drugs.com/pdr/FENOFIBRATE.html (accessed Mar. 29, 2006).
40. See http://www.niaspan.com/pdf/niaspan_PI_RI. pdf (accessed Mar. 29, 2006).
41. Davidson MH, Ballantyne CM, Kerzner B, et al. Efficacy and safety of ezetimibe coadministered with statins: randomized, placebo-controlled, blinded experience in 2382 patients with primary hypercholesterolemia. *Int J Clin Pract.* 2004;58(8):746–55.
42. Knopp RH, Dujovne CA, Le Beaut A. Evaluation of the efficacy, safety, and tolerability of ezetimibe in primary hypercholesterolaemia: a pooled analysis from two controlled phase III clinical studies. *Int J Clin Pract.* 2003;57:363–8.
43. Davidson MH, Dillon MA, Gordon B, et al. Colesevelam hydrochloride (Cholestagel): a new potent bile acid sequestrant associated with a low incidence of gastrointestinal side effects. *Arch Intern Med.* 1999;159;1893–900.

5

Managing Diabetes Mellitus and Thyroid Disease in the Elderly

CYNTHIA G. OLSEN

He who is of a calm and happy nature will not feel the pressures of age, but to him who is of an opposite disposition, age and youth are of an equal burden.

—Plato 428–328 BC

OVERVIEW

Diabetes mellitus and thyroid disease are the number one and number two most common disorders of the endocrine system that affect the elderly. Diabetes mellitus type 2 is presented in this chapter as a disorder of glucose metabolism and as a disease that must be taken seriously. But it is also a disease that can be managed by various and flexible means if elderly persons' needs are to be met, but unfortunately, in most cases, they are not. A review of the oral hypoglycemics and insulin use in the elderly is presented as the best intervention to help the elderly reach glycemic control. Thyroid disease (hyperthyroidism and hypothyroidism) are also presented and their control in the elderly by pharmacotherapeutic means is described.

Johnny Johnston, a 72-year-old feisty Irishman who looks "slightly obese," comes into the family medicine clinic for a follow-up visit. Diagnosed with type 2 diabetes mellitus 5 years ago and found to be "out of glycemic control" the past 6 months, he has been asked to maintain a record for the past 2 months, indicating whether or not he: (1) takes his blood glucose levels twice a day (he is looking for a blood glucose range of 125–135 mg/dL), (2) sticks to an 1800-calorie-per-day diet, and (3) walks on his treadmill at least twice a day for 30 minutes. Johnny enjoys his daily bottle of beer but was able to break his pack-a-day smoking habit when he learned he had diabetes. His medications include:

Rx: Glucophage® 0.5 g ii tabs BID
Lisinopril 5 mg i tab OD
Enteric-coated aspirin 81 mg, i tab each morning
Glynase® 6 mg, i tab each morning

Johnny tells the "new" physician he is feeling "fine," but when getting a refill prescription for his Glucophage at the clinic's pharmacy, he states, "My grandmother had diabetes, but in her day they never had medicines like this." Then he adds, "I am really feeling OK, but from time to time I have trouble with some blurry vision and leg pain. I figure that this must be old age."

- What do you think may be Johnny's drug-related problems?
- What should the goals of his treatment be?
- Are there any patient characteristics that would influence the goals of a treatment plan?
- What pharmacotherapy would you recommend to help Johnny?
- What would you monitor to watch for adverse drug reactions associated with diabetic drugs?
- How would you see the clinic involving a team of health professionals to help manage Johnny's diabetes and hypertension?

GLUCOSE REGULATION IN THE AGING

Diabetes mellitus not only is the most common chronic disease among the elderly but also is the most common endocrine disorder in the United States. Diabetes mellitus is characterized by an abnormality in insulin secretion, action, or both, resulting in hyperglycemia. It is estimated that the incidence of diabetes in those over 65 years of age is approximately 15% to 20%, and the incidence increases after the age of 75. Diabetes mellitus is the sixth leading cause of death in Caucasians over 65 years of age and the fourth leading cause of death among older blacks and Hispanics.[1] Older diabetics risk a 10-year life expectancy reduction compared to their nondiabetic cohorts. In addition to the increased mortality, the morbidity brought by diabetes complications is significant.

There is a strong genetic predisposition toward diabetes mellitus type 2. The UK Prospective Diabetes Study (UKPDS) group demonstrated that beta-cell function progressively declines over time in individuals, regardless of treatment, and that the decline occurs over a relatively short number of years. At the time of diagnosis, approximately 50% of beta-cells are still functional. The severity of illness among the elderly varies widely, depending on time of diagnosis and many other factors.[2]

DEFINING GLUCOSE REGULATION DISORDERS

The American Diabetes Association (ADA) recognizes three types of diabetes mellitus in the elderly: type 1, type 2, and exogenous (Table 1).

This chapter focuses primarily on type 2 diabetes mellitus, the most common form in the elderly. The diagnosis of diabetes is not adjusted for age. However, any of the three methods outlined by the ADA can be used to confirm the diagnosis. The three criteria are:

1. Symptoms of diabetes (i.e., excessive thirst or hunger, excessive urination, unexplained weight loss) plus a casual postprandial plasma glucose concentration (PPG) =/> 200 mg/dL (11.1 mmol/L). Casual is defined as any time of day without regard to the time of the last meal.
2. A plasma glucose concentration after an 8-hour fast (FPG) >/= 126 mg/dL (7.0 mmol/L).
3. A 2-hour PPG of =/> 200 mg/dL (11.1 mmol/L) after an oral glucose tolerance test (OGTT). This test, as described by the World Health Organization, uses a glucose load of 75 g of anhydrous glucose dissolved in 300 mL of water after an overnight fast. This test is not recommended for routine clinical use; it is reserved for difficult to diagnose and equivocal cases.

WHY DIABETES SHOULD BE TREATED SERIOUSLY

The impact of diabetes mellitus type 2 in the elderly is substantial because it will:

Table 1   American Diabetes Association classification of diabetes[3]

Type	Etiology	Prevalence	Treatment Considerations
Type 1	Autoimmune destruction of β-cells of the pancreas. Absolute deficiency in insulin secretion.	Infrequent	Insulin replacement. Typical diabetic care and prevention.
Type 2	Tissue resistance to the action of insulin. Relative insulin deficiency. Strong genetic predisposition.	90% of older diabetics	Management of life-style through the treatment of obesity, exercise, and diet. Begin with oral hypoglycemic medications. Advance to insulin to achieve glycemic control. Typical diabetic care and prevention.
Exogenous	Specific events such as trauma to the pancreas, chemical etiologies, alcoholism, infections damaging β-cells, or other endocrinopathies (hormone-secreting tumors, paraneoplastic syndromes, adrenal hyperplasia)	Infrequent	Careful medication review and adjustment or removal of drugs causing hyperglycemia (epinephrine, phenytoin, corticosteroids, diuretics). Treatment of underlying endocrinopathies such as exogenous hormone-secreting tumors. Treatment of alcoholism and pancreatitis. Insulin replacement. Typical diabetic care and prevention.

- Increase disability.
- Lower mortality.
- Reduce quality of life.
- Negatively impact comorbid illnesses.
- Result in financial and caregiver burden.
- Affect all other aspects of a patient's well-being, from cognition and mood, autonomy, and sense of dignity to level of functioning.[4]

Failure to recognize and treat diabetes has a great impact on the elderly. Oftentimes, however, presentation is masked. As many as one-third of older diabetics remain undiagnosed. Untreated diabetes may present in a number of ways, especially as geriatric syndromes (Table 2). Undiagnosed diabetes should always be considered during a physician's workup of new symptoms and presentations in an elderly patient.

Table 2 Relationship of abnormal glycemic control to syndromes in the elderly[a]

Syndrome	Effect of Poor Glycemic Control
Falls	Polyuria and resultant dehydration and orthostasis, poor nutrition, generalized weakness, peripheral neuropathy, autonomic dysfunction and orthostasis, dizziness, and visual impairment.
Urinary incontinence	Polyuria, polydipsia, neurogenic bladder, and loss of control.
Constipation	Dehydration and poor nutrition, diabetic gastroparesis, and lack of physical activity.
Depression	Hyperglycemia and electrolyte depletion and dehydration, loss of health status, feelings of inadequacy and low self-esteem, loss of autonomy, multiple stressors, fatigue, and other constitutional symptoms.
Cognitive impairment	A possible early warning sign of loss of glycemic control. Severe impairment is usually in the form of somnolence and delirium, seen in extreme dehydration and blood glucose levels > 800 mg/dL. Blurred vision, focal neurologic symptoms, seizures, and coma may develop. May contribute to preexisting dementia.
Adult failure to thrive	Ketosis causes anorexia and nausea, weight loss and weakness, increasing debility, and other syndromes.
Pressure ulcers	Excessive moisture due to urinary incontinence, poor nutrition, obesity and dehydration, immunocompromise and susceptibility to infection.

[a] Adapted from Reference 4.

A great deal of controversy exists concerning how tightly to manage blood glucose in the elderly, as they are especially susceptible to brain impairment from sustained or repeated episodes of hypoglycemia. Likewise, worsening of overall health and the advancement of cardiovascular disease, renal dysfunction, and neuropathic symptoms can be halted and improved by achieving glycemic control. Because older individuals vary widely in their health status, functional abilities, and prognosis, the primary health care provider, the patient, the family, and other caregivers should make an individualized glycemic goal and management expectation. Individualized patient-centered goals for HbA1c levels are critical because, for every 1% HbA1c increase over glycemic goal, the risk of diabetes complications increases. These complications include any diabetes-related endpoint (21%), myocardial infarction (14%), stroke (12%), and microvascular complications (37%). The risk of blindness is increased 40% in older diabetics. Thus, early diagnosis and aggressive treatment of insulin resistance is always a better intervention, as it may alter the natural course of the disease by preserving beta-cell function and by halting disease progression before serious complications develop.[5]

Table 3   ADA recommendations for glucose control in adult diabetic patients

Measurement	Normal Value	Goal Value	Additional Action Suggested
Whole blood values			
Average preprandial glucose (mg/dL)	< 100	80–120	< 80 or > 140
Average bedtime glucose (mg/dL)	< 110	100–140	< 100 or > 160
Plasma values			
Average preprandial glucose (mg/dL)	< 110	90–130	< 90 or > 150
Average bedtime glucose (mg/dL)	< 120	110–150	< 110 or > 180
Hemoglobin A1c	< 6	< 7	> 8

Loss of a lower extremity due to vascular compromise and neuropathy is the diabetic's worse fear. The incidence of polyneuropathy in diabetics ranges from 10% to 50%. This devastating complication of diabetes, especially poorly controlled diabetes, markedly diminishes function and quality of life. The combination of ischemia and sepsis leads to the development of gangrene and can result in death. These complications can be prevented and must be addressed immediately by the health care team.

DIABETIC MANAGEMENT IN THE ELDERLY

The treatment of diabetes mellitus type 2 requires a broad approach allowing flexibility to address the diverse needs of the elderly. Realistic goals should be set in collaboration with the patient and family. Glycemic control of the older, newly diagnosed diabetic or frail elder with a shortened life expectancy may be less strict than with younger patients. The benefits of tighter glycemic control for the type 1 diabetic and the younger type 2 diabetic are better established. As a heterogeneous group, the elderly must be approached and treated individually based on multiple factors. Some of these considerations include health status, functional status, support system, financial means, cultural factors, and level of commitment. Unfortunately, ADA recommendations for glucose control for adult diabetics (Table 3) are not being met and in the United States 50% of type 2 diabetics are not at the ADA-recommended goal for glycemic control. Additionally, specific recommendations for target glucose goals for the frail and elderly are not available, but the following stratification of fasting glucose levels to assess the severity of glycemic control in the type 2 diabetic has been proposed:[6]

- Mild (126–159 mg/dL)
- Moderate (160–239 mg/dL)
- Severe (240–350 mg/dL)

ORAL HYPOGLYCEMICS

If glycemic goals are not achieved after the initiation of nonpharmacologic treatment modalities such as diet and exercise, initiation of oral hypoglycemics should be considered. Monotherapy with any class of agent is suggested, and clear algorithms for medication choice are now available. Sulfonylureas are effective, have a long safety history, and are affordable.[7] This class of drugs stimulates the remaining beta-cells to release their insulin stores. Maximizing the dosage of a sulfonylurea may not be cost effective and may not even provide the best glycemic control. These agents have relatively flat dose–response curves at higher doses, so higher doses add little benefit. For example, there is no statistical difference in significant mean blood glucose among patients receiving glipizide at 10-, 20-, or 40-mg doses.[8] One such agent in this class, chlorpropamide, should not be used in the elderly due to its prolonged half-life and propensity toward life-threatening hypoglycemia.[9]

When glycemic goals are not achieved with monotherapy, combination regimens that provide complementary mechanisms should be considered and possibly started earlier in the treatment process. By treating the underlying causes of diabetes type 2, such as beta-cell dysfunction and loss and insulin resistance, a durable glycemic control can be obtained and ultimately slow disease progression. An example of a drug that improves insulin sensitization is the biguanide metformin. Metformin can be used as monotherapy or in combination with an oral sulfonylurea if 4 weeks of monotherapy fails to achieve the glycemic goal. It is contraindicated in the presence of renal disease or renal dysfunction as defined by:

- Males: serum creatinine =/> 1.5 mg/dL
- Females: serum creatinine =/> 1.4 mg/dL
- Creatinine clearance < 60 mL/minute

In the elderly, serum creatinine measurement is deceiving and oftentimes overestimates renal function. A quantitative creatinine clearance is a more effective means of determining function and the presence of insufficiency. Metformin should be discontinued when radiological procedures requiring intravenous iodized contrast material are anticipated. It should be withheld for 48 hours after the procedure and resumed only after renal function has been reassessed. The risk of lactic acidosis, a potentially life-threatening reaction, has been associated with this class of drugs, yet providers frequently fail to review renal function prior to prescribing metformin.[10]

The efficacy of combination drug therapy in diabetes mellitus type 2 is well established. The Rosiglitazone Early vs. SULfonylurea Titration study (RESULT) was a 2-year, randomized, double-blinded, parallel-group study that examined elderly type 2 diabetic patients who were inadequately controlled on a sulfonylurea alone. The early addition of rosiglitazone to one-half the maximum dose of sulfonylurea improved beta-cell function from baseline 10-fold, reduced HbA1c levels, and was well tolerated. Likewise, combination therapy of rosiglitazone and low-dose metformin is more effective and tolerable than metformin alone.[11]

Furthermore, the Troglitazone in the Prevention of Diabetes (TRIPOD) study revealed that troglitazone reduced progression to type II diabetes and preserved beta-cell function.

To meet this need, new combined formulations that also take into consideration patient cost and compliance are becoming available (Tables 4 and 5).

INSULIN THERAPY

When combinations of oral hypoglycemics are no longer effective in maintaining glycemic control, the addition or substitution of insulin therapy should be considered. The acceptable threshold of glycemic control may vary among clinicians, and a liberal view of accepting a fasting glucose of < 150 mg/dL for older patients may be reasonable. The initiation of insulin therapy need not follow maximal trials of oral hypoglycemics if the patient is very symptomatic or has severe hyperglycemia. Patients often see initiating insulin as the "last resort" in glycemic management and may perceive failure in their self-management. Many patients will barter with health care providers for "another chance" at lifestyle modification and medication adherence. Patients need to be educated about the progression of beta-cell decline and the chronicity of this disease. The availability of several insulin types that differ in the rate of onset and patient-friendly delivery systems have allowed for greater flexibility and ease in scheduling meals and injections (Table 6).

The elderly, as a group, vary widely in lifestyle needs and desire for activity and recreation. Medications and insulin regimens should be individualized to meet these needs and accommodate patients' functional level and comorbid conditions. Cultural beliefs and customs may present as barriers to the acceptance of insulin therapy. Race has been shown to affect antidiabetic medication usage, despite socioeconomic status, health system access, and health status factors.[17] Careful counseling is best provided prior

Table 4 Oral hypoglycemic agents[a] and special concerns in the elderly[12–16]

Class	Generic Name	Brand Name ($ cost)	Concerns for Elderly
Biguanide	Metformin	Glucophage® ($$$) Glucophage® XR® ($$) Riomet® oral solution ($$$$)	Renal clearance. Risk of lactic acidosis. Avoid if intravenous iodinated contrast material is present or planned. Avoid in severe CHF, hypotension, and sepsis. Liquid form available.
Sulfonylurea	Acetohexamide	Dymelor® ($)	>10% ADR. Hypoglycemia. Elderly may be more sensitive.
	Chlorpropamide	Diabinese®	Long half-life and high (>10%) ADR, especially hypoglycemia. Disulfiram-like reaction with alcohol. Avoid in the elderly.
	Glimepiride	Amaryl® ($)	No reported mental status effect. Low ADR. Elderly begin at 1 mg/day.
	Glipizide	Glucotrol® ($) Glucotrol XL® ($)	No reported mental status effect. Caution in presence of hepatic disease. Dose 30 minutes before meal. Initiate elderly dose at 2.5 mg/day.
	Glyburide	DiaBeta® ($) Glynase® PresTab® ($) Micronase® ($)	Dizziness common. Rapid and prolonged hypoglycemia in the elderly (>12 hours). Caution in hepatic and renal disease. Elderly dose is 1.25 mg/day.
	Tolazamide	Tolinase®	Dizziness common. Several drug interactions. Not studied in the elderly.
	Tolbutamide	Orinase®	Dizziness common. Several drug interactions. Risk of hypoglycemia.

Table 4 (continued) Oral hypoglycemic agents[a] and special concerns in the elderly[12-16]

Class	Generic Name	Brand Name ($ cost)	Concerns for Elderly
Thiazolidinedione	Pioglitazone	Actos® ($$$)	May cause fatigue, weight gain, and edema. Caution with atypical antipsychotics and in patients with NYHA class III or IV CHF. Several drug interactions. Dose adjustment not recommended in elderly.
	Rosiglitazone	Avandia® ($$$$)	May cause fatigue, weight gain, and edema. Caution with atypical antipsychotics and in patients with CHF, cardiac hypertrophy, and hepatic disease. Dose adjustment in the elderly not recommended.
	Troglitazone	Rezulin®	Was removed from the market due to cases of fatal liver failure.
Glucosidase inhibitor	Acarbose	Precose® ($$)	May cause drowsiness. Side effects with several psychotropic drugs. 10% ADR with GI complaints common. Dosed three times a day with meals.
	Miglitol	Glyset® ($$)	No mental status effect reported. 10% ADR with GI complaints common. Dosed three times a day with meals.
Nonsulfonylurea secretagogue; Meglitinides	Repaglinide	Prandin® ($$$$)	No mental status effects. Several drug interactions. Caution in hepatic disease. Dosed three or four times a day 15–30 minutes before meals. Combination with sulfonylurea of no added benefit.
	Nateglinide	Starlix® ($$$$)	Several drug interactions. Caution in hepatic disease. Dosed three or four times a day 15–30 minutes before meals. Combination with sulfonylurea of no added benefit.

[a] ADR = adverse drug reaction, CHF = congestive heart failure, GI = gastrointestinal, NYHA = New York Heart Association; relative cost comparison ($ = less expensive; $$$$ = more expensive).

Table 5 Oral hypoglycemic combination preparations and dosing

Classes Combined	Generic Names	Brand Name	Formulation Dosages Available	Maximum Dosage Approved
Thiazolidinedione/ biguanide	Rosiglitazone/ Metformin	Avandamet®	1 mg/500 mg 2 mg/500 mg 4 mg/500 mg 2 mg/1000 mg 4 mg/1000 mg	4 mg/1000 mg One tablet twice a day
Sulfonylurea/ biguanide	Glyburide/ Metformin	Glucovance®	2.5 mg/500 mg 5 mg/500 mg	5 mg/500 mg Two tablets twice a day
	Glipizide/ Metformin	Metaglip®		

to dispensing insulin and repeated on subsequent follow-up visits. Topics of discussion should include the onset of insulin action, times insulin should be administered, methods of administration, storage and safety, and recognition of signs of hypoglycemia.

Patients may find the cost of insulin can vary by several dollars between pharmacies and brands and may be tempted to switch during therapy. They should be warned that brands or types of insulin differ greatly and should not be switched without a physician's recommendation and close follow-up monitoring. Mail-order drug companies can offer considerable savings for quarterly supplies. The patient or caregiver may want to consider environmental concerns with shipping, such as extreme heat or freezing. Contacting the distributor to guarantee proper handling of the insulin is appropriate. Close inspection of bottles upon arrival is recommended.

The presence of neuropathy in the hands, arthritis, or stroke may interfere with the physical ability to perform a home glucose check and to administer insulin. Visual impairment, whether as a direct result of diabetes or another condition, interferes with these maneuvers and the safe measurement of the insulin dosage. Use of adaptive equipment, such as visual aids, and the assistance of an occupational therapist can improve confidence and success in mastering this procedure.

Insulin pens, with premeasured amounts of insulin, can be carried and can reduce patient inconvenience and lower the risk of error. Several brands provide a wide variety of insulin types. Autoinjectors are devices that hold the filled syringes and inject into the adjacent site with the push of a button.

Table 6 Types of injectable insulin and comparison by action[a]

Category	Brand Name (Company)	Approximate Onset Time	Approximate Peak Time	Approximate Duration
Rapid acting	Humalog® (lispro) (Lilly) NovoLog® (aspart) (Novo Nordisk)	5–15 minutes	45–90 minutes	3–4 hours
Short acting (regular)	Humulin® R (Lilly) Novolin® R Novolin® BR, Velosulin® (regular buffered) (Novo Nordisk).	30 minutes	2–5 hours	5–8 hours
Combination short/intermediate acting	Humulin 50/50 (Lilly) Humulin 70/30 (Lilly) Humalog 70/30 (Lilly) Humalog 75/25 (Lilly) NovoLog (Novo Nordisk)	30 minutes	N/A	16–24 hours
Intermediate acting (NPH)	Humulin-N (Lilly) Humulin Lente (Lilly) Iletin® II Lente (Lilly) Iletin II NPH (Lilly) Novolin N (Novo Nordisk) Novolin Lente (Novo Nordisk)	1–3 hours	6–12 hours	16–24 hours
Long acting	Humulin Ultralente (Lilly) Lantus® (Aventis Pharmaceuticals)	6–10 hours >1 hour	8–20 hours N/A	20–24 hours >24 hours

[a] Adapted from Reference 16. See also Diabetes Forecast Guide 2003, American Diabetes Association, 17–21.

These devices can be useful for those with impaired mobility and dexterity, are needle phobic, or have visual impairment. Several syringe magnifiers exist that clip onto the syringe and improve calibration on filling. Other devices are available to stabilize the syringe and bottle and guide the needle. Nonvisual insulin measurement devices that incorporate raised numbers or Braille exist. Jet injectors—a needle and syringe alternative—release a small stream of insulin forced through the skin with pressure rather than a puncture. The thin skin of the elderly has a loss of elasticity and may be prone to bruising with this delivery method.

As with insulin delivery systems and devices, home blood glucose monitors have evolved to improve ease of use and recording of data. All patients who are capable of measuring blood glucose should be encouraged to purchase and utilize a monitor. For the newly diagnosed diabetic, home monitoring offers a means of self-education and regulation as therapy is initiated. Oral medication and insulin users need a means of rapid detection of hypoglycemia. Machines with a voice synthesizer or large, lighted digital display are available for the visually impaired.

Urine glucose testing strips are still available in retail stores, but they do not adequately reflect the patient's current glycemic situation. The kidneys are less likely to spill glucose with aging, thus resulting in very high blood glucose levels that may culminate in hyperosmolar coma. Negative urine glucose is no reassurance of acceptable blood glucose levels and should not be used as a monitoring tool. The detection of microalbumin in the urine is an early sign of renal disease in diabetics. Its presence may warrant the addition of nephroprotective therapy or the elimination of potentially nephrotoxic medications. Sensitive methods of urine microalbumin detection are readily available in physicians' offices and clinical laboratories.[18] New home test kits for collection of urine and mail delivery to a testing laboratory are available and can be important for the care of the home-bound or rural diabetic patient.

Hypoglycemia

The central nervous system in the elderly is particularly sensitive to hypoglycemia. Older diabetics may be less likely to recognize low blood sugars and risk brain impairment with prolonged or repeated episodes of hypoglycemia. Symptoms of confusion, new onset depression, memory loss, or newly impaired function should alert the health care provider to possible hidden hypoglycemia. Liberalization of therapy, checking the hemoglobin A1c, and more frequent monitoring, including nocturnal checks, may be required to make this diagnosis. Hospitalization of the patient for 24-hour monitoring may be necessary. However, removal of the patient from their daily environment and home-based diet may not reflect exact blood glucose patterns once the patient is in a controlled setting. Medical identification of a patient's diabetic status can be life-saving in an emergency and should be encouraged. These identification systems come in many forms, including wallet cards, bracelets, watch charms, shoe tags, and necklaces.

Over-the-counter products for meal replacement and blood glucose stabilization can be used when hypoglycemia is a risk. Special meal bars and drinks for diabetics can provide or supplement nutrition when a healthy meal is not readily available. Special dietary bars that contain uncooked starch provide a continuous glucose supply and are particularly useful for low blood sugar at night or during exercise. Glucose tablets and gels are available for emergency use when food is unavailable. Sugar cubes and candy are less expensive but more tempting forms of a fast-acting carbohydrate. Regular use of these rapid sources of glucose may contribute to poor regulation and spikes in blood glucose. Reassessment of the patient's therapy and diet is warranted when these products are required often to reverse hypoglycemia.

Effects of Comorbid Conditions

Hypertension

Up to 60% of diabetic patients have hypertension. Hypertension is a component of the dysmetabolic syndrome X, which also includes central obesity and dyslipidemia. The combination of hypertension and diabetes accelerates the risk of diabetic nephropathy and renal failure and all-cause mortality from cardiovascular disease. Likewise, several studies have shown that blood pressure control significantly reduces both micro- and macrovascular disease and survival.[19] Tighter goals for blood pressure (< 130/80) were released in May 2003 by the Seventh Report of the Joint National Committee on Prevention, Detection, Evaluation, and Treatment of High Blood Pressure (JNC 7). Study on the further reduction in blood pressure in these individuals and further cardiovascular risk reduction is in progress.

Despite clear evidence on the benefits of blood pressure control in diabetic patients, only 11% of adult diabetics are at the goal of less than 130/80.[20]

The important Antihypertensive and Lipid-Lowering treatment to prevent Heart Attack Trial (ALLHAT) found that diuretics were superior as first-line treatment in type 2 diabetic patients with good renal function (serum creatinine of 1.0 mg/dL and no proteinuria).[21] However, these patients often required multidrug regimens for adequate control, with 66% of patients needing two drugs and 33% requiring at least three antihypertensive drugs. For combined therapy, a thiazide diuretic and either an angiotensin-converting enzyme (ACE) inhibitor or an angiotensin-II receptor blocker (ARB) is an excellent combination. The potential renoprotective effect of these two classes of drugs in diabetics has been shown.[22] For the one-third of diabetic hypertensive patients who have not reached goal, the addition of either a calcium channel blocker or a beta-blocker is the next reasonable approach.

Psychological Illness

Compared to older nondiabetics, older diabetics are at an increased risk of developing major depression or cognitive dysfunction. The presence of depression or cognitive decline in this group can result in poorer self-management, noncompliance, and poorer glycemic control. A new mood disorder or decrease in cognition can also be an explanation for loss of glycemic control in the previously controlled diabetic. Using brief screening tools in the initial history of the new diabetic and on subsequent occasions is a reasonable approach to identification of these disorders. Because the elderly respond to depression treatment with psychotherapy, pharmacotherapy, or both, identified patients should receive timely referral. Such referral and treatment becomes part of the overall careplan for the older diabetic.[23] Changes in cognitive function may present in different forms, such as memory loss, activities of daily living failure, and learning impairment, but hyperglycemia also can result in deterioration of cognitive function.[24] Immediate referral for proper assessment, treatment of potentially reversible causes, and adjustment of the careplan is imperative.

Antipsychotic medications are some of the most frequently prescribed drugs in the elderly, both community dwelling and in the long-term care setting. The use of newer atypical antipsychotics has gained popularity over the traditional antipsychotics in the elderly due to reduced side effects such as movement disorders, orthostatic hypotension, sedation, and cardiac conduction disturbances. Improvement in the recognition and treatment of mental illness, including the dementias, in this growing population will only result in increased use of these drugs. According to the Centers for Medicare and Medicaid Services, approximately 23.5% of almost 1.7 million long-term care patients receive antipsychotic medications.[25]

Recent observations and research have linked the use of the newer atypical antipsychotics and changes in glucose control. Significant increases of blood

Table 7 Recommendations for glucose monitoring in elderly patients receiving
atypical antipsychotics[a]

Determine baseline fasting blood glucose levels and possibly HbA1c.
Weigh monthly and evaluate glucose levels if there is a 5% weight gain over a month.
Check the fasting glucose level every 2 weeks for a month after initiation of therapy.
Check the fasting glucose level if symptoms of diabetes such as polyuria or polydipsia develop.
Consider the need for reassessment if the doses or class of antipsychotic changes.
If hyperglycemia is found, immediate medical evaluation and management is necessary. The risks and benefits of antipsychotic therapy should be considered.
Nursing facility policies concerning the monitoring of glucose and lipids in residents receiving atypical antipsychotic treatment should be developed.

[a] Adapted from Reference 28.

glucose and triglycerides may result in both new onset type 2 diabetes and ketoacidosis, even in the absence of weight gain.[26] Modest weight gain can occur with all of the atypical antipsychotics. Most cases of hyperglycemia have occurred within the first several weeks of drug treatment. Reports that document the worsening of preexisting diabetes over a 3-year period using atypical antipsychotic treatment have emerged.[27,28]

The mechanisms of atypical antipsychotic medications on glucose control are not understood. Possible mechanisms include:

- Dysregulation of the sympathetic nervous system.
- Serotonin antagonism of pancreatic beta-cells, leading to lower insulin production.
- Altered cellular insulin resistance.

When diabetic and elderly patients are taking atypical antipsychotics, the recommendations for glucose monitoring given in Table 7 should be utilized.

Fortunately, few drug–drug interactions exist between psychotropics and antidiabetic drugs. Concurrent use of metformin and some psychotropic medications may cause additive sedation. Tricyclic antidepressants and fluvoxamine (Luvox®) have been reported to decrease sulfonylurea metabolism and result in clinical hypoglycemia. Hypoglycemia may mimic the sedating effects of psychotropics and is deserving of immediate diagnosis.

Rheumatic Disease

Arthritis is the most common chronic medical illness in the elderly. Disability related to degenerative and inflammatory forms of arthritis results in chronic pain, depression, insomnia, and loss of function. The systemic effects of autoimmune disease such as lupus and rheumatoid arthritis are both crippling and life-threatening. Functional impairments may prevent sufferers from being able to perform the basics of diabetic care such as exercising, food preparation, medication administration, and blood glucose monitoring. Referral to occupational and physical therapists should be considered for assessment and management of these essential components of care. Additional services, including home health care, visiting nurses, and home-delivered meals, may assist the functionally disabled diabetic.

Nonsteroidal anti-inflammatory drugs are known to have significant renal effects and can worsen renal function in the diabetic with preexisting nephropathy. Possible renal complications may include elevations in serum creatinine and renal failure, edema, electrolyte disturbances, and elevated blood pressure. Oral and parenteral use of corticosteroids is known to cause hyperglycemia and can disrupt glycemic control in a previously controlled patient. The diabetic should be cautioned about this effect and should discuss their careplan and blood sugar monitoring with their primary care provider. A recent study by Blackburn et al.[29] demonstrated the onset of diabetes in elderly subjects receiving oral corticosteroids. The effect appeared quite early after initiation of the steroids, and 10% of the patients were diabetic after 3 years of oral steroid therapy. This study also showed that long-term use of inhaled corticosteroids did not cause diabetes in nondiabetic elderly subjects.

LIFESTYLE CHANGES FOR LIVING WITH DIABETES

Diabetes is a "patient-controlled" illness. Although many types of care providers will interface with the patient during the long course of management, ultimately the patient is responsible for the careplan. Special issues of the elderly that impact diabetic care might include financial constraints, health care accessibility, caregiver support, functional decline, education, recreational needs, cultural and personal health care beliefs, and environmental concerns. Diabetes education must be culturally sensitive and tailored to match the learning abilities of the patient. A focused interview and a brief cognitive screen of the elderly diabetic patient will help the educator determine the patient's abilities, special circumstances, and needs.[30] Ascertaining the new diabetic's beliefs about the illness and helping him or her gain confidence with the new information and careplan improve success in blood sugar control. The older diabetic patient may be challenged by the concept of diabetes as a long-term, chronic management illness, given their advanced age. Explanation about the goal of avoiding disability and improving quality of life, as opposed to the goal of extending the quantity of life, should be clarified.

Multiple health care providers may be involved in the management of the older diabetic patient. Understanding the roles of the care team members and actively communicating with each other improves patient care and helps avoid iatrogenic mishaps. Some members of the elderly diabetic patient's health care team and their roles are listed in Table 8. Chronic disease programs for diabetics often use a systems approach to ensure regular patient monitoring and delivery of services.[31]

MANAGEMENT OF COMORBID CONDITIONS

Diabetes is the leading cause of peripheral neuropathy in all groups in the United States. Neuropathy can develop with both idiopathic glucose intolerance (IGT), or "prediabetes," and frank diabetes mellitus.[32] Studies have confirmed the long-held belief that peripheral neuropathy is an early symptom resulting from chronic hyperglycemia. As many as 10%–18% of patients will have neuropathy at the time of diagnosis, well before the onset of other common symptoms. Of patients with IGT, 11% show signs of neuropathy. Long-term patients with at least 25 years of diabetes have a greater than 50% chance of the complication.[33,34] Symmetrical, sensory neuropathy is experienced as a burning pain. The pain can be extremely severe and tingling, and have associated hyperesthesia, where the lightest touch can be excruciating. The distribution is in a glove and stocking pattern on the distal extremities. Many of these patients complain of nocturnal worsening and sleep disturbance and are unable to have sheets or blankets on their feet. The loss of the ability to sense cold temperatures, vibration, and the position of joints can ensue, which places the patient at risk for accidents and trauma. Motor impairment is less common and is an advanced symptom. Diabetic foot ulcers are the result of both neuropathy and microvascular damage.

Treatment consists of achieving glycemic control, careful foot care and daily inspection, and pain management. Several drug classes have been used for the treatment of diabetic neuropathy. The pathophysiology of diabetic peripheral neuropathy is quite complex, and no one treatment can prevent or reverse its development or progression, as oxidative stress, formation of glycation end

Table 8 Diabetes health care team members and their roles[a]

Team Member	Possible Management Roles
Primary care physician	Oversight of the careplan. Setting of goals. Regular office visits with the patient for acute care, chronic disease care (e.g., laboratory monitoring), preventive care (e.g., immunizations), referral to and coordination with other team members and services, and interface with family and other important care providers. Interface with third-party payers for authorizations.
Endocrinologist or diabetes specialist	Consultation for management concerns, evaluation and treatment of comorbid conditions and diabetic complications, and patient education. Updates in new therapies and monitoring tools.
Medical subspecialists	For comorbid conditions and complications pertinent to their field (e.g., nephrologist for diabetic nephropathy, cardiologist for diabetic cardiomyopathy).
Ophthalmologist	Annual dilated retinal exam and treatment of complications. Monitoring of eye pressure. Assistance with existing low vision.
Podiatrist	Education on foot self-care, neuropathy screening, preventive care and treatment of complications (e.g., corns, infections, ulcers), and provision of specialized diabetic footwear.
Pharmacists	Medication education, dispensing, and monitoring. Medication reviews for potential interactions. Screening for adverse events. Provision of diabetic supplies (monitors, glucose test strips, needles, syringes). Interface with third-party payers for authorizations and suggested substitutions based on formularies.
Registered dietitian	Nutritional assessment. Dietary plan development and education. Consideration of family involvement and cultural needs. Weight management and ongoing dietary monitoring. Supplement recommendations.
Dentist and hygienist	Preventive oral care, treatment of complications, and dentures.
Nurses	Chronic disease monitoring, education (home glucose monitoring, administration of insulin, smoking cessation), wound care, assistance with medications (e.g., pill box set-up), home health care services, early detection of acute illness or decline, and family support.
Social workers	Case management and assessment of level of care needed. Environmental assessment. Bolstering of social supports and referral to community resources (e.g., Meals-on-Wheels, transportation, Senior Citizens Centers). Assistance with advanced directives and indigent drug programs.

Table 8 (continued)   Diabetes health care team members and their roles[a]

Team Member	Possible Management Roles
Nursing aides and home health aides	Assistance with bathing, grooming, and other activities of daily living (ADL). Early recognition of skin problems, acute illness, and changes in condition. Companionship and support. Light housework and errands. Medication reminder.
Physical therapist	Exercise plan, gait training, fall prevention and safety concerns, adaption of home environment, equipment (braces, walkers, canes, fitted elastic hose).
Occupational therapist	Assessment of ADLs, upper extremity function, and cognitive abilities. Adaption of home environment and use of equipment for deficits (specialized utensils, door handles, large print books, glucose meters).
Mental health provider	Cognitive assessment, recognition and treatment of mood disorders, counseling for bereavement and loss of health or roles, assistance in addressing medical noncompliance.

[a] These are only some of the providers involved in the routine care of the elderly diabetic. The column on roles provides some examples of tasks important to this specialty in caring for the elderly diabetic patient.

products, protein kinase C, and the polyol pathway are involved. Drug treatment guidelines are available from the Mayo Clinic and are tiered as:[35]

- Tier 1: duloxetine, oxycodone, tricyclics
- Tier 2: carbamazepine, lamotrigine, tramadol
- Tier 3: capsaicin, bupropion, citalopram, methadone, topiramate

These drugs are relatively safe in low doses and can be titrated to the patient's pain, but they may require metabolic monitoring. Tricyclic antidepressants have been a favorite choice for many years because of their affordability and sleep-enhancing qualities. Much lower doses than those used for depression usually achieve the desired effect. The dose-related anticholinergic effect of tricyclics, which the elderly are so sensitive to, prevents use in many older and frail patients and in those needing higher doses. Use of antiarrhythmics such as mexiletine and topical lidocaine has been shown to improve neuropathic pain, but use carries the risk of toxicity. Opiates and other analgesics, such as tramadol or nonsteroidal anti-inflammatory drugs, can be used as an adjunct to treating exacerbations of pain. The risks of long-term nonsteroidal anti-inflammatory drugs outweigh the benefits for this use. Topical capsaicin cream can be beneficial, but it requires multiple daily applications and is often associated with initial burning, reducing its acceptance.

Dysregulation of the autonomic nervous system can also result from hyperglycemia.[36] The symptoms are more systemic in nature and can be difficult to manage. Neurologic damage of the bladder and sphincter can result in urinary urgency and frequency, incontinence, and complete neurogenic bladder. Erectile dysfunction in males and anorgasmia and inadequate vaginal lubrication in females can be the result of both neurologic and vascular damage from diabetes. Furthermore, because of vascular damage from diabetes, the erectile drugs sildenafil, vardenafil, and tadalafil may have disappointing outcomes in affected diabetic men with advanced disease. Sweating is impaired and can lead to hyperthermia. Patients need to be precautioned about heat injury and should be encouraged to use cooling methods and adequate hydration in extreme climates.

Cardiovascular complications include heart rate abnormalities and orthostatic hypotension in response to posture changes. Cautious use of antihypertensives, isometric exercises, elastic support hose, and safety preparations before rising from a bed or chair can help avoid fainting episodes.

Gastrointestinal complications that affect motility of the digestive system are some of the most frustrating symptoms these patients experience. Gastroparesis, or delayed gastric emptying, manifests as nausea, vomiting, upset stomach, reflux, loss of appetite, and bloating. The motility drug metoclopramide is not recommended in the elderly due to anticholinergic side effects and extrapyramidal symptoms (tremors, rigidity, and tardive dyskinesia). Erythromycin has been shown to accelerate gastric emptying in healthy subjects and has been used for this purpose.[36] Botox® injection of the pyloric sphincter and implanted electric stimulation devices in the stomach are some of the more invasive treatments for this debilitating condition. Likewise, diarrhea and constipation are frequent symptoms seen in diabetics with autonomic involvement. Fiber supplementation and bulking agents can be of benefit.

THYROID DISEASE IN THE ELDERLY

Thyroid disease is the second most common endocrine disease in the elderly after diabetes mellitus. The prevalence of thyroid dysfunction increases with age and is estimated at about 4% or higher in the older population.[37] In another recent study, females, whites, and Mexican Americans experienced greater rates of thyroid dysfunction than males and blacks.[38] Finally, the frail and hospitalized population are at greater risk for thyroid disease.[39] Since minimally significant changes in thyroid production and thyrotropin stimulation occur with normal aging, hypothyroidism is more commonly found than hyperthyroidism. A slight reduction in thyroxine is balanced by a decrease in T4 clearance, thus maintaining normal levels. Changes in thyroid structure, both an increase and decrease in size, can be related to iodine intake over time. In addition, thyroid disease can have both a typical and an atypical presentation in the elderly.

Symptoms of thyroid illness are frequently mistaken for other disease processes and medication side effects or seen as due to normal aging. Normal physiologic changes of aging such as decreased skin elasticity, a diminishment in muscle strength, and a reduction in maximal heart rate make a clinical diagnosis of thyroid disease difficult and unreliable. For example, older people frequently associate fatigue, constipation, hair loss, joint aches and pains, and weight gain with a "slowing down" process that they attribute to aging. Metabolic disturbances can be precipitated by hypothyroidism (e.g., hyperlipidemia), glucose dysregulation, and electrolyte disturbances. Subclinical hypothyroidism is more common than overt hypothyroidism in the elderly, but it is commonly missed. These symptoms can sometimes be found in both extremes of thyroid illness, hypothyroidism and hyperthyroidism.

In the aged, hyperthyroidism may not have the classic symptoms seen in the young, such as weight loss, diarrhea, palpitations, and sweating. A syndrome of "apathetic thyrotoxicosis" exists when an elderly person becomes so weak and debilitated by hyperthyroidism that he or she paradoxically appears to be apathetic, depressed, and lethargic, and gains weight. Certain medications such as beta-blockers and sedatives may further confuse or mask these presenting symptoms for thyroid illness.

Nearly every body system is affected by thyroid regulation in some manner. Uncontrolled thyroid disease can often precipitate a decline in existing impaired organ systems. For example, depressed or demented patients will deteriorate more rapidly with the onset of thyroid illness. In addition to cardiac disease, hypothyroidism should be considered with the new onset of angina pectoris, myocardial infarction, atrial fibrillation, and congestive heart failure. The new onset of neuropathy, hearing loss, arthralgias, constipation, electrolyte disturbances, or edema likewise requires a consideration of hypothyroidism. Screening for thyroid dysfunction is an important part of the medical evaluation for memory loss, dementing illness, and depression. This is why some geriatricians consider the measurement of thyroid-stimulating hormone (TSH) a necessity for both periodic screening and in the assessment of new complaints for both men and women over 65 years of age.

Table 9 Laboratory findings in thyroid disorders

Hyperthyroidism	Suppressed TSH, elevated free T4 or T3
Subclinical hyperthyroidism	TSH level < 0.1 μIU/mL
	Normal free T4 and T3
Hypothyroidism	Elevated TSH
	Suppressed free T4 or T3
Subclinical hypothyroidism	TSH level > 5.0 – 10.0 μIU/mL
	Normal free T4 and T3
	Presence of thyroid antibodies or goiter strengthens diagnosis.
Euthyroid sick syndrome	TSH normal or < 10.0 μIU/mL
	Suppressed free T4 and T3 levels
Chronic thyroiditis	Normal or reduced free T4 and T3
	Normal or elevated TSH
	95% have thyroid antibodies

Hospitalized, frail, and chronically ill patients may display confusing thyroid function results. When the elderly become ill or undergo starvation, their body's normal response is to conserve energy by lowering the metabolic rate. This physiologic compensation may result in low serum thyroxine levels and normal or mildly elevated serum thyrotropin levels. This syndrome does not always warrant treatment; it is best managed with observation, and will correct itself upon restitution of health.[40]

Laboratory Measurements for Thyroid Disease

In healthy patients, repeated measurements of thyroid function are unnecessary because tests demonstrate a high level of consistency.[41] The laboratory assessment of thyroid disorder (Table 9) includes the measurement of thyroxine (T4), triiodothyronine (T3), thyrotropin (TSH), and a resin uptake (T3RU). Serum concentration of TSH has become the single best screening test for both hyperthyroidism and hypothyroidism. The accepted reference range for TSH in a euthyroid state is 0.4 to 4.0 milli-International Units per liter (mIU/L).

Hyperthyroidism is characterized by elevations in T4, T3, T3RU, and a lowered TSH. A case of "T3 thyrotoxicosis" will demonstrate an elevated T3 and suppressed TSH, despite a normal T4. The availability of a high sensitivity TSH test aids in the detection of subtly suppressed levels of thyrotropin. In cases of uncertainty, a 24-hour radioactive iodine uptake nuclear thyroid scan can delineate the thyroid gland's metabolic activity. The measurement of thyroid antibodies such as antithyroglobulin can assist in the diagnosis of subclinical thyroid disease and the identification of those who are at risk of developing disease.

Drugs Affecting Thyroid Function and Replacement Therapy

There are several drugs that should not be administered concurrently with levothyroxine because they bind to levothyroxine or impair its absorption. Calcium carbonate binds to form an insoluble chelate with levothyroxine. Ferrous sulfate binds to form a ferric–thyroxine complex. Antacids containing aluminum or magnesium, simethicone hydrochloride, sucralfate, bile salt sequestrants, and cation-exchange resins (e.g., Kayexalate®) impede levothyroxine absorption.

Certain medications can interfere with the diagnosis of thyroid disease, resulting in unexpected thyroid function tests.[42] By increasing thyroglobulin-binding hormone (TGB), estrogens have been recognized as causing elevated T4 and T3 levels and lower T3RU levels with a normal TSH in the euthyroid patient. Jodbasedow thyrotoxicosis is a syndrome of acquired and oftentimes transient hyperthyroidism. In this situation, a patient, often with a thyroid goiter, is affected by the high levels of iodine from a radiocontrast study. Table 10 lists some commonly used pharmacologic agents and their effects on thyroid function.

Treatment of Hyperthyroidism in the Elderly

The treatment of hyperthyroidism is aimed at reducing circulating thyroxine levels and controlling symptoms. Beta-blocking agents are used to suppress tachycardia, sweating, and tremor. A mild, short-acting anxiolytic can be useful short-term in this regard. Antithyroid drugs such as propylthiouracil can be used alone to reduce thyroxine production. Propylthiouracil can also be used to block a worsening of thyrotoxicosis prior to or during a more definitive treatment with radioactive iodine. The course of treatment is monitored during and afterward with serial TSH levels. The development of hypothyroidism can manifest in time. Once hyperthyroidism is relieved, the clearance of other drugs also decreases, possibly resulting in toxic levels.

Treatment of Hypothyroidism in the Elderly

The treatment of hypothyroidism in elderly patients is important for the avoidance of functional decline and improvements in quality of life. As in other treatment regimens in the elderly, the caveat of "start low and go slow" applies. Overly aggressive thyroid replacement may cause exacerbation of underlying cardiac disease, resulting in unstable angina, congestive

Table 10 Some common pharmacologic agents and their effects on thyroid function

Drug Categories	Drug Names	Thyroid Syndrome	Thyroid Function Tests
Estrogens Oral contraceptives Antiestrogen drugs	Conjugated estrogens, estradiol, endogenous estrogens, tamoxifen	Euthyroid	⇑ serum T4, ⇑ serum T3, ⇓ T3RU, normal TSH, ⇑ TGB
Perphenazine (high dose)		Euthyroid	⇑ TGB
β-Adrenergic blocker	Propranolol[a] (high dose)	Euthyroid	⇑ TGB, ⇓ T3, normal T3RU, normal TSH, ⇑ or normal serum T4
Iodine, radiocontrast dyes, and iodine-containing drugs	Amiodarone, ipodate, iopanoic acid	Hyperthyroid, euthyroid, or hypothyroid	⇑ TGB, ⇓ T3, ⇑ T3RU, ⇑ ⇓ or normal TSH, ⇑ or normal serum T4
Glucocorticosteroids	Hydrocortisone, dexamethasone	Euthyroid sick syndrome	⇓ or normal serum T4, ⇓ T3, ⇓ TSH, ⇓ TBG, ⇑ or normal T3RU
Dopamine		Euthyroid sick syndrome	⇓ serum T4, ⇓ T3, ⇓ TSH, ⇓ TBG, normal T3RU
Bile salt sequestrant	Clofibrate, cholestyramine	Euthyroid hypothyroxinemia	⇑ TGB
Cytokines	Interferon alfa, interferon-2	Hyperthyroidism, transient hypothyroidism	Antithyroid microsomal antibodies in 20% of cases
Androgens	Testosterone	Euthyroid	⇓ TBG
Asparagine inhibitor	L-Asparaginase	Euthyroid	⇓ TBG[b]
Growth hormone (high doses)	Somatrem, somatropin	Euthyroid	⇓ TBG
Anticonvulsants	Phenytoin, carbamazepine	Euthyroid hypothyroxinemia	⇓ serum T4, normal or ⇓ T3, normal or ⇑ T3RU, normal or ⇓ TSH
Salicylates		Euthyroid hypothyroxinemia	⇓ or normal serum T4, ⇓ T3, ⇓ TSH, ⇓ TBG, ⇑ or normal T3RU

Table 10 (continued) Some common pharmacologic agents and their effects on thyroid function

Drug Categories	Drug Names	Thyroid Syndrome	Thyroid Function Tests
Lithium	Lithium carbonate	Hypothyroidism[c]	⇓ serum T4, ⇓ TSH
Opiates	Methadone, heroin	Euthyroid	⇑ TGB

[a] This effect is not found with other beta-blocking drugs.

[b] Rapid reduction in serum concentration of TBG within first 2 days of administration; pretreatment values return to baseline 4 weeks after discontinuation.

[c] Through the inhibition of thyroid synthesis and release, goiter may develop.

heart failure, and atrial fibrillation. Initial doses of levothyroxine sodium should begin at 12.5 to 25 mcg daily and titrated slowly to avoid these complications.

Levothyroxine sodium preparations have a narrow therapeutic range, that is, the difference between plasma levels that produce the desired effect and levels that induce toxicity. Small incremental changes of even 25 mcg can result in out-of-range serum TSH levels and physiologically significant subclinical hypothyroidism or hyperthyroidism. A physiologically decreased T4 clearance in the elderly results in about a one-third lower T4 requirement for replacement compared to younger patients. The average dosage for elderly patients is 110 mcg daily. The therapeutic target for replacement is a TSH level of 0.5 to 2.5 mIU/L.

Up to one-fourth of treated patients may have levels above or below the accepted reference range for TSH (0.4 to 4.0 mlU/L). Over extended periods, failure to maintain accurate control can result in adverse physiologic changes, such as osteoporosis in subclinical hyperthyroidism.[43] Atherogenesis and cardiac functional changes have been recognized in elders with subclinical hypothyroidism.[44,45] Contraindications to thyroid replacement include acute myocardial infarction, untreated thyrotoxicosis, uncorrected adrenal insufficiency, or hypersensitivity to any of its inactive ingredients. Food–drug interactions that can affect absorption include soy products and fiber supplements. Intrinsic gastrointestinal dysfunction, including postsurgical states, inflammatory colitis, or peptic ulcer disease, can interfere with thyroid absorption. Adjustments in the levothyroxine sodium dose should be made based on TSH measurements, and incremental adjustments should be made no more often than every 6 weeks. Close patient followup and patience during titration are suggested. Once stabilized, the patient should be monitored every 6–12 months with a serum TSH level.[46]

Other less frequent indications for treatment with thyroid replacement include chronic thyroiditis, the suppression of thyroid cancer, and multinodular goiter.

The management of thyroid disease in the nursing home setting requires some special considerations. Approximately 12% of nursing home patients receive thyroid replacement. Patients of advanced age may have been on thyroid replacement for many years. The background history of the original diagnosis and laboratory testing may not be known to the medical staff and may be irretrievable. Oftentimes the initiation of this drug was for nonspecific symptoms or euthyroid sick syndrome.[47] Up to 50% of patients have been withdrawn from thyroid replacement therapy but still maintained a normal TSH.[48] Due to the prevalence of these disorders, the initial measurement of TSH for new admissions to long-term care is prudent when the status is not known. Annual measurement of TSH on the patient's written careplan is an appropriate approach for those on replacement therapy.

Thyroid Preparations

Most endocrinologists agree that a high-quality levothyroxine sodium preparation should be used. The U.S. Food and Drug Administration (FDA) determines bioavailability by pharmacokinetic studies. Bioequivalence is based on total T4 measurements, not on serum TSH levels. Bioequivalence is not the same as therapeutic equivalence and does not take into consideration the pharmacodynamic properties of the different levothyroxine preparations. The therapeutic difference between two different levothyroxine products with the same dosage may be as much as 25%.

Switching levothyroxine preparations is not advised. It results in more frequent laboratory testing, more physician office visits, new prescriptions, greater cost to the patient, and possible emergence of clinical symptoms. Automatic formulary changes between products should be questioned. Nursing home formularies may switch brands of medications without prior authorization. Desiccated thyroid hormone, combinations of thyroid hormone, and triiodothyronine therapy should not be used for replacement.[49]

KEY POINTS

- Diabetes is the most common chronic disease among the elderly; it is found in 15%–20% of persons over 65 years of age.
- Diabetes is categorized as type 1, type 2, or exogenous.

- Failure to recognize and treat diabetes has a great impact on the elderly, but treatment must be flexible to meet the needs of the elderly.
- Oral hypoglycemics and insulin are the mainstays of treatment but must be tailored to specific concerns relative to the elderly patient.
- Hypertension can be found in 60% of diabetic patients, and together with diabetes accelerates diabetic nephropathy and renal failure and all-cause mortality from cardiovascular disease.
- Psychological illness such as depression occurs in older diabetics.
- Antipsychotic medications are some of the most frequently prescribed drugs in the elderly and can affect glucose control.
- Rheumatic disease is also common in the elderly, and some pharmacological agents used can affect renal function.
- The team approach is critical to maintaining the elderly diabetic patient.
- Hypothyroidism is more common than hyperthyroidism in the elderly.
- Given the broad effects of thyroid dysfunction, screening should be a component of any evaluation of memory loss, dementing illness, or depression.

REFERENCES

1. Health, United States, 1999. *With Health and Aging Chartbook.* Hyattsville, MD: U.S. Department of Health and Human Services, National Center for Health Statistics; 1999:156 (table 33).
2. United Kingdom Prospective Diabetes Study 16. *Diabetes.* 1995;44:1249–58.
3. American Diabetes Association (ADA). Diagnosis and classification of diabetes mellitus. *Diabetes Care.* 2005;28:537–42.
4. Gregg EW, Brown A. Cognitive and physical disabilities and aging-related complications of diabetes. *Clin Diabetes.* 2003;21(3):113–8.
5. Stratton IM, Adler AL, Neil HA, et al. Association of glycaemia with macrovascular and microvascular complications of type 2 diabetes (UKPDS 35): prospective observational study. *BMJ.* 2000;321(7258):405–12.
6. Wyne KL, Drexler AJ, Miller JL, et al. Constructing an algorithm for managing type 2 diabetes. Focus on role of the thiazolidinediones. *Postgrad Med.* 2003;May, Spec No:63–72.
7. Ramsdell JW, Braunstein SN, Stephens JM, et al. Economic model of first-line drug strategies to achieve recommended glycaemic control in newly diagnosed type 2 diabetes mellitus. *Pharmacoeconomics.* 2003;21(11):819–37.
8. Stenman S, Melander A, Groop PH, et al. What is the benefit of increasing the sulfonylurea dose? *Ann Intern Med.* 1993;118:169–72.
9. Paice BJ, Paterson KR, Lawson DH. Undesired effects of the sulfonylurea drugs. *Adverse Drug React Acute Poisoning Rev.* 1985;4:23–36.

10. Hurley D, Bronstein D. Metformin contraindications not being heeded. *Pharmacy Practice News.* August 2003;18–20.
11. Rosenstock J. Management of type 2 diabetes mellitus in the elderly: special considerations. *Drugs Aging.* 2001;18:31–44.
12. Fuller MA, Sajatovic M. *Drug Information for Mental Health 2001.* Hudson, OH: Lexi-Comp; 2001.
13. Kelley DB, Anderson RM, Freeman JC, et al., eds. *Medical Management of Type 2 Diabetes.* 4th ed. Alexandria, VA: American Diabetes Association; 1998.
14. Reuben DB, Herr K, Pacala JT, et al. *Geriatrics at Your Fingertips: 2001 edition.* Belle Mead, NJ: Excerpta Medica, Inc. for the American Geriatrics Society; 2001:46–8.
15. Nesto RW, Bell D, Bonow RO, et al. Thiazolidinedione use, fluid retention, and congestive heart failure: a consensus statement from the American Heart Association and American Diabetes Association, October 7, 2003. *Circulation.* 2003;108(23):2941–8.
16. Weiss PM, Finch FG, Hess LW. Insulin delivery system options in diabetes: novel approaches to an old disease. *The Female Patient.* 2003;28:14–9.
17. Lindblad CI, Hanlon JT, Artz MB, et al. Antidiabetic drug therapy of African American and white community dwelling elderly over a 10 year period. *J Am Geriatr Soc.* 2003;51:1748–53.
18. Comper WD, Osicka TM, Jerums G. High prevalence of immuno-unreactive intact albumin in urine of diabetic patients. *Am J Kidney Dis.* 2003;41(2):336–42.
19. United Kingdom Prospective Diabetes Study (UKPDS) Group: Tight blood pressure control and risk of macrovascular and microvascular complications in type 2 diabetes: UKPDS 38. *BMJ.* 1998;317(7160):703–13.
20. Burt VL, Whelton P, Roccella EJ, et al. Prevalence of hypertension in the US adult population. Results from the Third National Health and Nutrition Examination Survey, 1988–1991. *Hypertension.* 1995; 25(3):305–13.
21. Appel LJ. The verdict from the ALLHAT trial—thiazide diuretics are the preferred initial therapy for hypertension. *JAMA.* 2002;288:3039–42.
22. Lewis EJ, Hunsicker LG, Clarke WR, et al. Renoprotective effect of the angiotensin-receptor antagonist irbesartan in patients with nephropathy due to type 2 diabetes. *N Engl J Med.* 2001;345(12):851–60.
23. Lustman PJ, Clouse RE. Treatment of depression in diabetes: impact on mood and medical outcome. *J Psychosom Res.* 2002;53(4):917–24.
24. Stewart R, Liolitsa D. Type 2 diabetes mellitus, cognitive impairment and dementia. *Diabet Med.* 1999;16(2):93–112.
25. Weinberg AD, Weinberg JD. Antipsychotic medications and diabetes mellitus: risk management in the geriatric population. *ElderCare.* 2003 March;3(1):1–4.
26. Wirshing DA, Spellberg BJ, Erhart SM, et al. Novel antipsychotics and new onset diabetes. *Biol Psychiatry.* 1998;44(8):778–83.
27. Ramankutty G. Olanzapine-induced destabilization of diabetes in the absence of weight gain. *Acta Psychiatr Scand.* 2002;105(3):235–7.
28. Goldstein LE, Henderson DC. Atypical antipsychotic agents and diabetes mellitus. *Primary Psychiatry.* 2000;7(5):65–8.
29. Blackburn D, Hux J, Mamdani M. Quantification of the risk of corticosteroid-induced diabetes mellitus among the elderly. *J Gen Intern Med.* 2002;17(9):717–20.
30. Ryan CM, Geckle M. Why is learning and memory dysfunction in type 2 diabetes limited to older adults? *Diabetes Metab Res Rev.* 2000;16(5):308–15.

31. Hummel J, Norris TE, Gibbs K. Introduction of an electronic registry to improve diabetes outcomes in a primary care network. *J Clin Outcomes Manag.* 2003;10(10): 541–6.

32. Polydefkis M, Griffin JW, McArthur J. New insights into diabetic polyneuropathy. *JAMA.* 2003;290(10):1371–6.

33. Singleton JR, Smith AG. Painful sensory neuropathy in patients with impaired glucose tolerance: Part II—treatment. *Clin Geriatr.* 2003;11(4):21–6.

34. Singleton JR, Smith AG. Painful sensory neuropathy in patients with impaired glucose tolerance: part I—diagnosis and pathophysiology. *Clin Geriatr.* 2003;11(3):28–34.

35. Poncelet AN. Diabetic polyneuropathy: risk factors, patterns of presentation, diagnosis, and treatment. *Geriatrics.* 2003;58(6):16–30.

36. Boivin MA, Carey MC, Levy H. Erythromycin accelerates gastric emptying in a dose-response manner in healthy subjects. *Pharmacotherapy.* 2003;23(1):5–8.

37. Ladenson PW, Singer PA, Ain KB, et al. American Thyroid Association guidelines for detection of thyroid dysfunction. *Arch Intern Med.* 2000;160(11):1573–5.

38. Hollowell JG, Staehling NW, Flanders WD, et al. Serum TSH, T(4), and thyroid antibodies in the United States population (1988 to 1994): National Health and Nutrition Examination Survey (NHANES III). *J Clin Endocrinol Metab.* 2002;87(2):489–99.

39. Mohandas R, Gupta KL. Managing thyroid in the elderly. *Postgrad Med.* 2003;113: 54–6.

40. AACE Thyroid Task Force. *Endocrine Pract.* 2002;8:459–61. Available at: www.aace. com.

41. Andersen S, Pedersen KM, Bruun NH, et al. Narrow individual variations in serum T(4) and T(3) in normal subjects: a clue to the understanding of subclinical thyroid disease. *J Clin Endocrinol Metab.* 2002;87(3):1068–72.

42. Surks MI, Sievert R. Drugs and thyroid function. *N Engl J Med.* 1995;353(25): 1688–94.

43. Foldes J, Tarjan G, Szathmari M, et al. Bone mineral density in patients with endogenous subclinical hyperthyroidism: is this thyroid status a risk factor for osteoporosis? *Clin Endocrinol.* 1993;39(5):521–7.

44. Hak AE, Pols HA, Visser TJ. Subclinical hypothyroidism is an independent risk factor for atherosclerosis and myocardial infarction in elderly women: the Rotterdam Study. *Ann Intern Med.* 2000;132(4):270–8.

45. Charib H, Tuttle MR, Baskind H, et al. Subclinical thyroid dysfunction, a joint statement on management from the American Association of Clinical Endocrinologists. *Endocrine Pract.* 2004; 10:497–501.

46. Coll PP, Taxel P. The management of thyroid disorders in long-term care. *Ann Long-term Care: Clinical Care and Aging.* 2004 March;12(3):26–32.

47. Coll PP, Abourizk NN. Successful withdrawal of thyroid hormone therapy in nursing home patients. *J Am Board Fam Pract.* 2000;13(6):403–7.

48. Hennessey JV. Levothyroxine a new drug? Since when? How could that be? *Thyroid.* 2003;13(3):279–82.

49. Clyde PW, Harari AE, Getka EJ, et al. Combined levothyroxine plus liothyronine compared with levothyroxine alone in primary hypothyroidism: a randomized controlled trial. *JAMA.* 2003;290(22):2952–8.

6

Issues Concerning Common Infections in Community-Dwelling Elderly

CYNTHIA G. OLSEN AND WILLIAM N. TINDALL

You know you are getting old when all the names in your little black book have MD after them.

—Arnold Palmer

OVERVIEW

This chapter discusses important aspects of how a health professional can help an elderly person with an infectious disease. Health care professionals must first realize that the elderly respond to infections differently than younger adults. In addition, general problems such as diminished homeostasis, diminished physiological and organ system reserves, diminished immunity, blunted febrile response, chronic comorbid diseases, polypharmacy, decreased mobility, and malnutrition contribute to the seriousness of infections in the elderly. Several common infections in the community-dwelling elderly are discussed in order to further understanding of the seriousness of infections and to promote the realization that most infections could be prevented with a little care and attention. Special emphasis is given to upper and lower respiratory infections, urinary tract infections, diarrhea-causing infections, and viral infections that are a common cause of death in the elderly. Emphasis is also given to the use of pneumonia vaccines and antiviral medications. Because fever is often blunted in the elderly, the first sign of an infection is usually acute confusion. Health care professionals must keep this in mind and provide caring and compassionate care to the elderly, who are often alone, frightened, and unable to fully comprehend an untenable situation.

Your small pharmacy provides and delivers prescriptions to the local Senior Citizens Center for its residents, a valuable service for those seniors who lack transportation. The center runs an adult day care program for 14 men and women, most of whom have mild-to-moderate dementia but still reside with their families. There has been a sharp increase in prescriptions for antibiotics for urinary tract infections. Four of the program participants have had recurrent infections and several rounds of treatment. One was hospitalized.

- What variables may be contributing to this increase in antibiotic use?
- What nonpharmacologic interventions may reduce or prevent this problem?
- What medical considerations should be explored?

IMMUNITY CHANGES IN AN AGING BODY

Despite all the advances made in antibiotic therapy, infectious diseases still account for one-third of all deaths in persons 65 years and older.[1] In fact, more than 60% of persons 65 years of age and older are admitted to a hospital because they have pneumonia.[2] Patient factors such as altered immune function or comorbid illnesses as well as social factors all contribute to the emergence of infectious disease in this vulnerable population. Diagnosis is frequently difficult because many signs and symptoms of infection that are common in younger adults, particularly fever and leucocytosis, present less frequently or not at all in adults.[3] Additionally, vaccine shortages, trends in antibiotic usage, increases in the number of invasive procedures being performed, and the increasing rate of hospitalization and long-term care placement contribute to the problems of failing to manage preventable infectious illnesses. Also, the emergence of antibiotic-resistant microbes requires the control of these microbes to be quite specific and based on where the patient was residing when the infection was acquired.

Normal aging has a marked effect on immunity, and evidence indicates that cell-mediated immunity consistently shows age-related decreases in function.[4] Thus, important barriers to invasion by microbial agents become increasingly impaired with advancing age, and more and more evidence shows that those barriers are impaired by stress.[5] The body's first defense barrier is the skin, which demonstrates considerable physiologic change: thickness is reduced and the skin becomes dryer. Likewise, the mucous membranes undergo thinning, and there is a minor reduction in the functional reserve of the salivary glands, thus reducing moisture. Systemic illnesses, including diabetes mellitus, Sjögren syndrome, hypothyroidism, malnutrition, and peripheral vascular disease, compromise the integrity of this important first barrier, and xerostomic medications, in particular anticholinergics, and poor hydration contribute to the drying and diminishment of mucus and oral secretions.

Mucosal surfaces in the oral cavity, respiratory tract, gastrointestinal tract, and urogenital tract also undergo compromise, which results in colonization with gram-negative bacilli.[6-8] Physiologic changes such as diminished antibody levels and estrogen deficiency alter the antiadherence mechanisms of urogenital epithelial cells, which increases the rates of bladder colonization and urinary tract infections. Another aspect of this defense barrier is the body's gag-reflex and cough mechanism in the prevention of pulmonary infection. Disease-related contributors to the impairment of these important safety mechanisms include neuromuscular diseases that impair swallowing (such as stroke, Parkinson's disease, and Alzheimer's disease) and chronic lung disease, which produces small airway collapse (emphysema), inflammation, mucous plugging, and loss of lung tissue elasticity (restrictive airway disease). Reduced gastric pH interferes with the normal microbial flora of the gastrointestinal tract.

Research over the past few decades has repeatedly confirmed the role of "immunosenescence" in human aging and the accompanying evidence that many of the so-called diseases of aging are initiated by a deregulation of immune function and inflammation.[9] One such example is Alzheimer's disease, in which patients demonstrate a correlation between mental function and T-cell telomere length.[10] The on-going analysis of the Swedish geriatric population has added to the knowledge that a series of immune dysfunctions leads to all-cause mortality in the elderly.[11]

It is not uncommon for the elderly to have a reduced or absent fever in the face of infection, which in turn delays diagnosis and treatment. Compromised and frail elders, such as those found in long-term care settings, may have relative hypothermia at baseline and a "normal temperature" of 98.6° F. Even a "low-grade temperature" can signify serious, life-threatening illness such as sepsis. Presenting symptoms of serious infection in the elderly might include a change in mental status (confusion, drowsiness), new onset in impairments in functioning (incontinence, falls), and lassitude (diminished appetite, lack of interest). Leukocytosis, or an elevated white blood cell count, is oftentimes suppressed. To ensure that important changes in the patient's condition are recognized, these atypical presentations must be familiar to any health care provider caring for the elderly.

Consider the following case:

> An 85-year-old Cuban-American woman is brought to the physician's office by her niece, with whom she lives. Three days ago this elderly woman complained of being fatigued and her niece noticed she was eating very little. Yesterday she developed a dry cough and slept all day, only consuming scant amounts of fluids. Upon rising this morning, she seemed a bit disoriented and fell on her way to the bathroom. She has been healthy and active. She does not smoke or use alcohol. Her only medications are a multivitamin, aspirin 81 mg daily, and an herbal supplement "for occasional constipation."
>
> On examination she has a temperature of 100.2° F orally, a resting pulse of 112, respirations is 18 and unlabored, and her blood pressure is 108/68. She is alert and oriented, but she needs help rising from a chair. She is not diaphoretic, and her oral membranes are tacky but pink. She is not cyanotic; her oxygen saturation is 92% on room air. On auscultation, dry rales are discovered in the right lung base. A chest radiograph confirms a right lower lobe infiltrate. A complete blood count is 12,100 without increased neutrophils.
>
> Following the physical exam, her niece asks, "Can my aunt be treated at home, or should she go to the hospital?"

- What is happening here?
- What would you tell the niece?
- What would be a likely course of treatment?
- What antibiotics could be used empirically?

UPPER RESPIRATORY INFECTIONS COMMON IN COMMUNITY-DWELLING ELDERLY

Upper respiratory infections are the most common infections among the community-dwelling and institutionalized elderly. As with younger patients, common illnesses such as upper respiratory infection (URI), acute sinusitis, conjunctivitis, and otitis media are frequently limited to viral agents and select bacterial etiologies. The possible viral agents include influenza A and B strains, parainfluenza, respiratory syncytial virus, adenovirus, and rhinovirus. The most common respiratory bacterial agents found include streptococcal species, *Haemophilus influenzae, Staphylococcus aureus,* and *Moraxella catarrhalis.*

Guidelines exist for the treatment of such infections in healthy elders without serious comorbidities. The Centers for Disease Control and Prevention (CDC) and the American Academy of Family Practice (AAFP) suggest symptomatic care for otherwise healthy patients when a viral etiology is suspected (Table 1). By avoiding treatment of nonspecific URIs with antibiotics, the possibility of emergence of resistant organisms is reduced. The health care provider must demonstrate concern for the patient and avoid telling the patient that "it's just a simple virus," which tends to trivialize a serious situation. When antibiotics are requested, the patient should be informed as to the potential risks and harm of promoting resistance, and alternative management of the illness should be discussed. Providing preprinted instructions that give patients guidance on symptomatic care and when to return to the clinician is a strategy that helps alleviate the patient's concerns about not receiving an antibiotic.

A second upper respiratory infection that often affects the elderly is acute bacterial rhinosinusitis (ABRS). It can present with a wide range of symptoms and can vary in severity from mild to life-threatening. This entity is a transient inflammation of the mucosal lining of the paranasal sinuses and typically lasts less than 4 weeks. Environmental agents such as fumes, cigarette smoke, dust, and common allergens can play an etiologic role. Symptoms may include nasal drainage, postnasal drip, throat irritation, nasal congestion, facial pressure or pain, and sneezing. More serious symptoms include fever, chills, and loss of appetite and generalized malaise, which in the elderly would warrant close consideration of a more serious process such as abscess, sepsis, or dehydration. In addition to the clinical presentation and exam, the diagnosis is supported by radiographic studies of the paranasal sinuses. The mere changing in color of nasal secretions does not warrant a diagnosis of a bacterial etiology.

Antibiotics are warranted for moderate-to-severe cases, when a mild case worsens over 5–7 days, when the illness persists 10 days or more, when there are comorbidities, or when the patient is immunocompromised. Patients

Table 1 Treatment summary for minor respiratory illness in healthy adults

Diagnosis	CDC/AAFP Principles of Appropriate Antibiotic Use
Nonspecific upper respiratory infection (URI)	• Antibiotic treatment does not enhance illness resolution and is not recommended. • Life-threatening complications are rare. • Purulent secretions from nares or throat do not predict bacterial etiology and do not benefit from antibiotics. • Symptomatic treatment only is suggested.
Acute bacterial rhinosinusitis (ABRS)	• Most ambulatory cases are caused by uncomplicated viral upper respiratory tract infections. • Acute bacterial rhinosinusitis may not require antibiotics if symptoms are mild. • Watchful waiting and symptomatic care are indicated.
Acute pharyngitis	• Limit antibiotics to patients likely to have group A beta-hemolytic streptococcus (GABHS); symptoms include fever, tonsillar exudates, tender anterior cervical adenopathy, and the absence of cough. • GABHS is the causative agent in 10% of adult cases. • When available, rapid antigen testing and follow-up confirmatory throat culture can help delineate positive cases. • Offer analgesics, antipyretics, and supportive care. • Preferred antibiotic treatment for acute GABHS pharyngitis is penicillin or erythromycin (in penicillin-allergic patients).
Acute bronchitis	• The evaluation of adults should rule out pneumonia or respiratory complications. • Routine antibiotic use in otherwise healthy adults is not recommended. • Symptomatic treatment of cough with antitussives, bronchodilators, supportive care, and education is helpful.

who have underlying lung disease, renal failure, diabetes, or steroid dependency may have a lower threshold for antibiotic treatment. Choice of antibiotic should include knowledge of the patient history, recently prescribed antibiotics, and the local setting and its trends in microbial resistance. The drugs of choice for ABRS usually include a cephalosporin, amoxicillin–clavulanate, a macrolide, or a respiratory quinolone (e.g., levofloxacin, gatifloxacin, moxifloxacin).[12]

LOWER RESPIRATORY INFECTIONS COMMON IN COMMUNITY-DWELLING ELDERLY

Lower respiratory infections (LRI) affecting the elderly commonly include tracheitis, acute and chronic bronchitis, community-acquired pneumonia (CAP), and lung abscess. The usual causative agents are bacteria (i.e., streptococcal species, *H. influenzae*, *M. catarrhalis*, and *S. aureus*) and respiratory viruses. Atypical microbes may be present in up to one-fourth of patients, and they may include *Mycoplasma pneumoniae*, *Legionella*, *Chlamydia pneumoniae*, and *Bordetella pertussis*. Most of these microbes are treatable with antibiotics on an outpatient basis. Anaerobic and gram-negative bacteria are also seen more often in the frail elderly and the institutionalized elderly.

Community-Acquired Pneumonia

Diagnosis of pneumonia or CAP is challenging in older patients due to their presentation of blunted or atypical symptoms; however, these patients tend to have a worse prognosis and higher mortality rates than younger adults, and their initial chest radiographs can be negative. Thus, they require continuous monitoring by their clinicians to ensure that the infection does not progress. Older adults tend to be more susceptible to CAP because of the following changes[13] in their physiology, changes that can leave them with a diminished cough reflex and diminished airway patency:

- Changes in pulmonary reserve.
- Decreases in cough reflex.
- Decreases in mucociliary transport.
- Decreases in elasticity of alveoli.
- Poorer ventilation.

The choice to hospitalize an elderly person with CAP becomes a serious question, since adverse drug reactions (ADRs), nosocomial infections, and delirium are possible risks of being institutionalized.[14] Hospitalization of the elderly with CAP should only be considered when the elderly person has a compromised cardiopulmonary system or demonstrates symptoms such as tachypnea, tachycardia, lowered oxygen saturation, hypotension, severe dyspnea, or chest discomfort. An unstable home situation and the lack of an adequate caregiver may warrant hospitalization of an elder who is temporarily unable to care for himself. Algorithms based on demographic and clinical factors have been published that stratify patients in order to determine the most appropriate setting for treatment (Table 2).

Table 2 Predictive clinical criteria for hospitalization of elderly patients with pneumonia

Demographic Factors	Points
Age	
Male	Age in years
Female	Age in years −10
Nursing home resident	+10
Specific comorbidities	
Malignancy	+30
Congestive heart failure	+10
Renal insufficiency	+10
Hepatic dysfunction	+10
Cerebrovascular disease	+10
Altered mental status	+20
Vital sign abnormalities	
Respiratory rate > 30 breaths/minute	+20
Systolic blood pressure < 90 mm Hg	+20
Heart rate > 125 beats/minute	+10
Body temperature < 35° C or > 40° C	+15
Laboratory abnormalities	
Arterial pH < 7.35	+30
Blood urea nitrogen > or equal to 30 mg/dL	+20
Serum sodium < 130 mg/dL	+20
Serum glucose > or equal to 250 mg/dL	+10
Hematocrit < 30 %	+10
Arterial blood gas oxygen tension < 60 mm Hg	+10
Pleural effusion	+10

Total Points	Site of Care
< or equal to 70 points	Outpatient
71–90 points	Brief inpatient
> or equal to 91 points	Inpatient

[a] Adapted from Fine MJ, Auble TE, Yealy DM, et al. A prediction rule to identify low-risk patients with community-acquired pneumonia. *N Engl J Med.* 1997;336(4):243–50.

Timely administration of the first dose of an antibiotic has been shown to improve outcome and lessen the length of stay in hospitalized patients with CAP. Supportive care with fluid resuscitation, supplemental oxygen, early mobilization, and pulmonary toilet are all traditional modalities in the care of the hospitalized pneumonia patient. Numerous pathways and recommendations for antibiotic choice can be found. The Infectious Disease

Table 3 Antibiotic choice based on IDSA risk and treatment setting[a]

Outpatient IDSA Risk Class I, II	Inpatient IDSA Risk Class III, IV	ICU Patient IDSA Risk Class V
Doxycycline Amoxicillin + advanced macrolide, e.g., azithromycin Levofloxacin Amoxicillin–clavulanate + advanced macrolide, e.g., azithromycin In patients with suspected aspiration: amoxicillin–clavulanate + clindamycin	Ampicillin–sulbactam + azithromycin IV for 2 days, then oral for 8 days Levofloxacin IV and switch to oral when possible Ceftriaxone + azithromycin IV for 2 days, then switch to oral cefuroxime and azithromycin	When *Pseudomonas* is not suspected: • Piperacillin–tazobactam + levofloxacin IV • Cefepime + levofloxacin IV • For penicillin-allergic patients: aminoglycoside single daily dose + high-dose levofloxacin IV When *Pseudomonas* is suspected: • An antipseudomonal agent[b] + ciprofloxacin ± an aminoglycoside • Aztreonam + quinolone ± an aminoglycoside

[a] Adapted from Gleason PP, Meehan TP, Fine JN, et al. Association between initial antimicrobial therapy and medical outcomes for hospitalized elderly patients with pneumonia. *Arch Intern Med.* 1999;159(11):2562–72, and Conference Summaries: ICAAC 2001, IDSA 2001, and ASTFM 2001. American Health Consultants/Infectious Disease Alert. 2002; 21(13):97–104.

[b] Antipseudomonal agents include piperacillin, piperacillin–tazobactam, imipenem, meropenem, and cefepime.

Society of America (IDSA) bases its recommendations on the level of risk to the patient, setting of treatment, and understanding of antibiotic-resistant organisms (Table 3).

Aspiration Pneumonia

Aspiration pneumonia is the result of two distinct processes: the aspiration of gastric contents and the aspiration of oropharyngeal contents. The former process results in a chemical inflammatory response sometimes called pneumonitis. The latter process results in oral flora contaminating the respiratory tree and causing a bacterial pneumonia. Differentiation of these two types of aspiration may be difficult.[15] Elderly who are frail, debilitated, have dysphagia or neurodegenerative disease, or reside in a nursing facility are susceptible to aspiration pneumonia. Clinical features include dyspnea, fever, hypoxemia, and a chest radiographic demonstration of an infiltrate in a dependent section. Aspiration pneumonitis is not an infectious process and can be treated with supportive care and without antibiotics initially. Many clinicians who choose to treat with antibiotics consider the possibility of anaerobic microbes found in the oral cavity.

Several strategies for the prevention of aspiration pneumonia have been suggested. Feeding tubes do not reduce the risk of aspiration and may even increase the risk. Oral hygiene practices have not been shown to reduce the rate of pneumonia. Common maneuvers such as the use of soft diets, thickened liquids, and positioning are often suggested by speech therapists who regularly perform swallowing evaluations using video fluoroscopy.[16] The patient who experiences recurrent bouts of pneumonia should be studied for the possibility of aspiration.

Tuberculosis

Tuberculosis has long been a public health issue due to the morbidity and mortality of the disease. The elimination of the infective agent *Mycobacterium tuberculosis* has been one strategy for the control of this disease. The elderly are susceptible to this infection for the same reasons they are susceptible to other respiratory illness. In addition, reactivation of previously quiescent infection in susceptible patients and exposure in crowded settings such as the domiciliary or nursing home setting warrants a strategy for tuberculosis control. Gathering a history of previous tuberculosis infection or possible exposure, admission testing of new facility residents, annual testing of health care staff, and heightened awareness of signs and symptoms of infection are all necessary for the control of this pathogen. Known risk factors include HIV infection, incarceration, and international travel or residency in known endemic areas.

All pharmacists, nursing personnel, and other medical staff should be familiar with the principles behind the two-step tuberculin skin test and its interpretation. Proper intradermal administration of the tuberculin material is essential, and practitioners should be trained and their technique assessed. This serial tuberculin testing boosts the diminished immunity of an immunocompromised individual, eliminating a false-negative result. Identification of the person responsible for the proper recording of test results and reporting of positive results to the local health department is essential for any program.[17]

Using Pneumococcal Vaccine in the Elderly

Invasive pneumococcal disease includes (1) pneumonia with positive blood cultures or (2) isolates from other sterile sites such as cerebrospinal fluid and joint fluid. Approximately one-third of the cases of pneumococcal pneumonia in the elderly will involve this bacteremia. The rates of invasive pneumococcal disease are greater in institutionalized elderly than community-dwelling elderly, and its high rate of mortality is about 30%. Furthermore, emerging quinolone resistance to pneumococcus in both settings increases the fatal outcome of the infection.[18] The recommendation to vaccinate the elderly and those with chronic illnesses with pneumococcal polysaccharide vaccine is a safe and cost-effective strategy in primary prevention. Studies of the effectiveness against pneumococcal pneumonia without bacteremia show mixed conclusions. Recent studies have shown that the vaccine does not reduce the rate of any-case of CAP.[19]

The duration of initial immunity from pneumococcal vaccine is not known, and reimmunization does not induce a response that is any longer lasting than the initial immunization.[20] If a patient under 65 years of age was once immunized, and it has been at least 5 years since that immunization, it is reasonable to revaccinate if the individual is now over 65. One side effect of pneumococcal vaccination is a local reaction at the injection site.

Consider the following case:

> As the consulting pharmacist at the local nursing home, you are asked to sit on the Infection Control Committee. This 80-bed facility has both skilled and permanent residents. The director of nursing shares that last year the facility had a high rate of respiratory infections despite 95% of the residents having received the influenza vaccine in September. You have recognized that the facility's usage of antibiotics last fall and winter seemed extraordinarily high. The facility does not offer staff influenza vaccine but recommends that the staff go to the County Health Department for immunization. Review of past patients' orders reflects that the nursing staff frequently called the attending physician and received an empiric phone order for antibiotics when the patient demonstrated a low-grade temperature, runny nose, or cough.

- What other questions need to be asked?
- What suggestions can be made to help curtail flu during the upcoming flu season?

VIRAL INFECTIONS COMMON IN COMMUNITY-DWELLING ELDERLY

Viral Influenza

Viral influenza results in 35,000 deaths and more than 110,000 hospitalizations annually in the United States and, while it is a common respiratory infection, its impact is enormous and is felt worldwide. In the United States, it is responsible for more than $1 billion in Medicare expenditures. And, when deaths result from viral influenza, 80%–90% of them occur in adults more than 65 years of age.[21]

Influenza A and B are the two viruses that are known to infect humans. The A subtype tends to cause a more severe clinical course and to demonstrate antigenic shift. The B subtype generally causes a milder course and also demonstrates antigenic shift. Antigenic shift is the phenomenon that occurs when two strains of influenza virus infect a single host and exchange RNA segments, creating a newly reconstructed virus. Antigenic shift poses the potential for high infectivity due to the lack of immunity in humans to the new virus. This is why a new influenza vaccine needs to be researched, formulated, and distributed for each annual flu season. This tedious process improves the likelihood that the selected vaccine will protect against that year's anticipated strain(s) of virus.

The clinical presentation of viral influenza is extremely broad, but its classical symptoms include high-grade fever, chills, muscle aches, headache, sore/dry throat, general malaise, and photophobia, all with sudden onset after an incubation period of 1–2 days. Viral respiratory symptoms include a nonproductive cough, pharyngitis, and clear rhinitis. The elderly may not present with the high fever usually seen in younger patients. Caregivers must realize that viral influenza may not be well characterized in the elderly. In fact, anorexia, confusion, and unsteady gait are common presenting symptoms in the frail and those of advanced age.

Rapid identification of infected individuals can now be expedited by the use of rapid diagnostic tests, which entail the use of a nasopharyngeal swab and provide an answer in 30 minutes.[22] These tests aid in decisions about treatment but are only one part of the challenge, as the accuracy rate for influenza A is only 65%–81%. Although follow-up and confirmatory testing is required, this should not prevent the clinician from using empiric treatment in highly suspicious cases.

Table 4 Antiviral influenza medications[a]

	Amantadine	Rimantadine	Zanamivir	Oseltamivir
Type effective	A	A	A and B	A and B
Route	Oral	Oral	Inhaled	Oral
Usage type	Treatment and prevention	Treatment and prevention	Treatment only	Treatment and prevention
Side effects	CNS and GI	CNS and GI, but milder	< 5% diarrhea, nausea, headache, and cough	Nausea and vomiting
Dosage for the elderly	100 mg/day	100 mg/day	10 mg twice daily	75 mg twice daily
Duration of therapy	Until 24–48 hours after symptom resolution	Until 24–48 hours after symptom resolution	Five days	Five days
Cost per 5-day course	$2	$10	$48	$60

[a] Adapted from Kingston BJ, Wright CV. Influenza in the nursing home. *Am Fam Physician.* 2002;65(1):75–8.

Primary treatment with anti-influenza drugs includes the use of amantadine and neuraminidase inhibitors, as they are known to decrease flu symptoms when initiated early. While most cases of the flu are self-limiting, the elderly may have other comorbidities that would warrant treatment with the available antivirals (Table 4). Although amantadine is quite affordable, the high incidence of side effects limits its use in the elderly population. Clinicians and caregivers should keep in mind that use of antiviral drugs is an adjunct to any vaccine for controlling and preventing influenza, but such drugs are not a substitute for vaccination. Currently, four antiviral agents are approved by the FDA: amantadine (Symmetrel®), rimantadine (Flumadine®), zanamivir (Relenza®), and oseltamivir (Tamiflu®). To achieve any degree of effectiveness, these agents must be administered within 48 hours of onset of symptoms.[23] Amantadine, and to a lesser extent rimantadine, is excreted via the kidneys; thus when amantadine is given to elderly patients or anyone with renal insufficiency, its dose should be reduced to 100 mg/day. Using antiviral drugs for treatment and prophylaxis is a key component of controlling influenza in institutions such as hospitals and nursing homes. Should an outbreak occur, the CDC recommends that all residents should receive these agents for a minimum of 2 weeks whether or not they received an influenza vaccine the previous flu season (fall).[24]

Uncomplicated viral infections usually resolve in a few days, with fatigue and weakness possibly lingering for a week or two. General supportive care, antipyretics, antitussives, hydration, and a gradual return to daily activities are beneficial. Complications of viral influenza in the elderly include pneumonia, myositis, rhabdomyositis, cardiac compromise, pulmonary distress, hypoxemia, central nervous system problems, and bacterial superinfections. Bacterial superinfections are serious situations and, as they have high mortality rates, require consideration of hospitalization for additional respiratory support and antibiotic coverage with either a beta-lactam or a respiratory quinolone.

The primary method of prevention of viral influenza in the elderly is immunization. Persons 50 years of age or older or those with a chronic medical problem (cardiac, renal diabetes, lung disease) should be vaccinated annually. Anyone residing in a nursing or chronic care facility, regardless of condition, and those who are immunocompromised, regardless of age, should also be considered for vaccination. Persons who would likely transmit influenza to high-risk patients, such as health care personnel, caregivers, and household members, should also be vaccinated. In fact, it is best if both nursing home residents and staff be immunized at the same time prior to the flu season, which starts in October and November. A common barrier to health care staff getting vaccinated is the belief that they will contract a milder form of the illness through the vaccine itself. This myth should be dispelled and staff should be educated to the fact that they cannot get the flu from an inactivated vaccine. Vaccinated persons who do get a respiratory flu-like illness may be experiencing a mild illness from the actual virus itself, or from another noninfluenza virus, or they may have received vaccine with absent antigens due to genetic drift.

Contraindications for viral influenza vaccine are few and include those who have had a previous severe reaction (such as anaphylaxis) to the vaccine or to eggs. Inactivated vaccine is preferred in persons who have contact with immunocompromised patients. The most common side effect is soreness and redness at the injection site which lasts a day or two.

Strategies for the control of an outbreak in a nursing facility or residential home for the elderly should be part and parcel of mandated written policies and procedures and should be available for rapid access and implementation. A clinical outbreak is defined as at least three infected residents with flu-like symptoms and an oral temperature of 100° F or greater within a 3-day period. Immediate confirmation, with rapid testing, should be sought, and ill residents should be isolated and their activities (recreational, dining, visitation) should be decentralized. Symptomatic staff should take sick leave, while the remaining staff should be offered respiratory masks and reminded of strict hand-washing technique. Staff and residents should be restricted from moving between units if possible. Unvaccinated residents and staff should be reoffered an opportunity to be vaccinated. The medical director should consult with the facility pharmacist as to the availability and rapid dissemination of chemoprophylaxis. Visitors to the facility should be made aware of the outbreak and the measures being taken and should see signs posted to remind them. In addition, local and state public health officials should be notified of the outbreak.[25]

Respiratory Syncytial Virus Infection

Human respiratory syncytial virus (RSV) is an enveloped virus recently recognized as a cause of lower respiratory infections in elderly patients, especially those in long-term care facilities, adult day-care centers in the community, and homes that have children. In long-term care facilities, these infections occur at a rate of 5%–10%, with 10%–20% of those occurrences resulting in pneumonia and 2%–5% resulting in death.[26] RSV is among the three most common viruses detected in elderly patients hospitalized with pneumonia. RSV is transmitted by the spread of large droplets containing the virus and by direct contact with nasal secretions. RSV manifests in the elderly with a variable and wide range of symptoms, from a mild cold to severe respiratory distress. The typical presentation is nasal congestion, nasal discharge, and a nonproductive cough, with fever in about 50% of patients. Rales and wheezing are also common. The clinician will use these signs to differentiate RSV infection from bacterial influenza.[27] Although there are a number of diagnostic tests, their sensitivity is suspect. Therefore, clinicians use a viral culture and a rapid RSV antigen detection method as better means for identifying RSV.[28]

The treatment of RSV infection in the elderly calls for a supportive regimen which includes administration of fluids, oxygen, bronchodilators, and in some cases aerosolized ribavirin (Virazole®). Even though the literature lacks any evidence that ribavirin is effective in the elderly, many clinicians do use it for elderly patients with a severe case of RSV.

URINARY TRACT INFECTIONS COMMON IN COMMUNITY-DWELLING ELDERLY

Urinary tract infections (UTIs) are the most frequent nosocomial bacterial infection and the most common source of bacteremia in the elderly population. UTIs can be classified as acute or chronic, hospital-acquired (nosocomial) or community-acquired, complicated or uncomplicated, upper or lower, and symptomatic or asymptomatic. But, however UTIs are labeled, the elderly are more susceptible to them because of the following:

- Obstruction from prostatic hypertrophy in males.
- Use of urethral or condom catheters.
- Neurogenic bladders or prolapsed bladders in females that result in poor bladder emptying, which then allows residual urine to serve as a reservoir for bacteria.
- Fecal incontinence in demented patients.
- Neuromuscular disease, including strokes.

As a result of the enhanced susceptibility to UTIs, the ratio of UTIs in women to men is approximately equal in those over 65 years of age. In women, it is usually sexual intercourse which triggers a UTI, although the reason is unclear. In men, prostatitis syndromes (i.e., the enlarged prostate obstructs the flow of urine) is the trigger for 25% of UTIs.[30] Whether male or female, a UTI patient will likely present with dysuria, fever, increased urinary frequency, and some pain, discomfort, and tenderness over the bladder area. The special challenge for a clinician is that a UTI may be asymptomatic, or its symptoms may be vague, or it may be difficult to distinguish from other common illnesses when all that a patient has as a chief complaint is a general lack of well-being.

The difficulty in making a diagnosis has resulted in an advisory that antibiotics should be withheld from patients who are asymptomatic until a urinalysis and a gram stain and culture are complete so the clinician can better target antibiotic therapy.[31] Treatment of asymptomatic UTIs with antibiotics does not appear to reduce morbidity and mortality and in fact may increase drug-resistant microorganisms and ADRs. The best antibiotic for a UTI is one directed at a microorganism identified by gram stain. Unfortunately, in about 30% of cases, the problem is a polymicrobial infection. Polymicrobial infections occur quite frequently if the UTI is associated with use of a catheter. For empiric prescribing, broad-spectrum antibiotics remain the drugs of choice; elderly women receive 7 days of therapy and elderly men receive 14 days of therapy. The duration of therapy is usually doubled if the infection is considered serious. For the general management of a UTI, the patient should be counseled to:

- Drink plenty of water, as it helps cleanse the urinary tract of bacteria.
- Drink cranberry juice and take vitamin C supplements; both inhibit the growth of some bacteria by acidifying the urine.
- Avoid coffee, alcohol, and spicy foods.
- If feeling discomfort in the abdomen, use a heating pad or take a mild analgesic, either of which can bring relief.

ACUTE INFLAMMATORY DIARRHEA COMMON IN COMMUNITY-DWELLING ELDERLY

For most elderly persons diarrhea is a short-lived, unpleasant experience, but for some it can be dangerous as "diarrhea can impact on the ability of the body to process and absorb necessary water, salts and nutrition and in some cases can lead to dehydration, shock, and even death."[32] Diarrhea can be a symptom of many chronic conditions the elderly have, including irritable bowel syndrome (IBS) and Crohn's disease. In the United States, acute infectious diarrhea accounts for 250,000 hospital admissions and nearly 8 million office visits to physicians each year.[33] It may be an acute condition having rapid onset and lasting for only a brief time. Among the elderly, acute diarrhea is often caused by food allergies, various antibiotics, changes in eating habits, viruses (such as rotavirus), bacteria (e.g., *Salmonella* or *Campylobacter*), parasites (e.g., *Giardia lamblia*), and microorganisms (e.g., *Escherichia coli*).

Escherichia coli

E. coli is a growing cause of food-borne diarrhea. While most strains of *E. coli* are harmless and live as part of the common flora of the large intestine, strains can produce bacteriophages or plasma DNA-encoded enterotoxins that can become virulent and cause plain watery diarrhea or result in inflamed dysentery with bloody diarrhea and occasionally kidney failure. *E. coli* diarrhea is most often associated with eating undercooked or contaminated ground beef, but it can be spread person to person. Infection can also occur after drinking raw milk or swimming in or drinking contaminated water. Usually little or no fever is present, and the illness resolves in 5–10 days; however, among the elderly its complications can be serious and deadly.[34] Interestingly, enterotoxigenic *E. coli* (ETEC) is the most common pathogen in travelers' diarrhea; it puts the elderly at great risk if they have a lowered gastric pH from using antacids, H_2-blockers, or proton pump inhibitors.[35]

Salmonella

In the United States, *Salmonella*-induced diarrhea affects approximately 800,000 to 4 million persons per year, resulting in about 500 deaths per year.[36] The elderly and those with a weakened immune system are most likely to acquire *Salmonella* bacteria, which are usually transmitted to humans through the eating of foods that look and smell fine, although they are actually contaminated with feces. All foods, including vegetables, may become contaminated, although most cases involve foods from animal sources such as meat, poultry, eggs, or milk.

Symptoms of *Salmonella*-induced diarrhea typically start 12 to 72 hours after infection and include severe diarrhea, fever, and abdominal cramps lasting 4–7 days, with most persons recovering without treatment. In some, the diarrhea is so severe that they need to be hospitalized, especially when the *Salmonella* spreads from the intestine to the bloodstream and if the patient becomes severely dehydrated. Persons with severe diarrhea may require rehydration, often with intravenous fluids. Antibiotics are not usually necessary unless the infection spreads from the intestines; in that case, it can be treated with ampicillin, gentamicin, trimethoprim–sulfamethoxazole, or ciprofloxacin.[37] Warnings are being issued, however, against exposing *Salmonella* to the fluoroquinolones, as some *Salmonella* bacteria have become resistant to these drugs.[38] During the last decade, the World Health Organization, the American Medical Association, and the CDC have called for an end to the practice of giving feed animals low doses of antibiotics to promote growth. The United States is the only developed nation that still allows important human antibiotics to be used for "therapeutic purposes" in livestock. Some manufacturers, however, are heeding the call.[39]

Campylobacter

Campylobacter is the most common bacterial organism associated with diarrheal illness in the United States. Virtually all cases occur as isolated, sporadic events, not as a part of large outbreaks. Many cases go undiagnosed or unreported, and campylobacteriosis is estimated to affect more than 2 million persons every year. Infants and young adults are the groups hit the most often by the bacteria, but the elderly can acquire it. Most persons who become ill with campylobacteriosis get diarrhea, cramping, abdominal pain, and fever within 2–5 days after exposure to the organism. The diarrhea may be bloody and can be accompanied by nausea and vomiting. The illness typically lasts 1 week. Most persons recover without any treatment within 2–5 days. Most cases of campylobacteriosis are associated with handling raw poultry or eating raw or undercooked poultry. Even one drop of liquid from raw chicken meat can infect a person. Persons become infected when they cut poultry on a cutting board and then use the unwashed board or utensil to prepare vegetables or other raw or lightly cooked foods, permitting *Campylobacter* organisms from the raw meat to spread to other foods.[40]

Clostridium difficile

C. difficile is a gram-positive anaerobic bacterium responsible for most inflammations of the colon, especially antibiotic-associated colitis, an inflammation of the intestines that occurs following antibiotic treatment. Antibiotic-associated colitis, also called antibiotic-associated enterocolitis, occurs when the normal population of *C. difficile* (the population normally found in the intestines of 5% of healthy adults) finds that surrounding normal flora have been killed by antibiotics. With fewer bacteria to compete with, this normally harmless bacterium grows rapidly and produces two toxins. These toxins damage the inner wall of the intestines and cause inflammation and diarrhea. Although all antibiotics can cause this disease, the most common culprits are clindamycin (Cleocin®), ampicillin (Omnipen®), amoxicillin (Amoxil®), Augmentin®, and any antibiotic in the cephalosporin class (such as cefazolin and cephalexin).[41] Symptoms can occur during antibiotic treatment or within 4 weeks after the treatment has stopped.

In approximately one-half of the incidents of antibiotic-associated colitis, the condition progresses to a more severe form of colitis called pseudomembranous enterocolitis, in which pseudomembranes are excreted in the stools. Pseudomembranes are membrane-like collections of white blood cells, mucus, and the protein that causes blood to clot (fibrin) that are released by the damaged intestinal wall. *C. difficile* can be spread easily from one person to another, especially among residents of nursing homes, causing the elderly, the severely ill, the frail, those with poor hygiene, those institutionalized for a long time, and those who are immunocompromised to be at high risk.[42]

The *C. difficile* toxin is found in the stools of persons older than 60 years of age 20–100 times more frequently than in the stools of persons who are 10–20 years old. As a result, the elderly are more prone to develop this serious antibiotic-associated colitis which in most cases manifests as a watery diarrhea containing mucus but no blood 10 to 20 times a day, and which develops 4–9 days after antibiotic therapy starts. A full-blown case of *C. difficile* may result in pseudomembranous colitis, but a lower crampy abdominal pain, low-grade fever, dehydration, and nonspecific colitis are the most common manifestations. *C. difficile* can complicate Crohn's disease and HIV and can be seriously life-threatening to elderly persons who are debilitated from other diseases.[43]

Therapy for *C. difficile* is directed at eradicating the microbe from the intestinal flora. In uncomplicated cases, simple discontinuation of the antibiotic(s), if possible, is enough to alleviate the symptoms and halt the diarrhea. But if the diarrhea is severe and colitis is present, two drugs are supported by Guidelines of the American Society of Gastroenterology[44] and the Society for Healthcare Epidemiology of America:[45] metronidazole (Flagyl®) and vancomycin (Vancocin®). When either drug is used, therapy should be given for 10–14 days; both drugs have been shown to be 95% effective, with improvement after 1–4 days and complete resolution in about 2 weeks. However, while patients respond well to either metronidazole or vancomycin, 15%–20% of patients will experience a relapse weeks or even months after therapy has stopped, a situation that requires repeating the metronidazole or vancomycin for another 10–14 days or switching to the other antibiotic.[46] The issue with vancomycin is that it causes serious side effects.

Miscellaneous Causes of Diarrhea in the Elderly

Giardiasis, a common form of poisoning acquired from drinking water contaminated with the protozoan *Giardia lamblia*, was once thought to be harmless. Outbreaks in travelers returning to the United States from endemic areas have proved this assumption incorrect. Now about 2.5 million cases occur annually in the United States. Persons pick it up while drinking water from a stream, river, pond, or other such source and pass it along. The diarrhea starts a week after ingesting the contaminated water. It lasts for 1–2 weeks, but there are cases of chronic infections lasting months to years.

Treatment of giardiasis includes both measures to prevent dehydration and a 5–10-day course of metronidazole (Flagyl® 250 mg PO TID). Metronidazole is not the only drug approved by the FDA; it also recommends treating giardiasis with a course of furazolidone (Furoxone® 400 mg PO QID) for 7–10 days. Newer agents are albendazole (Albenza® Tiltab® 400 mg PO QD for 3 days), nitazoxanide (Alinia® 500 mg PO BID for 3 days), and tinidazole (Tindamax® 2 g PO once with food). The newer drugs are nitrofurans with antiprotozoal activity; while effective, they may be less effective than metronidazole. Should the first course of treatment fail, the clinician is likely to try a second course using either another drug, the same drug but at a higher dose or longer duration, or a combination of two drugs.[47]

Shigellosis, another acute diarrhea-causing infection of the bowel, is induced by a group of bacteria called *Shigella*. The source of the infection is excreta of contaminated individuals who can spread it indirectly through contaminated food. When the elderly are infected with *Shigella,* it causes diarrhea, fever, and stomach cramps starting a day or two after exposure to the bacterium. The diarrhea is often bloody, showing mucus and pus, yet shigellosis usually clears up in 5–7 days. In some elderly, however, the diarrhea is so severe, with high fever and seizures, that hospitalization is necessary.[48] Treatment is use of fluid replacement, ampicillin, tetracyclines, and sulfamethoxozole–trimethoprim.

Cryptosporidiosis is a diarrheal disease caused by a microscopic parasite, *Cryptosporidium parvum.* It can live in the intestine of humans and animals and is passed in the stool of an infected person or animal. Both the disease and the parasite are also known as "Crypto." The parasite is protected by an outer shell that allows it to survive outside the body for long periods of time, making it very resistant to chlorine disinfection. During the past two decades, Crypto has become widely recognized as a disease easily acquired from ingesting drinking and recreational water infested with this parasite, which can be found in every region of the United States and the world. Symptoms include loose, watery bowel movements, stomach cramps, nausea, and a slight fever, with symptoms generally beginning 2–10 days after being infected. In persons with average immune systems, the disease lasts about 2 weeks; however, it may occur in cycles in which the person feels better for a few days and then feels worse again, before the illness ends. Since most people with a healthy immune system recover on their own, there is no effective treatment for Crypto. An elderly person who is in poor health or has a weakened immune system is at higher risk for a more severe and more prolonged illness.[49]

Pharmacotherapy and Prevention of Acute Diarrheal Infections

Should an elderly person develop a case of mild diarrhea, he or she will typically recover without treatment. However, the biggest danger for an elderly person with a serious case of diarrhea is dehydration, when the body loses more fluid and electrolytes than it takes in. Signs and symptoms of mild, moderate, and severe dehydration are given in Table 5.

Severe dehydration is a medical emergency requiring immediate care, starting with oral rehydration fluids. Most commercially available oral rehydration therapies are either packages of salts and glucose available to mix in water or "sports drinks" ready to drink (e.g., Gatorade®). The World Health Organization and UNICEF have agreed to a standard formula for oral rehydration therapies. It is a package of salts and glucose designed to be mixed with a liter of water. The formula is:[51]

Table 5   Signs and symptoms of dehydration[50]

Mild Dehydration

Increased thirst.

Dry mouth and sticky saliva.

Reduced urine output, with dark yellow urine.

Moderate Dehydration

Extreme thirst.

Dry appearance inside the mouth and eyes that do not tear.

Decreased urination, or half the usual number of urinations in 24 hours
  (usually three or fewer); urine dark amber or brown.

Lightheadedness that is relieved by lying down.

Irritability or restlessness.

Arms or legs that feel cool to the touch.

Rapid heartbeat.

Severe Dehydration (even if only one sign is present)

Altered behavior such as severe anxiety, confusion, or not being able to stay awake.

Faintness that is not relieved by lying down or lightheadedness that continues after standing
  for 2 minutes.

Inability to stand or walk.

Rapid breathing.

Weak, rapid pulse.

Cold, clammy skin or hot, dry skin.

Little or no urination.

Loss of consciousness.

Glucose	20.0 g
Sodium chloride	3.5 g
Potassium chloride	1.5 g
Trisodium citrate	2.9 g

Use of oral electrolyte solutions, such as Cera Lyte 50 (mild dehydration), Cera Lyte 70 (mild-to-moderate dehydration, travelers' diarrhea), and Cera Lyte 90 (severe diarrhea), are designed to replace fluid loss of 18%–30% and will typically shorten the length of an acute diarrheal illness by as much as 2 days. Although oral electrolyte solutions are effective, the elderly who cannot get them or are home bound often find that a salted drink or salted soup works as well as the commercial products.

The best advice for any caregiver is to take preventive measures that allay and hinder acute diarrheal episodes from being initiated in the elderly. Such preventive measures[52] include:

- Washing hands carefully and often, particularly after using the toilet or helping the elderly use the toilet and before preparing or serving any meal or snack.
- Frequently disinfecting bathrooms and food preparation surfaces, especially if a sick elderly person has recently been in the house or facility.
- Containing bodily fluids—if the elderly use pads or sanitary diapers—by using ones with waterproof outer covers, disposing of all such items promptly and safely.
- Washing all raw fruits and vegetables thoroughly before serving them.
- Cooking meats (especially ground beef), fish, eggs, and poultry thoroughly.

SEXUALLY TRANSMITTED DISEASES COMMON IN THE COMMUNITY-DWELLING ELDERLY

Throughout the United States about two-thirds of all cases of sexually transmitted diseases (STDs) occur in people under 25 years of age. But, since any infection, including STDs, is associated with physiological changes that enhance the risk of acquiring them and since sexual activity still occurs among a high proportion of elderly men and women, health professionals should not be surprised that sexually active seniors are just as likely as younger persons to contract a sexually transmitted disease, even HIV.[53]

Issues that make STDs among the elderly problematic for the clinician include the following:

- A high percentage of STDs in the elderly is asymptomatic or minimally symptomatic, causing the elderly to be diagnosed later in the disease and to experience its progression at a faster rate.[54]
- The elderly are only one-sixth as likely to use condoms for protection against STDs during sexual intercourse.[55]
- Younger people share one risk factor with older people; when it comes to contracting STDs, the risk increases as the number of sexual partners increases.[56]
- There is considerable risk for drug interactions between medications taken for HIV treatment and those commonly used for treating chronic conditions in the elderly.
- The number of cases of HIV is expected to rise along with the increasing number of elderly in whom HIV-associated dementia—

a manifestation of the later stages of HIV—will be the presenting symptom.[57]

- The elderly tend to survive for a shorter period of time than younger persons with HIV.[58]

Discussing specific treatments for the many STDs is beyond the scope of this text, especially since clinical guidelines for such treatments are always in flux. Thus, the reader is directed to the best source for current treatment guidelines, the CDC and its excellent Web site.

Health professionals need to be familiar with and able to differentiate among the cognitive impairment due to Alzheimer's, HIV-associated dementia, and normal senescence dementia. They also need to recognize and help prevent or correct drug interactions in older patients with HIV. In fact, since prevention is a better paradigm, it would behoove any and all professionals who know a sexually active elderly person to remind them of the long-honored precautions of (1) remaining monogamous; (2) using condoms, spermicides, and vaginal barriers; and (3) avoiding exposure to bodily fluids, especially semen.

A better understanding of the sexual preferences, habits, and activities of the elderly and how STDs occur and are transferred not only may help to improve care but will do much to reduce the mortality and morbidity associated with these dreaded diseases.

BACTERIAL RESISTANCE TO ANTIBIOTICS

Antibiotic resistance is a problem of global proportions, as the easy nature of international travel contributes to the rapid dissemination of resistant microorganisms. In the United States, antimicrobial resistance is not only an institutional issue but also a community issue, and in both situations it is an issue tied to the inappropriate use of antibacterial drugs in matters such as the following:[59]

- Not having a valid indication for an antibiotic (e.g., for an uncomplicated viral illness).
- In the treatment of fever that does not appear to be due to bacterial infection. Without strong evidence of bacterial invasion, antibiotic therapy should be delayed, if possible, until clinical and laboratory studies confirm the infection.
- Underdosing, overdosing, or improper route of administration.

- Continuing antibiotic use after bacterial resistance has developed.
- Continuing antibiotic use in the presence of a serious toxic or allergic reaction.
- Prematurely stopping an effective antibiotic therapy.
- Using antibiotics in inappropriate combinations.
- Relying on antibiotics, or prophylaxis therapy, to the exclusion of surgical interventions (e.g., drainage of localized infection, removal of a foreign body).

It is important that every health professional have a heightened awareness of the continual emergence of resistant bacteria, the clinical consequences, and how best to manage the changes.

In the United States, two situations of antibiotic-resistant bacteria are of particular concern: vancomycin-resistant *Enterococcus* (VRE) and methicillin-resistant *Staphylococcus aureus* (MRSA). Either may infect the seriously ill elderly, causing life-threatening situations. These two infections have evolved largely due to the overuse of broad-spectrum antibiotics, the use of antibiotics in food animals, and the inappropriate dosing of many antibiotics; however, it was well known that antibiotic-resistant genes existed in bacteria long before the introduction of the first antibiotic.[60] Other resistant bacteria are penicillin-resistant *Streptococcus* pneumonia (PRSP), multi-drug-resistant gram-negative bacilli (MDR-GNB), and multidrug-resistant *Mycobacterium tuberculosis* (MDR-TB).

Vancomycin-Resistant Enterococcus (VRE)

Enterococcus is a gram-positive coccus that colonizes the lower gastrointestinal and genital tracts, abdomen, and endocardium and can be found in about 95% of any population. In general, these are not harmful bacteria, but when they become invasive they cause UTIs, wound infections, septicemia, and endocarditis. VRE is a strain that is resistant to many common antibiotics, but when it is resistant to vancomycin it hinders the ability of vancomycin to be used in situations where other antibiotics have failed. Enterococci can easily develop resistance to cephalosporins, semisynthetic penicillins (nafcillin, oxacillin), trimethoprim–sulfamethoxazole, clindamycin, tetracycline, erythromycin, and sometimes aminoglycosides.[61] This resistance to vancomycin and other antibiotics occurs when the enterococcus acquires from other bacteria several genes that help it encode a bacterial cell wall peptide. A change in this cell wall peptide reduces the binding capacity of an antibiotic so it is unable to act as a bacteriocidal drug.[62] Thus, finding another antibiotic that is active against the bacterial cell wall is the logic behind finding optimal therapy for these serious infections. Some success has been realized in fighting VRE with a synergistic combination of ampicillin and piperacillin, or a combination of vancomycin and gentamicin, or with the newer agents such as quinupristin and dalfopristin. Quinupristin and dalfopristin, the first parenteral streptogramin antibacterial agent, is a 30:70 (w/w) ratio of two semisynthetic pristinamycin derivatives.[63]

But again, the real message is clear: the health professional who is involved with caring for the elderly should be looking for and implementing protocols that prevent VRE from happening in the first place.

Methicillin-Resistant *Staphylococcus aureus*

When penicillin was introduced in the 1940s, its main use as a bacteriocidal agent was against *S. aureus*. However, within a few years, *S. aureus* demonstrated resistance to penicillin, and a battle has been waged ever since. Several antibiotic surveillance studies have now shown that the prevalence of MRSA has steadily increased to a worldwide problem, causing as much as 50% of the mortality occurring in intensive care units and institutions. Its presence in institutions has resulted in it being called health care associated MRSA or HA-MRSA, due to its significant role as the source of nosocomial infections.

MRSA is now a factor in the rising percentage of mortality seen in the community due to infections. The presence of MRSA in the community is growing, causing its elderly to be at great risk if:

- They are or have been residents of long-term care facilities or nursing homes.
- They have had a hospital admission within 6 months.
- They have had surgery within 6 months.
- They have a skin disease.
- They have a recent burn or an extensive wound.

This new form of MRSA in the community, which is called community-acquired MRSA, or CA-MRSA, is emerging as a major source of CAP, causing the prevalence of CAP to quickly double and sometimes triple between 2001 and 2004.[64] A significant difference between it and hospital-acquired MRSA is that the community form expresses a potent toxin, called panton–valentine leukocidin, which attacks leucocytes and results in the terrible life-threatening skin infection known as necrotizing fasciitis.[65]

S. aureus is common to the nares and the skin of 30%–80% of the population, but it can cause various infections, from minor skin conditions to life-threatening conditions such as wound infections, pneumonia, carbuncles, abscesses, impetigo, and sepsis. During the past five decades, the inappropriate use of antibiotics has allowed *S. aureus* to develop its ability to resist all types of β-lactam antibiotics from penicillin to methicillin, as well as aminoglycosides such as gentamicin.[66] This resistance to antibiotics by staphylococci is caused when a penicillin-binding protein (PBP) is acquired from fragments of other bacteria and these fragments are then incorporated into the *S. aureus* genetic material, to be encoded as an alteration in its own PBP. When incorporated into new cell wall structures, this altered PBP confers resistance to the β-lactams and their derivatives.[67]

What the optimal pharmacotherapy for an MRSA infection would be remains in question, but most clinicians select vancomycin as their drug of first choice. Beyond the use of vancomycin, the options are few. Clindamycin is one alternative and, if the infection is in a soft tissue, oral rifampin, clindamycin, ciprofloxacin, trimethoprim–sulfamethoxazole, doxycycline, and topical bacitracin are often treatment choices for mild-to-moderate infection. Susceptibility testing should be performed on all isolates, because in vitro susceptibility testing may not always correlate with in vivo efficacy. Rifampin and trimethoprim–sulfamethoxazole in combination may provide increased efficacy, but rifampin should not be used as monotherapy, as resistance to it develops rapidly.

Should treatment failure occur with the described antibiotics, additional treatment choices include newer antibiotics such as linezolid (Zyvox®), daptomycin (Cubicin®), and quinupristin and dalfopristin (Synercid®). Linezolid is active against MRSA, although resistant isolates have been reported. Linezolid is available as an oral dosage form (tablet and suspension), but it is relatively costly and has many significant drug–drug interactions, including selective serotonin reuptake inhibitors. Daptomycin is active against MRSA but is costly and available only as a parenteral. Quinupristin and dalfopristin is also active against MRSA, although it is costly, only a parenteral, and not well tolerated, and inducible resistance may occur.[68] Unfortunately, the professional literature is reporting that resistance to vancomycin is starting to develop.[69] Fortunately, CA-MRSA remains susceptible to several antibiotic classes outside the β-lactam group, such as clindamycin, although hospital-MRSA remains resistant to macrolides, aminoglycosides, fluoroquinolones, tetracyclines, and lincosamides. Within 5 years, however, CA-MRSA resistance rates may be as high as 25%, causing even more issues for the community-dwelling elderly.[70]

KEY POINTS

- Infections in the elderly are complicated by diminished homeostasis, diminished physiological and organ system reserves, diminished immunity, blunted febrile response, chronic comorbid diseases, polypharmacy, decreased mobility, and malnutrition.
- Infections in the elderly are more common than in younger persons, and more complex, providing the clinician special challenges.
- With an elderly patient, one special challenge may be combining antibiotics with other drugs the patient is taking for chronic conditions.
- Antibiotics have been improperly used over the last half century, promoting the development of resistant bacteria, including vancomycin-resistant *Enterococcus* and methicillin-resistant *Staphylococcus aureus*.
- New classes of antibiotics, such as ketolides, oxazolidinones, and streptogramins (Synercid®), have been developed for the treatment of multidrug-resistant gram-positive infections. However, the efficacy and the side effect profile in the elderly have yet to be determined.
- Health professionals must work together and build programs to stop the spread of opportunistic infections.
- Programs promoting hand-washing and adherence to protocols that help keep the elderly from spreading microbes to each other and their helping professionals can be successful if a concerted effort is prioritized, promoted, and maintained.
- As a health professional, remember that:
  - Most infections do not require the use of antibiotics.
  - Antibiotics may harm helpful bacteria in the body.
  - Bacteria often develop unnecessary resistance to an antibiotic, rendering it useless.

REFERENCES

1. Pinner RW, Teutsch SM, Simonsen L, et al. Trends in infectious disease mortality in the United States. *JAMA*. 1996;275(3):189–93.
2. Crossley KB, Peterson PK. Infections in the elderly. *Clin Infect Dis*. 1996;22(2):209–15.
3. Norman DC. Special infectious disease problems in geriatrics. *Clin Geriatr*. 1999;(Suppl 1):3–5.

4. Castle SC. Clinical relevance of age related immune dysfunction. *Clin Infect Dis.* 2000;31(2):578–85.

5. Ader R, Felten DL, Cohen N, eds. *Psychoneuroimmunology.* 3rd ed. San Diego: Academic Press; 2000.

6. Weinberg JM, Vafaie J, Scheinfeld NS. Skin infections in the elderly. *Dermatol Clin.* 2004;22(1):51–61.

7. Laube S, Farrell AM. Bacterial skin infections in the elderly: diagnosis and treatment. *Drugs Aging.* 2002;19(3):331–42.

8. Weinberg JM, Scheinfeld NS. Cutaneous infections in the elderly: diagnosis and management. *Dermatol Ther.* 2003;16(3):195–205.

9. Caruso C, Candore G, Colonna-Romano G, et al. Inflammation and life-span. *Science.* 2005;307(5707):208–9.

10. Panossian LA, Porter VR, Valenzuela HF, et al. Telomere shortening in T cells correlates with Alzheimer's disease status. *Neurobiol Aging.* 2003;24(1):77–84.

11. Pawelec G, Akbar A, Caruso C, et al. Is immunosenescence infectious? *Trends Immunol.* 2004;25(8):406–10.

12. Fine MJ, Smith DN, Singer DE. Hospitalization decision in patients with community-acquired pneumonia: a prospective cohort study. *Am J Med.* 1990;89(6):713–21.

13. Riedinger JL, Robbins LJ. Prevention of iatrogenic illness: adverse drug reactions and nosocomial infections in hospitalized older adults. *Clin Geriatr Med.* 1998;14(4):681–98.

14. Anon JB, Jacobs MR, Poole MD, et al. Executive Summary: Antimicrobial treatment guidelines for acute bacterial rhinosinusitis. *Otolaryngol Head Neck Surg.* 2004;130 (1 Suppl):1–45.

15. Kupronis BA, Richards CL, Whitney CG, et al. Invasive pneumococcal disease in older adults residing in long-term care facilities and in the community. *J Am Geriatr Soc.* 2003;51(11):1520–5.

16. Jackson LA, Neuzil KM, Yu O, et al. Effectiveness of pneumococcal polysaccharide vaccine in older adults. *N Engl J Med.* 2003;348(18):1747–55.

17. Jackson LA, Benson P, Sneller VP, et al. Safety of revaccination with pneumococcal polysaccharide vaccine. *JAMA.* 1999;281(3):243–8.

18. Mylotte JM, Goodnough S, Naughton BJ. Pneumonia versus aspiration pneumonitis in nursing home residents: diagnosis and management. *J Am Geriatr Soc.* 2003;51(1):17–23.

19. Loeb MB, Becker M, Eady A, et al. Interventions to prevent aspiration pneumonia in older adults: a systematic review. *J Am Geriatr Soc.* 2003;51(7):1018–22.

20. National Tuberculosis Controllers Association; Centers for Disease Control and Prevention (CDC). Guidelines for the Investigation of Contacts of Persons with Infectious Tuberculosis: recommendations from the National Tuberculosis Controllers Association and CDC. *MMWR Recomm Rep.* 2005 Dec 16;54(RR-15):1–47.

21. Kuhle C, Evans JM. Prevention and treatment of influenza infections in the elderly. *Clin Geriatr.* 1999;7(2):27–35.

22. Couch RB. Prevention and treatment of influenza. *N Engl J Med.* 2000;343(24):1778–87.

23. Harper SA, Fukuda K, Uyeki TM, et al. Prevention and control of influenza: recommendations of the Advisory Committee on Immunization Practices (ACIP). *MMWR Recomm Rep.* 2004 May 28;53(RR-6):1–40.

24. Zhanel GG, Harding GK, Guay DR. Asymptomatic bacteriuria. Which patients should be treated? *Arch Intern Med.* 1990;150(7):1389–96.

25. Gomolin IH, Kathpalia RK. Influenza. How to prevent and control nursing home outbreaks. *Geriatrics.* 2002;57(1):28–34.

26. Falsey AR, Walsh EE. Diagnosis of respiratory syncytial virus in adults. *N Clin Microbiol Rev.* 2000;13(3):371–84.

27. Dowell SF, Anderson LJ, Gary HE, et al. Respiratory syncytial virus is an important cause of community-acquired lower respiratory infection among hospitalized adults. *J Infect Dis.* 1996;174(3):456–62.

28. Falsey AR, McCann RM, Hall WJ, et al. Evaluation of four methods for the diagnosis of respiratory syncytial virus infection in older adults. *J Am Geriatr Soc.* 1996;44(1): 71–3.

29. Lipsky BA. Urinary tract infections in men. Epidemiology, pathophysiology, diagnosis, and treatment. *Ann Intern Med.* 1989;110(2):138–50.

30. Boscia JA, Kobasa WD, Abrutyn E, et al. Lack of association between bacteriuria and symptoms in the elderly. *Am J Med.* 1986;81(6):979–82.

31. McCue JD. Treatment of urinary tract infections in long-term care facilities: advice, guidelines and algorithms. *Clin Geriatr.* 1999(Suppl 1):11–7.

32. Berkow R, ed. *Merck Manual.* 16th ed. Rahway, NJ: Merck Research Labs; 1992: 806–8.

33. Friedman LS, Isselbacher KJ. Diarrhea and constipation. In: Isselbacher KJ, Braunwald E, Wilson JD, eds. *Harrison's Principles of Internal Medicine.* 13th ed. New York: McGraw-Hill; 1994:213–21.

34. Mayo Clinic Staff. *E. coli:* the raw and the cooked. Available at: http://www.mayoclinic.com/health/e-coli/DG00005 (accessed April 6, 2006).

35. Dial S, Delany JA, Barkun AN, et al. Use of gastric acid-suppressive agents and the risk of community-acquired *Clostridium difficile*-associated disease. *JAMA.* 2005; 294(23):2989–95.

36. Available at: http://www.cdc.gov/ncidod/dbmd/diseaseinfo/salmonellosis_g.htm (accessed April 5, 2006).

37. Vila J, Vargas M, Ruiz J, et al. Quinolone resistance in enterotoxigenic *Escherichia coli* causing diarrhea in travelers to India in comparison with other geographical areas. *Antimicrob Agents Chemother.* 2000;44(6):1731–3.

38. McCusker ME, Harris AD, Perencevich E, et al. Fluoroquinolone use and *Clostridium difficile*-associated diarrhea. *Emerg Infect Dis* [serial online] 2003 Jun. Available at: http://www.cdc.gov/ncidod/EID/vol9no6/02-0385.htm (accessed April 5, 2006).

39. Weise E. 'Natural' chickens take flight. *USA Today.* Available at: http://www.usatoday.com/news/health/2006-01-23-natural-chickens_x.htm (accessed April 10, 2006).

40. Available at: http://www.cdc.gov/ncidod/dbmd/diseaseinfo/campylobacter_g.htm (accessed April 10, 2006).

41. Yassin SF, Young-Fadok T, Zein NN, et al. *Clostridium difficile*-associated diarrhea and colitis. *Mayo Clin Proc.* 2001:76:725–30. Available at: http://www.mayoclinicproceedings.com/Abstract.asp?AID=1239&Abst=Abstract (accessed April 12, 2006).

42. Gorbach SL. Antibiotics and *Clostridium difficile. N Engl J Med.* 1999;341(22): 1690–1.

43. Simor AE, Bradley SF, Strausbaugh LJ, et al. *Clostridium difficile* in long-term-care facilities for the elderly. *Infect Control Hosp Epidemiol.* 2002;23(11);696–704.

44. Fekety R. Guidelines for the diagnosis and management of *Clostridium difficile*-associated diarrhea and colitis. American College of Gastroenterology, Practice Parameters Committee. *Am J Gastroenterol.* 1997;92(5):739–50.

45. Gerding DN, Johnson S, Peterson LR, et al. *Clostridium difficile*-associated diarrhea and colitis. *Infect Control Hosp Epidemiol.* 1995;16(8):459–77.

46. Johnson S, Homann SR, Bettin KM, et al. Treatment of asymptomatic *Clostridium difficile* carriers with vancomycin or metronidazole (fecal excretors). A randomized, placebo-controlled trial. *Ann Intern Med.* 1992;117(4):297–302.

47. Cash BD, Johnson M. Giardiasis, updated June 23, 2005. Available at: http://www.emedicine.com/med/topic868.htm (accessed April 12, 2006).

48. Available at: http://www.cdc.gov/ncidod/dbmd/diseaseinfo/shigellosis_t.htm (accessed April 12, 2006).

49. Available at: http://www.cdc.gov/od/oc/media/pressrel/R2K0306.htm (accessed April 12, 2006).

50. Available at: http://www.webmd.com/hw/health_guide_atoz/std120726.asp (accessed March 31, 2006).

51. WHO. New formula for oral rehydration will save millions of lives. 2002 press release. Available at: http://www.who.int/mediacentre/news/releases/release35/en/index.html (accessed April 7, 2006).

52. Available at: http://www.cdc.gov/ncidod/dbmd/diseaseinfo/escherichiacoli_g.htm (accessed April 7, 2006).

53. Davidson JM. Sexuality and aging. In: Hazzard WR, Andres R, Bierman EL, eds. *Principles of Geriatric Medicine and Gerontology.* 2nd ed. New York: McGraw-Hill; 1990:108–14.

54. Knodel LC. Sexually transmitted diseases. In: DiPiro JT, Talbert RL, Yee GC, et al., eds. *Pharmacotherapy: A Pathophysiologic Approach.* 5th ed. New York: McGraw-Hill; 2002:1997–2015.

55. Goodroad BK. HIV and AIDS in people older than 50. A continuing concern. *J Gerontol Nurs.* 2003;29(4):18–24.

56. McLennon SM, Smith R, Orrick JJ. Recognizing and preventing drug interactions in older adults with HIV. *J Gerontol Nurs.* 2003;29(4):5–12.

57. Beers MH, Berkow R, eds. *The Merck Manual of Geriatrics.* 3rd ed. Whitehouse Station, NJ: Merck & Co.; 2000:1378–82.

58. Whitehouse PJ, Lanska DJ. Less common dementias. In: Hazzard WR, Andres R, Bierman EL, eds. *Principles of Geriatric Medicine and Gerontology.* 2nd ed. New York: McGraw-Hill; 1990:949–53.

59. Sherman M. An overview of antibiotic resistance. *US Pharm.* 2006;1:HS-24–HS-28.

60. Salyers AA, Whitt DD. Revenge of the microbes: How bacterial resistance is undermining the antibiotic miracle. Washington, DC: ASM Press; 2005.

61. Murray BE. Vancomycin-resistant enterococcal infections. *N Engl J Med.* 2000;342(10):710–21.

62. Rice LB. Emergence of vancomycin-resistant enterococci. *Emerg Infect Dis.* 2001;7(2):183–7.

63. Lamb HM, Figgitt DP, Faulds D. Quinupristin/dalfopristin: a therapeutic review of its use in the management of serious gram-positive infections. *Drugs.* 1999;58(6):1061–7.

64. Foley L. CA-MRSA saw three-fold increase between 2001 and 2004: results of a three year study. *Infectious Disease News.* 2005;10:8.

65. Jones RN. Resistance patterns among nosocomial pathogens: trends over the past few years. *Chest.* 2001;119(2 Suppl):397S–404S.

66. Chambers HF. The changing epidemiology of *Staphylococcus aureus? Emerg Infect Dis.* 2001;7(2):178–82.

67. Stratton CW, Gelfand MS, Gerberding JL, et al. Characterization of mechanisms of resistance to beta-lactam antibiotics in methicillin-resistant strains of *Staphylococcus saprophyticus. Antimicrob Agents Chemother.* 1990;34(9):1780–2.

68. Hirsh A. New treatment option for gram-positive bacteria. Available at: http://www.clevelandclinicmeded.com/medical_info/pharmacy/julyaug2004/daptomycin.htm (accessed April 12, 2006).

69. Sieradzki K, Roberts RB, Haber SW, et al. The development of vancomycin resistance in a patient with methicillin-resistant *Staphylococcus aureus* infection. *N Engl J Med.* 1999;340(7):517–23.

70. Kuehnert MJ, Kruszon-Moran D, Hill HA, et al. Prevalence of *Staphylococcus aureus* nasal colonization in the United States, 2001–2002. *J Infect Dis.* 2006;193(2):172–9.

7

Issues in Geriatric Dermatology

ALICE A. HOUSE

Pharmacists are well placed to promote skin treatments for older people such as they do with acne treatments for the young.

—Dr. Roger Woodford, Hampshire, UK

OVERVIEW

The world's population is aging more rapidly now than at any other time in history, resulting in an increased demand for appropriate care and treatment of skin problems in the elderly. This chapter addresses issues related to changes in the physiology of skin and how sun exposure is clearly implicated in the formation of many skin problems, with health risks increasing with cumulative exposure. It outlines how the elderly population is more likely to not only have multiple chronic medical problems, but also to have an increased incidence of skin neoplasms and increased risk of dermatologic reactions to medications. Changes in the skin of the elderly are described as a contributing factor both to the etiology of dermatologic problems and to their treatment. Common adverse drug reactions of medications that manifest as skin issues and some commonly used dermatological agents also are covered.

Jane Prickle is an 82-year-old retired artist who lives alone despite her family's encouragement to move into an assisted living home due to worsening dementia and decreased ability to care for herself or her home. She also has a history of hypertension, seasonal allergies, and hypothyroidism, all under good control at this time. Six weeks ago Jane began to have intense itching under her breasts, and when she noted some "red bumps" that spread to both of her arm pit areas, she decided it was time to treat this "rash" with some steroid cream she bought in a pharmacy. But since it is not "clearing up," she has now decided to go to her family physician. Her urge to scratch is getting much worse at night and is interfering with her sleep. It has also been getting worse after her weekly soak in a tub of warm water. She tells her physician that she has gone through several tubes of nonprescription steroid cream which seemed to help at first, but then the rash recurred. She also tried a tube of an expired prescription antifungal cream that her late husband had used for an itchy rash, but that cream did not alleviate her symptoms either.

Her physician notices excoriated areas with scabbing under both breasts and has difficulty determining the nature of the original rash due to damage from Jane's scratching. The axillary area has several small red papules with minimal excoriation, about which Jane states that "the rash started up only 1 week ago and it resembles the original rash under my breasts." The physician then examines the intertriginous areas of Jane's hands and notes "burrows." He then makes a diagnosis of scabies and decides to treat Jane with permethrin (Nix®) rather than hexachlorocyclohexane (Lindane) because of the decreased chance of neurotoxicity with permethrin. He then asks her to follow up in 1 week. On her return, Jane reports that the itching has resolved and the excoriations are nearly healed.

- Why is scabies something to be addressed in the elderly? Is it because of delays in diagnosis? Is Jane Prickle's dementia a factor to consider?
- What role would a weakened immune system in the elderly play with regard to an infectious skin disease caused by barely visible mites?
- Might the intense itching that often worsens at night be any kind of clue to Jane's problem?
- What makes treatment difficult?

IMPACT OF DERMATOLOGIC PROBLEMS IN THE ELDERLY

Skin disease in the elderly is very common, with the vast majority of elders having at least one skin problem per year that results in a physician visit. Nonprescription medications or home remedies applied prior to the visit often result in an alteration of the original lesion, making diagnosis more difficult. The presentation of the typical geriatric patient is changing as the Baby Boomer population ages. These patients, who may be unwilling to accept suffering as inevitable, are more likely to seek medical attention for skin problems. Patients of today are also less likely to grow old gracefully, and many have the time and money to invest in slowing the aging process. In many social circles, it is no longer acceptable to grow old. And with the advent of sun-blocking agents, it is possible to reach old age with a much younger looking appearance.

Treatment to slow aging as well as to cure diseases of the skin is becoming more important to the general well-being of the elderly. This is especially true for an aging population that is increasingly more active in both the workplace and in social situations. Infections and infestations of the skin lead to decreased quality of life, decreased satisfaction with appearance, increased burden of illness, and, rarely, death.[1]

NORMAL STRUCTURE AND FUNCTION OF THE SKIN AND APPENDAGES

The skin is normally composed of two principal layers: the epidermis and its various appendages and the dermis, along with the underlying fat layer. The main functions of the skin are protection, thermoregulation, vitamin production, and water regulation. The hair serves mainly to protect and to help regulate temperature, and the nails serve primarily as protection. The epidermis is composed of four layers: the basal layer, the prickle cell layer, the granular cell layer, and the keratin layer. It takes approximately 30 days for a cell in the basal layer to transform into a keratinized cell in the outer skin layer. Other structures found in the epidermis include the apocrine glands, eccrine glands, Langerhans cells, melanocytes, Merkel cells, and sebaceous glands, as well as hair and nails. The dermis supports the epidermis and is composed of collagen, elastin, fibroblasts, and various inflammatory cells; its two layers are the papillary dermis and the reticular dermis. Subcutaneous fat is associated with the dermis and has thermoregulatory and nutritional functions.

Hair follicles can extend down into the subcutaneous fat layer; while hair serves chiefly as a thermoregulator, these structures can also serve as touch receptors. Hair grows while in the anagen phase (90% of hair's life span) and is shed while in the telogen phase. In general, hair grows at a rate of 1 cm per month, and an average of 50–100 telogen-phase hairs are lost per day.

Nails, like hair, are formed by an invagination of the epidermis into the dermis, but they are very highly keratinized. The nail is composed of three parts: (1) the root, which is under the proximal nail fold, (2) the nail plate, which merges into the lateral nail folds, and (3) the free edge, whose under-surface is continuous with the hyponychium. Nails grow approximately 0.1 mm/day, but growth varies based on the season of the year, the nutritional status of the patient, and the location of the nail on the body.[2-5]

EFFECTS OF AGING

The effects of aging on the normal structure and function of the skin and appendages are impacted by gene-regulated (biologic) aging, the damaging effects of sun exposure, and the damage incurred by other substances (caffeine, tobacco, etc.). Atrophy, freckles, pigmentation changes, telangiectasia, and xerosis are seen with increasing frequency as sun exposure accumulates. Changes due to normal aging (not sun exposure dependent) include:

- Fine wrinkling.
- Decreased elasticity of skin.
- Diffuse loss of body and scalp hair.
- Dryness (often associated with itching).
- Loss of subcutaneous fat in the extremities.
- Seborrheic keratoses.
- Skin tags.

Other normal changes seen in aging include decreased rete ridges; decreased subcutaneous fat pads; decreased sweat production, resulting in impaired thermoregulation; decreased vascularity of skin; and thinning of both layers of the skin. These changes result in decreased barrier function, an increased incidence of blistering lesions, and increased fragility (resulting in an increase in skin tears). Onychogryphosis, a dysmorphic thickening of the nails, occurs as one ages and can result in an increased risk of ingrown nails as well as difficulty in performing adequate nail care.[4-9]

TREATMENT CONSIDERATIONS

Because of the decreased function of many organ systems, oral and topical medications are often more potent and toxic in the elderly, resulting in decreased clearance of medications and their byproducts. In addition, topical medications are more potent and often more toxic due to increased absorption in the elderly. The older patient often has difficulty with mobility due to pain or joint restriction, which can make the application of topical medications difficult. The size and location of the treatment area as well as the potency of the topical agent must be considered prior to treating dermatologic problems in the elderly.

COMMON DERMATOLOGIC PROBLEMS AND THEIR TREATMENT

In general, conditions may be classified as either chronic or acute, with chronic lesions having the properties of lichenification, scaling, and xerosis, and acute lesions having the properties of crusting, oozing, and vesiculation. Treatment should be directed toward the underlying etiology, with formulation of the medication in a vehicle that facilitates cutaneous application. Vehicles, in decreasing order of moisture-trapping ability, include ointments, creams, pastes, powders, aerosols, gels, lotions, wet dressings, and tinctures. Chronic lesions should be treated with moisturizing agents such as ointments and creams, whereas more acute lesions should be treated with drying agents such as wet dressings and tinctures. Hairy areas, scalp lesions, and lesions covering large areas require treatment with lotions, gels, and aerosols in order to aid in the delivery of the medication, whereas emulsified creams work well in intertriginous areas to help avoid maceration. Information on commonly used products is given in Tables 1–3.

Senile Pruritus or Xerosis

The strong desire to scratch—the basic definition of pruritus—can be mediated by many mechanisms. Pruritus is very common in the elderly and may be due to internal or external factors. Despite careful evaluation, the etiology of pruritus in the elderly is often unknown. Senile pruritus is the condition in the elderly of a persistent desire to scratch despite no discernable etiology. Care should be taken to eliminate known causes of pruritus, including medications (aspirin, opiates, quinidine), dermatoses (eczema, scabies, urticaria), contact with infested animals, and exposure to skin irritants. Multiple internal factors can be responsible for pruritus, with histamine release being the most common.

Use of antihistamine (H_1) medications may relieve symptoms of pruritus, but caution must be taken in the elderly due to increased risk of drowsiness and possible falls. A counterstimulus such as cool water, cool compress, or mild pressure applied to the affected area may temporarily relieve the desire to scratch. These measures may decrease the secondary effects of scratching, which include excoriation, infection, and lichenification. Moisturizing the skin may help relieve itching. Use of urea-containing preparations may lead to stinging in excoriated areas and should be avoided unless the underlying skin is intact.[3,4,10]

Eczematous Dermatitis

Inflammatory dermatoses, including allergic dermatitis, atopic dermatitis, eczema, psoriasis, and seborrhea, can all be characterized by erythema, pruritus, and scaling in the acute or early stage and by lichenification, plaque formation, or scarring in the late stage. Treatment of these disorders is difficult due to the need for treatment of large areas of the body (Table 1). The large area of treatment increases the risk of side effects due to medication absorption. Moisturizing the skin is the cornerstone of treatment in order to avoid pruritus and further skin damage due to scratching.

Allergic Dermatitis

Allergic dermatitis or contact dermatitis (type IV hypersensitivity) remains fairly constant throughout life, although it is seen less in the elderly, perhaps due to less exposure to offending agents or to a decrease in cell-mediated immunity as one ages. Atopic dermatitis is not common in the elderly, possibly due to diminished immediate hypersensitivity reactions. Psoriasis remains active in the elderly, despite a decrease in T-cell immunity. Although the onset of psoriasis is more common in the younger population, psoriasis may still have its onset in old age. Psoriasis is characterized by plaque formation and can be a contributor to skin infection or breakdown. Seborrhea is quite common in the elderly and becomes more common with increasing age. It is characterized by the formation of scaling lesions in the ears, eyebrows, nasolabial folds, and scalp. There may be an association with *Pityrosporum ovale* (yeast), but the exact cause is still uncertain.[6,10]

Infections and Infestations

In general, decreased skin barrier function, decreased immunity, and decreased mobility resulting in decreased ability to bathe properly or to complete domestic chores may lead to an increased risk for infections and infestations in the elderly.

Table 1 Topical treatment of eczemous and related conditions

Generic Name (Brand Name)	Application Instructions[a] (How Supplied)
Dandruff/seborrheic dermatitis	
Ketoconazole 1% shampoo (Nizoral A-D®)	Shampoo into hair, then lather and rinse. Repeat every 3–4 days for up to 8 weeks. (4 ounce, 7 ounce)
Selenium 2.5% lotion (Selsun®)	Massage into scalp, rinse, repeat. Use two times a week for 2 weeks. (120 mL)
Pruritus	
Doxepin 5% cream (Zonalon®)	Apply TID to QID ≤ 8 days. (30 g, 45 g)
Psoriasis	
Calcipotriene 0.005% cream/ointment (Dovonex®)	Apply QD to BID for up to 8 weeks. (60 g, 120 g)
Tazarotene 0.05%, 0.1% cream/gel (Tazorac®)	Apply to stable plaques every evening.
Rosacea	
Azelaic acid 15% gel (Finacea®)	Apply BID for up to 12 weeks for mild-to-moderate rosacea. (30 g)
Metronidazole 0.75% cream (Metrocream®)	Apply BID to clean skin. (45 g)
Metronidazole 0.75% gel (Metrogel®)	Apply BID to clean skin. (45 g)
Metronidazole 0.75% lotion (MetroLotion®)	Apply BID to clean skin. (59 mL)
Metronidazole 1% cream (Noritate®)	Apply QD to clean skin. (30 g, 60 g)

[a] Dosages from: *Physicians' Desk Reference.* 59th ed. Monvale, NJ: Thompson PDR; 2005.

Bacterial

Cellulitis, erysipelas, and impetigo may be caused by group A streptococcus (most commonly) or *Staphylococcus aureus*. Cellulitis is a rather superficial infection of the skin, but erysipelas includes involvement of the lymphatic vessels. Patients with erysipelas may be ill-appearing, and the infection may spread rapidly. Cellulitis and erysipelas may occur concomitantly. Impetigo is seen at times in previously damaged skin, especially if the initial pruritic lesions lead to infection during scratching.[1]

Fungal

Normally the skin provides a barrier against low virulent fungi, but with aging the skin is more likely to have diminished barrier function, providing an entry to the superficial layers of the skin and hair. Yeast is more likely to grow in a moist and warm environment; in skin folds, which are more common with obesity; and in patients with decreased mobility. A decrease in mobility leads to the creation of moist, warm areas normally kept dry by exposure of the skin during normal movement. Treatment should begin with topical preparations, but fungal infections should not be treated with corticosteroids. Continuing corticosteroid agents will decrease the inflammation but will allow for continued spread of the infection. Nail fungus is difficult to treat and difficult to diagnose, as it can be confused with onychogryphosis, which is commonly seen in this age group.[7] Table 2 provides additional product information.

Viral

The virus most responsible for skin disease in the elderly is varicella, especially when manifested as herpes zoster. As cell-mediated immunity decreases with age, the likelihood of herpes zoster increases, although certain medication regimens (corticosteroids, neoplastic treatments) also contribute to an increased risk for shingles. Herpes zoster rarely occurs more than once in the immune-competent elderly. There are often symptoms that herald the onset of herpes zoster infection, including pain and paresthesia. Herpes zoster, or shingles, manifests as vesicular rash in a unilateral dermatomal distribution and then gives rise to its characteristic girdle-like band around the midline of the torso. The presence of lesions bilaterally or in multiple dermatomes rarely occurs with herpes zoster; if they appear, prompt investigation for immune compromise is called for. Although unusual, the symptoms of pain and paresthesia may persist for several months.

Treatment entails topical or oral antiviral medication including acyclovir. To avoid herpes ophthalmica, drug therapy should be started as soon as possible. Risk of herpes ophthalmica is increased when lesions are located near the eyes. Early treatment may also decrease the duration of the illness and help prevent postherpetic neuralgia, a persistent state of pain after all lesions have cleared.[11,12]

Parasites

Lice infestations become increasingly less common in the elderly, perhaps due to decreasing density of hair follicles and less contact with those who

Table 2 Topical treatment of common fungal infections

Generic Name (Brand Name)	Application Instructions[a] (How Supplied)
Candidiasis	
Nystatin 0.1% cream/ointment (Mycolog-II®)	Apply BID for 25 days maximum. (15 g, 30 g, 60 g)
Fungal infection of nails	
Ciclopirox 8% solution (Penlac®)	Apply to affected nail and surrounding skin daily, with application over previous coat, for 7 days. Remove with alcohol once a week. May continue for 48 weeks. (6.6 mL)
Tinea pedis	
Sertaconazole 2% cream (Ertaczo®)	Apply BID to affected area for 4 weeks. (15 g, 30 g)
Tinea pedis/cruris/corporis	
Betamethasone/clotrimazole cream (Lotrisone®)	Apply BID for 2 weeks for cruris/corporis and 4 weeks for pedis. (15 g, 30 g)
Butenafine 1% cream (Mentax®)	Apply BID for 7 days or QD for 4 weeks for pedis and QD for 2 weeks for corporis/cruris. (15 g, 30 g)
Naftifine 1% cream/gel (Naftin®)	Apply QD (cream) or BID (gel) for 4 weeks. Wash hands afterward. (15 g, 30 g, 60 g)
Terbinafine 1% cream (Lamisil®)	Apply BID for 1 week for pedis, QD for 1 week for cruris/corporis. (12 g, 24 g)
Tinea pedis/cruris/corporis/versicolor and candidiasis	
Ciclopirox 0.77% cream/lotion/gel (Loprox®)	Apply BID for up to 4 weeks. (15 g, 30 g)
Econazole 1% cream (Spectazole®)	Apply QD to BID for 2–4 weeks. (15 g, 30 g)
Miconazole 2% cream (Monistat®)	Apply QD to BID for 2–4 weeks. (15 g, 30 g, 85 g)
Oxiconazole 1% cream/lotion (Oxistat®)	Apply QD to BID for 1–2 weeks. (15 g, 30 g)
Tinea versicolor	
Ketoconazole 2% shampoo (Nizoral®)	Apply to damp scalp. Rinse after 5 minutes. One application is enough. (120 mL)
Selenium 2.5% shampoo (Selsun®)	Apply QD for 7 days. Rinse after 10–20 minutes.
Tinea versicolor/candidiasis	
Clotrimazole 1% cream/lotion (Lotrimin®)	Apply BID for 4 weeks. (15 g, 30 g)

[a] Dosages from: *Physicians' Desk Reference.* 59th ed. Monvale, NJ: Thompson PDR; 2005.

are infested. Scabies, however, is a concern, as it remains common. Scabies may be transmitted by fomites and may be improperly diagnosed, leading to further spread of the mites. Typical burrows and intense pruritus are the hallmarks of scabies infestation; if found, it requires simultaneous treatment of all contacts (including staff of a nursing facility) and all bedding. Due to the higher incidence of dementia or other psychological disorders in the elderly, there is a higher incidence of delusional parasitosis. Although there is no infestation present, the patient with delusional parasitosis exhibits all the symptoms of infestation, including itching and secondary lesions. Treatment is difficult, as patients will refuse to believe that no infestation is present.[9,13] Table 3 provides information on specific products.

Ulcerations

Although wound-healing mechanisms appear to be intact in the elderly, healing of ulcerated lesions is slower and more complicated. Venous ulcers are the most common type of ulceration in the elderly and are strongly associated with venous thrombosis, although the exact etiology is still uncertain. Treatment of venous ulcers is complicated but should include pressure dressings. Differentiating venous ulcer lesions from pressure ulcer lesions is imperative to choosing appropriate therapy. Pressure dressings aid in the healing of venous ulcers, but pressure should be eliminated in the treatment of pressure ulcers. Pressure ulcers become more common as elderly patients become increasingly immobile. Removal of pressure and attention to adequate nutrition are the key to healing this type of ulceration. Arterial ulcerations are related to atherosclerotic disease and are characterized by painful lesions that are best treated by correcting arterial blood flow problems. Irritation caused by exudates may result in eczema developing in the area surrounding vascular changes. All ulcerations may become complicated with infection. If infection is present, treatment should be initiated to ensure healing and to reduce the risk of systemic infection.[3,8,13–16]

Neoplasms

Basal cell carcinoma, melanoma, and squamous cell carcinoma are common in the elderly, as the primary risk factor is cumulative sun exposure and the resulting skin damage. Although increasing in frequency, melanoma is the least common of the three, with nonmelanoma skin cancers accounting for at least half of all newly diagnosed cancers. Treatment of melanoma is solely surgical, while treatment of basal cell carcinoma or squamous cell carcinoma is usually surgical. Some squamous cell carcinomas (Bowen's disease) may be treated medically. Squamous cell carcinoma can arise from

Table 3 Topical treatment of common skin infections and infestations

Generic Name (Brand Name)	Application Instructions[a] (How Supplied)
Cellulitis, impetigo, lacerations	
Gentamicin 0.1% cream/ointment (Garamycin Topical®)	Apply gently TID to QID.
Mupirocin 2% cream/ointment (Bactroban®)	Apply TID for up to 10 days. (cream 15 g, 30 g or ointment 22 g)
Neomycin/polymyxin/hydrocortisone (Cortisporin®)	Apply BID to QID for 7 days. (7.5 g, 15 g)
Herpes labialis (cold sores)	
Acyclovir 5% cream (Zovirax®)	Apply five times a day for 4 days. (2 g)
Penciclovir 1% cream (Denavir®)	Apply every 2 hours for 4 days at earliest sign of lesion. (1.5 g)
Lice	
Lindane 1% shampoo	Apply (if other treatment failed) to clean hair without water. Add water after 4 minutes and then lather and rinse immediately. (60 mL, 480 mL)
Malathion 0.5% lotion (Ovide®)	Apply to dry hair until wetted. Allow to dry naturally. Shampoo after 8–12 hours. May repeat in 7–9 days. (59 mL)
Permethrin 1% cream rinse (Nix®)	Apply to affected area. Rinse after 10 minutes. May repeat in 7 days. (60 mL)
Scabies	
Crotamiton 10% cream (Eurax®)	Apply to skin from chin to toes. Reapply in 24 hours. Wash off 48 hours after last application. May use for pruritus prn. (60 g, 60 mL)
Lindane lotion	Apply to dry skin from neck down. Wash off after 8–12 hours. Use only once. (60 mL, 480 mL)
Permethrin 5% cream (Elimite®, Acticin®)	Apply to skin from head to soles of feet. Wash off after 8–14 hours. May repeat in 14 days if living mites noted. (60 g)

[a] Dosages from: *Physicians' Desk Reference*. 59th ed. Monvale, NJ: Thompson PDR; 2005.

sun-exposed or trauma-exposed areas. Solar damage in the form of actinic keratosis may also be a precursor to squamous cell carcinoma. Actinic keratosis and Bowen's disease may be treated with fluorouracil as well as with cryosurgery.[3,6,17]

SYSTEMIC CONDITIONS THAT AFFECT THE SKIN

Many systemic conditions that affect the skin are often vague and nonspecific in nature. Side effects from medications that treat systemic conditions may include acne, bullous pemphigoid, erythema multiforme, lichen planus, psoriatic dermatitis, rosacea, and seborrheic dermatitis. Autoimmune disorders, diabetes, inflammatory bowel disorders, lymphoma, and vascular disease may exhibit diverse skin manifestations. Diffuse rashes or eczemous lesions often occur secondary to viral illnesses, including HIV. Acne can occur with Cushing's syndrome and pruritus can occur with many neoplasms. A full discussion of all etiologies is beyond the scope of this chapter. Attention focuses on the common manifestations of diabetes and vascular disease.[8]

Diabetes

Skin manifestations of diabetes result from a complex combination of microangiography and metabolic changes leading to an increased risk of infection and decreased healing or injury due to vascular changes. Acanthosis nigricans is a velvety, hyperpigmented plaque most often seen in the axilla, the back of the neck, and in other flexural folds. Glucose control is the best treatment, but keratolytic agents may help. Cutaneous infections are more common in the diabetic patient and the prevalence increases with decreasing glucose control. *Candida, Staphylococcus, Streptococcus, Echerichia coli,* and *Pseudomonas* are common infectious agents found in diabetic patients. Treatment includes both medications specific for the type of infection and improved glucose control. Diabetic dermopathy is common in the elderly, especially in men, and is manifested by hyperpigmented, raised lesions ranging from 0.5 to 1 cm that are brown and are located primarily on the pretibial and lateral leg. No treatment is needed, as spontaneous resolution is the norm. Thickening of the skin is common in diabetes and may restrict movement if located on the hands, but there is no treatment for this condition. Yellowing of the skin and nails occurs due to glycosylation of proteins. Since no significant adverse sequelae have been documented, no treatment is necessary.[9,14,18]

Vascular Disease

Complications of vascular disease that manifest in the skin include venous and arterial ulcers. Any patient found to have an ulceration, especially of the lower extremity, should undergo an evaluation for vascular disease to ensure the underlying cause is treated. Care of these ulcers should include optimal control of the vascular disorder and care for the ulcer itself. Treatment may include antibiotics, compression, debridement, skin graft, surgical correction of vascular deficit, and wound dressings. Treatment depends on the stage of the ulcer and the underlying cause.

ADVERSE DRUG REACTIONS

An adverse drug reaction (ADR) is any reaction to a drug given at an appropriate dose that leads to an undesirable or unintended response. Reactions that are predictable are related to the pharmacologic properties of the drug and are dose-dependent. Unpredictable reactions are often allergic in nature and unrelated to dose or pharmacologic properties. Drug reactions affecting the skin account for only 2%–4% of all ADRs, and only 0.1% of these reactions are severe enough to require hospitalization. Although most ADRs are benign, several reactions can be life-threatening (e.g., Stevens–Johnson syndrome, anticoagulant necrosis, toxic epidermal necrosis, vasculitis, and angioedema). Fixed drug eruptions, a specialized form of delayed hypersensitivity, are caused by nonprescription and prescription drugs. They are especially hard to diagnose because so many people, especially the elderly, do not consider over-the-counter products to be "drugs." The most common cause of fixed drug eruptions are NSAIDs, barbiturates, sulfonamides, phenolphthalein, and tetracyclines.[19] Table 4 lists the more common reactions and the medications most likely to cause them.

Less commonly seen reactions include acne-like lesions, alopecia, aphthous ulcers, bullous eruptions, exfoliative dermatitis, pityriasis-like eruptions, pruritus, purpura, and xerostomia. Treatment of ADRs affecting the skin and the appendages consists of withdrawing the offending agent and providing supportive care aimed at minimizing symptoms.[1]

COMMON MEDICATIONS USED IN THE ELDERLY

Corticosteroids

A cornerstone of dermatologic treatment is topical corticosteroid therapy, but multiple considerations must be made when choosing which agent is appropriate for geriatric patients. Dose of the medication is directly related to the efficacy, with higher concentration medications generally being more efficacious. Potency of the fluorinated corticosteroids has greatly increased the efficacy of these medications, but it has also increased both the cost to the patient and possibility of side effects. Potency to decrease inflammation is measured by a medication's ability to vasoconstrict and thereby to decrease the erythema of the affected area of skin (also known as blanching).

Table 4 Common adverse drug reactions

Adverse Skin Reaction	Associated Medications
Anticoagulant skin necrosis	Coumadin®
Erythema multiforme (Stevens–Johnson syndrome)	Allopurinol, anticonvulsants, barbiturates, estrogen, NSAIDs, sulfonamides, tetracycline
Exanthems	Amoxicillin, ampicillin, captopril, carbamazepine, naproxen, phenytoin
Fixed drug eruption	Ampicillin, aspirin, barbiturates, metronidazole, NSAIDs, phenytoin
Photodermatitis	NSAIDs, sulfonylureas, tetracycline, thiazides
Pigment changes	Anticonvulsants, antimalarials, hormones, tetracycline
Systemic lupus erythematosus	Beta-blockers, estrogen, hydralazine, isoniazid, phenytoin, procainamide, testosterone
Toxic epidermal necrolysis	Allopurinol, amoxicillin, anticonvulsants, NSAIDs, phenobarbital, sulfonamides
Urticaria	Antibiotics, captopril, NSAIDs, quinine, sulfonamides
Vasculitis	ACE inhibitors, ampicillin, Coumadin, NSAIDs, sulfonamides, thiazides

Low-potency formulations are better suited for atopic dermatitis, seborrheic dermatitis, irritant contact dermatitis, and some eczemas. Psoriasis, lichen planus, discoid lupus, and allergic contact dermatitis respond better to high-potency formulations.

Table 5 lists several common preparations according to potency and common dosages. Several vehicles are available for delivery of corticosteroids, including creams, ointments, aerosol sprays, lotions, and gels. Due to greater need for moisturization of chronic lesions, heavy (thicker and greasier) creams and ointments are used for chronic lesions and lighter creams, gels, and lotions are used for acute lesions. Creams are the mainstay of topical treatment due to the nonocclusive, convenient, and cosmetically acceptable nature of these medications. Ointments are more effective due to better absorption but are messy and unacceptable to many elders because of their greasy feel. Aerosol sprays are cosmetically acceptable, cooling, and easier to use on the scalp and on weeping lesions. Lotions are easier to spread over larger skin areas, but clear preparations may contain alcohol and therefore lead to a stinging sensation that may not be tolerated by the patient. Gels spread like lotions but are easier to manage than lotions due to a thicker formulation that makes them similar to creams in application.[3]

Table 5 Comparison of corticosteroids and dosages

Potency	Medication	Dosage[a]
I: Superhigh potency (maximum = 45 g/week)	Betamethasone dipropionate gel and ointment 0.05% (Diprolene®)	Apply QD to BID ≤ 2 weeks.
	Clobetasol propionate (all preparations) 0.05% (Temovate®)	Apply BID for 2–4 weeks maximum.
	Diflorasone diacetate ointment 0.05% (Psorcon®)	Apply QD to TID.
	Halobetasol propionate cream & ointment 0.05% (Ultravate®)	Apply QD to BID for 2 weeks maximum.
II: High potency	Amcinonide ointment 0.1% (Cyclocort®)	Apply QD to BID for 2 weeks maximum.
	Betamethasone dipropionate ointment 0.1% (Diprosone®)	Apply QD to BID for 2 weeks maximum.
	Desoximetasone cream and ointment 0.25%, gel 0.05% (Topicort®)	Apply QD to BID for 2 weeks maximum.
	Diflorasone diacetate cream and ointment 0.05% (Florone®)	Apply QD for 2 weeks maximum.
	Fluocinonide (all preparations) 0.05% (Lidex®)	Apply BID to QID.
	Halcinonide cream 0.1% (Halog®)	Apply QD to TID.
III: High potency	Betamethasone dipropionate lotion 0.05% (Diprosone®)	Apply QD to BID for 2 weeks maximum.
	Betamethasone valerate ointment 0.01% (Valisone®)	Apply BID for 2 weeks maximum.
	Diflorasone diacetate cream 0.05% (Florone, Maxiflor®)	Apply QD for 2 weeks maximum.
	Mometasone furoate ointment 0.1% (Elocon®)	Apply QD for 2 weeks maximum.
	Triamcinolone acetonide cream 0.5% (Aristocort®)	Apply QD to TID for 2 weeks maximum.
IV: Medium potency	Desoximetasone cream 0.05% (Topicort®)	Apply QD to BID for 2 weeks.
	Fluocinolone acetonide cream 0.2%, ointment 0.025% (Synalar®)	Apply BID to QID.
	Flurandrenolide ointment 0.05% (Cordran®)	Apply QD to QID.
	Triamcinolone acetonide ointment 0.1% (Aristocort®, Kenalog®)	Apply QD to TID for 2 weeks maximum.

Table 5 (continued)   Comparison of corticosteroids and dosages

Potency	Medication	Dosage[a]
V: Medium potency	Betamethasone valerate cream and lotion 0.1% (Valisone®)	Apply BID for 2 weeks maximum.
	Fluocinolone acetonide cream 0.025% (Synalar®)	Apply BID to QID.
	Flurandrenolide cream 0.05% (Cordran®)	Apply QD to QID.
	Hydrocortisone butyrate cream 0.1% (Locoid®)	Apply BID to TID.
	Hydrocortisone valerate cream 0.2% (Westcort®)	Apply BID to TID.
	Prednicarbate emollient cream 0.1% (Dermatop®)	Apply BID to TID.
	Triamcinolone acetonide cream and lotion 0.1% (Kenalog®)	Apply QD to TID for 2 weeks maximum.
VI: Medium potency	Triamcinolone acetonide cream 0.1% (Aristocort®)	Apply QD to TID for 2 weeks maximum.
	Alclometasone dipropionate cream and ointment 0.05% (Aclovate®)	Apply BID to TID for 2 weeks.
	Betamethasone valerate lotion 0.1% (Valisone®)	Apply QD to TID.
	Desonide cream 0.05% (Tridesilon®)	Apply QD to TID.
	Desonide lotion 0.05% (DesOwen®)	Apply BID to TID.
	Fluocinolone acetonide cream and solution 0.01% (Synalar®)	Apply BID to QID.
VII: Low potency	Hydrocortisone cream, ointment, and lotion 1% and 2.5% (Hytone®)	Apply BID to QID.

[a] Dosages from: *Physicians' Desk Reference.* 59th ed. Monvale, NJ: Thompson PDR; 2005.

The location and extent of the affected area is an important consideration. For example, because the axilla, face, groin, and neck have greater percutaneous absorption, less medication should be used in these areas. Highly potent formulations placed over large areas can lead to significant absorption and therefore can lead to significant side effects similar to those seen with oral corticosteroid use. Finally, cost is also an important consideration when treating large areas.

Side effects of corticosteroid medication use increase with:

- The extent of the treatment area.
- The length of treatment.
- The location of the lesions to be treated.
- The potency of the formulation.

The most common ADR of corticosteroid use is cutaneous atrophy, manifested by thinning of the skin in the epidermal and dermal layers, accompanied by telangiectasia. Atrophy becomes increasingly more common with prolonged medication use and with increased medication potency. Topical steroids should be applied no more than twice a day (BID), as frequent use provides no advantage and may induce tachyphylaxis. Fluorinated steroids such as betamethasone, dexamethasone, flumethasone, and fluocinolone used on the face, around the eyes, in flexural folds, and on the groin lead to development of striae very quickly; use of the more potent fluorinated formulations such as 0.05% fluocinonide should usually be avoided in these areas. A midpotency steroid such as 0.1% triamcinolone (Kenalog®) is indicated in patients with more persistent dermatitis. When used on the face, the fluorinated preparations may cause a rosacea-like dermatitis when they are withdrawn. Because this rosacea-like reaction may last for months after discontinuation of the fluorinated preparations, clinicians should use non-fluorinated preparations when treating dermatological conditions on the face. Prolonged use on the anterior chest or the thighs may lead to striae and prolonged use of any topical steroid preparation may lead to adrenal suppression. Less common side effects of topical steroids include acne-like lesions, alopecia, folliculitis, hypopigmentation, and even glaucoma when these preparations are used on the eyelids.[4,5,8,17]

Antibacterial Agents

Topical antibacterial formulations can be useful for treatment of superficial infections of skin and prevention of infections in the case of wounds, including skin tears common in the elderly. Use of certain topical antibiotics (bacitracin) in the nares can help decrease or eliminate carrier status with staphylococcal organisms, including methicillin-resistant *Staphylococcus aureus* (MRSA), which may help decrease spread of this infection in the nursing home setting. The addition of a corticosteroid to an antibiotic preparation does not appreciably alter the efficacy of the antibiotic and can significantly decrease inflammation in cases of eczemous lesions with bacterial superinfection. Since most of the topical antibiotic preparations are not absorbed well, systemic toxicity is seldom seen. Selection of an antibacterial agent depends on the presumed cause of the infection as well as the location.

Topical bacitracin is a peptide antibiotic that is active against gram-positive organisms (pneumococci, staphylococci, and streptococci), several anaerobic cocci, tetanus bacilli, diphtheria bacilli, and *Neisseriae*. Bacitracin, which is often found in an ointment base compounded alone or in combination with polymyxin B and neomycin, is useful for many skin infections but can cause resistance when used for prolonged periods. Use of combination products may lead to less resistance and possibly better coverage when the specific causative agent is not known. Allergy to bacitracin is common and most often is exhibited as a contact dermatitis. Much less commonly it is exhibited as urticaria or anaphylaxis.

Topical metronidazole has an unknown mechanism of action but may be effective against rosacea, a common problem in the aging population. Side effects of this medication include burning, dryness, and painful stinging. To avoid irritation of the conjunctiva, use near the eyes should be avoided.

Topical mupirocin is active against most gram-positive bacteria and is useful in the treatment of MRSA topically, but it can irritate the nostrils when used to eliminate carrier status. Mupirocin's spectrum makes this agent an ideal choice for the treatment of impetigo and other superficial skin infections.

Topical neomycin, an aminoglycoside, is active against gram-negative organisms and is available in many topical preparations, both alone and in combination with bacitracin and polymyxin. Reactions to neomycin are more common than with any other topical antibiotic. Reactions are particularly common when used on eczematous skin lesions and when neomycin is used in ointment formulations. Toxic levels of neomycin may occur when used on extensive areas of broken skin. Decreased renal clearance may contribute to elevated levels of neomycin and increases the risk of nephrotoxicity, neurotoxicity, and ototoxicity.

Topical polymyxin B is also a peptide antibiotic, but it is more active against gram-negative bacteria, including *E. coli, Klebsiella,* and *Ps. aeruginosa.* Because gram-positive organisms are resistant to polymyxin, a combination preparation including this agent is preferred. Topical absorption through intact skin is minimal but absorption through broken skin can be significant. To avoid nephrotoxicity or neurotoxicity, topical absorption should be avoided in the elderly, especially in the treatment of skin tears or ulcers.[1,17]

Antifungal Agents

Fungal infections are common in the elderly and can be treated with either oral or topical preparations. Oral agents include the azole derivatives and griseofulvin, which is an inhibitor of hyphal wall synthesis. Topical agents have markedly less toxicity than their oral counterparts, although for some infections they may also have decreased efficacy. Topical preparations have been packaged with corticosteroids to decrease inflammation associated with fungal infections and to promote quicker healing. Some preparations may contain a fluorinated corticosteroid and should not be used in areas where increased absorption is a concern.

The oral azole derivatives fluconazole, itraconazole, and ketoconazole are effective against systemic mycosis. The oral azole derivatives can be used when topical therapy for skin infections fails. Adverse effects of this class include alterations of the metabolism of concomitantly used medications, including astemizole, cisapride, or terfenadine. Toxicity seen with these medications may lead to an increased risk of cardiac dysrhythmias. The use of this class of medications with midazolam or triazolam may increase the hypnotic side effects of the benzodiazepines.

Fluconazole (Diflucan®) has a long half-life (>30 hours) and is rapidly absorbed. A single dose of this agent may lead to complete resolution of a cutaneous infection.

Griseofulvin, which is used orally for dermatophyte infections, is not useful for *Candida* or *Pityrosporum orbiculare*. The normal adult dose is 500 mg/day either in a single dose or divided but always given with meals to avoid gastric upset. It must be given for 12–18 months for response to be seen in fungal infections of the toenails, 6 months for fungal infections of the fingernails, 4–6 weeks for fungal infections of the scalp, and 3–4 weeks for fungal infections of the nonhairy areas of the skin. There is an increased possibility of adverse effects with longer treatment. Adverse effects include diarrhea, gastric upset, hepatic dysfunction, leukopenia, mental confusion, peripheral neuritis, photosensitivity reactions, and proteinuria. A complete blood count (CBC), liver function tests (LFTs), and renal function tests (BUN/creatinine) should be made periodically in patients taking this medication for prolonged periods.

Itraconazole (Sporonax®), which has a half-life equally as long as that of fluconazole, is effective against onychomycosis when taken daily for 3 consecutive months. Ketoconazole (Nizoral®) was the first of the azoles developed for oral use and is effective against cutaneous infections, although hair and nail infections require higher doses for longer periods of time in order to reach therapeutic response.

The topical azole derivatives clotrimazole, ketoconazole, and miconazole are also effective against fungal agents and yeast infections. Clotrimazole (Lotrimin®, Mycelex®) is effective against candidal infections that are common in elderly patients, especially those in the skin folds and vaginal area. It is available as a cream or lotion formulation for topical use and as a cream or tablet for vaginal use. Ketoconazole (Nizoral®) is useful as an agent against *Candida* and dermatophytosis; it is also available as a shampoo for the treatment of seborrheic dermatitis of the scalp. Miconazole (Micatin®, Monistat®) is used topically as a cream or lotion and vaginally as a cream or suppository. It is useful in the treatment of *Candida*.

The allylamine naftifine (Naftin®) is very active against dermatophytes but is rather ineffective against yeast organisms. Adverse effects include irritation; to limit mucosal irritation patients should be careful to avoid mucous membranes. Other adverse effects include burning and erythema.

Nystatin is useful for the treatment of *Candida* only. It is ineffective in the treatment of dermatophytosis. Due to low absorption in the GI tract and its narrow spectrum of antifungal activity, nystatin is not used systemically. It is useful for oral candidiasis however when used as a suspension. It is used by holding the suspension in the mouth for 2–5 minutes before swallowing (swish and swallow). Topically, it is useful for intertriginous and paronychial infections. Adverse effects include mild nausea and diarrhea when used orally. When used topically, it has virtually no adverse effects and irritation is very rare.

Terbinafine (Lamisil®) is also an allylamine. It is used as a cream for topical dermatophyte infections, although it must be used for at least a week to elicit positive effects. Improvement may take as long as 4 weeks after cessation of the medication. The chief adverse effect is irritation; contact with mucous membranes should be avoided.

Tolnaftate (Aftate®, Tinactin®) is effective against dermatophytes but not yeast and is available topically in many preparations, including creams, powders, solutions, and sprays. Recurrence is common; this medication may need to be used as a preventative measure after the initial infection is resolved.[17]

Antiviral Agents

Illness with viral agents is becoming increasingly more common in the elderly as the Baby Boomer generation ages and herpes simplex I and II infections become more prevalent and as human papilloma virus infections increase.

Acyclovir (Zovirax®), famciclovir (Famvir®), penciclovir (Denavir®), and valacyclovir are all synthetic guanine analogs that affect members of the herpes family by inhibiting DNA replication. Topical preparations of acyclovir and penciclovir can decrease viral shedding and decrease healing time. Although use of these medications may lead to local pain, stinging, burning, and pruritus, most of these symptoms are transient and resolve with continued use.

Imiquimod (Aldara®) treatment for human papilloma virus infections has a mechanism of action thought to stimulate interferon, interleukins, and tumor necrosis factors from local cells by an uncertain mechanism of action. This increased immune response leads to the destruction of the papilloma virus and the resolution of verrucal lesions. Side effects include local inflammation with itching, redness, and ulcerations.[17]

Antiparasiticides

Crotamiton (Eurax®) has an unknown mechanism of action, but it is useful for infestations with scabies and is available as a cream and as a lotion. It often must be applied twice, which increases the risk of an irritant skin reaction. Crotamiton is much safer than hexachlorocyclohexane (Lindane), however, and has less neurotoxicity.

Hexachlorocyclohexane (Lindane), which is used in the treatment of scabies and lice, is a neurotoxin that acts on both the parasite and the host. Although banned in several countries, it is still used widely in the United States. Percutaneous absorption is fairly rapid, and the product is found in the urine for at least 5 days after application. It is stored in fatty tissues, including the brain, which furthers the concern for neurotoxicity, especially in the elderly and the very young. Lindane is available as a cream, lotion, and shampoo; directions vary based on treatment area and parasite type. Some local irritation has been noted at the site of application. Permethrin (Elimite®, Nix®) is also a neurotoxin, although much less of this medication is absorbed compared to Lindane. Residual amounts of this medication are found for more than 10 days following application. Adverse reactions include only transient irritation and some itching. Permethrin is useful in the treatment of lice and scabies, although the treatment regimen for each varies.[15]

Sunscreens

This class of products is worthy of increased attention. Use should be emphasized most in children, teens, and young adults in order to prevent the development of sun-exposure-related disease later in life. The damage caused by excessive sun exposure is the chief factor in the development of skin cancers and premature aging of the skin. Limiting sun exposure is the most important preventative action a person can take. Benzophenone, dibenzoyl methanes, and p-aminobenzoic acid (PABA) are the most common compounds used in sunscreens. In general, these agents absorb ultraviolet light in the range most responsible for skin damage. Local irritation may occur in some individuals, and caution should be taken to avoid the use of these preparations on mucous membranes and around the eyes. Many cosmetic products contain sunscreen, and in general the use of these preparations should be encouraged.

Psoriatic Medications

Acitretin (Soriatane®) is related to the retinoids and is especially effective for pustular forms of psoriasis. The mechanism of action, which is similar to all retinoids, is thought to be related to stabilization of lysosomes and the medication's effect on keratinization and desquamation. Side effects are similar to hypervitaminosis A and similar to those seen with use of isotretinoin. Acitretin is given orally, therefore increasing the risk of side effects, with elevation in the lipid profile, hepatotoxicity, and teratogenicity of most concern. To decrease hepatotoxicity, alcohol should be avoided. Blood donations should be avoided for 3 years after discontinuation of this medication in order to avoid the teratogen risk to the unborn children of those receiving the blood.

Calcipotriene is a synthetic vitamin D_3 derivative in an ointment base that is most effective in the plaque form of psoriasis because of its absorption through the plaque. This medication often leads to transient elevations in serum calcium levels. Adverse effects are burning, drying, and irritation. To avoid irritation, patients should avoid application to the eyes and mucous membranes.

Tar compounds may be used in psoriasis as an alternative to corticosteroids. However, they contain thousands of compounds, including many toxic substances, and commonly lead to skin irritation and pustule formation. Coal tar solutions can be formulated in shampoos, creams, and ointments in concentrations from 2% to 10% and are available over the counter as well as by prescription. The messiness of these preparations may inhibit their use in the elderly.

Tazarotene (Tazorac®), a prodrug, is hydrolyzed to an active retinoid by an esterase. The active form binds to retinoid receptors and alters gene expression, resulting in improvement in psoriasis symptoms by an unknown mechanism. The mechanism is thought to be both anti-inflammatory and antiproliferative in nature. Adverse effects are also irritating in nature, and this medication can also lead to photosensitivity. Sun protection should be worn at all times during treatment with tazarotene.[15]

Antipruritic Agents

Calamine and Caladryl® are useful for relief of skin irritation, especially if there is oozing, as both products are drying agents. Caladryl also contains pramoxine hydrochloride, which is a topical anesthetic. Pramoxine hydrochloride is also available as a single agent and may allow for some relief of pruritus associated with mild eczematous skin reactions.

Diphenhydramine (Benadryl®) and Atarax® are effective antipruritic medications. These antihistamines should be avoided in the elderly, however, due to their sedating effects and the increased risk for falls due to the anticholinergic effects of this class of medications.[10,17]

Hair Loss Products

Finasteride (Propecia®) is a 5α-reductase inhibitor that blocks the androgens responsible for androgenic hair loss, although no evidence is available for its use in women.

Minoxidil (Rogaine®) is useful in the treatment of androgenic hair loss, especially in the vertex, although the exact mechanism of action on the hair follicle is not known. Side effects rarely include low blood pressure, but blood pressure should be monitored more carefully in patients with heart disease.

Miscellaneous

Urea has a moisturizing effect on the stratum corneum and can soften skin. Urea decreases the greasy sensation of medications when added to heavy cream medication preparations. Urea is keratolytic and increases moisture content, making it helpful in decreasing the symptoms of ichthyosis, keratosis pilaris, and xerosis.

KEY POINTS

- Normal changes of the skin and nails of the elderly contribute to the burden of dermatologic skin disease.
- Damage inflicted by overexposure to the sun leads to rapid aging of the skin and an increased risk for malignant skin disease. Practitioners must remain sensitive to these changes and their effect on the treatment of skin disorders.
- Oral and topical medications are often more potent and more toxic in the elderly due to decreased function of organ systems.
- Topical corticosteroid therapy is the cornerstone of dermatologic treatment but involves many considerations.
- Medication strength, site of application, and medication vehicle must be considered when treating elders.
- Many medications taken by the elderly may contribute to disease burden, either directly or indirectly.
- Certain disease states, such as diabetes, have dermatologic manifestations that may also require treatment.
- Attention to proper skin care, proper nutrition, and proper treatment of skin disease can help the elderly lead more enjoyable and productive lives.

REFERENCES

1. Hutchison LC. Antimicrobial therapy and resistance in dermatologic pathogens of the elderly. *Dermatol Clin.* 2004;22(1):63–71.
2. DuVivier A, McKee PH, eds. *Atlas of Clinical Dermatology.* 2nd ed. London: Mosby-Wolfe Times Mirror International; 1993: chapter 2, chapter 9.
3. Dahl MV. *Common Office Dermatology.* New York: Grune & Stratton; 1983: chapter 9, chapter 20.
4. Gay C, Thiese MS, Garner E. Geriatric dermatology. *Clinics in Family Practice.* 2003;5(3):771–89.
5. Norman RA, ed. *Geriatric Dermatology.* New York/London: The Parthenon Publishing Group, Limited; 2001: chapters 3–9.
6. Chung JH, Hanft VN, Kang S. Aging and photoaging. *J Am Acad Dermatol.* 2003; 49(4):690–7.
7. Keehn CA, Morgan MB. Clinicopathologic attributes of common geriatric dermatologic entities. *Dermatol Clin.* 2004;22(1):115–23.
8. Norman RA. Geriatric dermatology. *Dermatol Clin.* 2004;22(1):ix.
9. Brocklehurst JC, Tallis RC, Fillit HM, eds. *Textbook of Geriatric Medicine and Gerontology.* 4th ed. New York: Churchill Livingston; 1992: chapter 69.
10. Charlesworth EN, Beltrani VS. Pruritic dermatoses: overview of etiology and therapy. *Am J Med.* 2002;113(Suppl 9A):25S–33S.

11. Stulberg DL. Dermatology through the ages. *Clinics in Family Practice.* 2003;5(3): xi–xii.
12. Abrams W, Beers M, Berkow R, eds. *The Merck Manual of Geriatrics.* 2nd ed. Whitehouse Station, NJ: Merck Research Laboratories; 1995: chapter 101.
13. Besdine RW, Rubenstein LZ, Snyder L, eds. *Medical Care of the Nursing Home Resident: What Physicians Need to Know.* Philadelphia: American College of Physicians; 1996:77–88.
14. Schneider JB, Norman RA. Cutaneous manifestations of endocrine-metabolic disease and nutritional deficiency in the elderly. *Dermatol Clin.* 2004;22(1):23–31.
15. Theodosat A. Skin diseases of the lower extremities in the elderly. *Dermatol Clin.* 2004;22(1):13–21.
16. Elgart ML. Skin infections and infestations in geriatric patients. *Clin Geriatr Med.* 2002;18(1):89–101.
17. Kalant H, Roschlau WH, eds. *Principles of Medical Pharmacology.* 6th ed. New York: Oxford University Press; 1998:120–34.
18. New York State Department of Health. *Dermatologic Manifestations.* New York: New York State Department of Health; 2004.
19. Berlin JM, Lipshitz OH, Taylor JS. The clinical picture. *Cleveland Clin J Med.* 2002;69: 745–9.

8

Dealing with the Dread of Dementia and Alzheimer's Disease

KATHY KEMLE AND JONIE FAWLEY

OVERVIEW

This chapter covers two issues feared by most people as they age, Alzheimer's disease and dementia, both being cognitive deficits that affect daily living. While dementia in the elderly is commonly caused by Alzheimer's disease, vascular dementia, and Lewy body disease, evaluating its true cause requires great clinical skill and finesse. As there is no way to prevent dementia, once it is diagnosed the goal of management is to use both pharmacological and nonpharmacological support for prevention of injury secondary to dementia. Because caring for people afflicted with dementia is a tremendous burden, support for the caregivers, in the form of better education and information about Alzheimer's disease, is also needed. Two clinical pearls presented in this chapter are (1) the key to a dementia diagnosis is the patient's family history and (2) a thorough search for potentially reversible underlying conditions is required.

Zelda White, who is 78 years old, is brought to the office of her primary care provider by her husband because she has become "irritable and forgetful" over the past 3 months; he proclaims that she "has just gotten worse about her memory." She recently misplaced her purse and accused her son of stealing it. On three occasions, she has left the stove on and boiled a pot dry, nearly causing a fire. And she recently put a container of ice cream into the washing machine instead of into the freezer. Zelda says her family wants to take her money and leave her with nothing, "No matter what they say, there is nothing wrong with me," she proclaims.

- What do you suspect is happening to Zelda?
- How should an evaluation of her cognitive abilities proceed?
- What do you think can be done for Zelda?

DEMENTIA

Dementia is a clinical syndrome characterized by cognitive deficits and disturbances in the activities of daily living. Typical symptoms are amnesia, apraxia, and eventually anomia. As the population of the industrialized world ages, dementia is becoming increasingly prevalent. Dementia has many causes, but the most common causes behind its general deterioration of the cerebrum and diencephalon are Alzheimer's disease, vascular dementia, and Lewy body disease. The depression and dementia associated with Parkinson's disease and its variants is covered in another chapter. Mild cognitive impairment has recently been recognized as a possible prodromal state that often precedes dementia.

As in any encounter between clinician and patient, the evaluation of dementia should begin with a thorough history and physical examination, with emphasis on cognitive abilities. An inquiry regarding the onset and timeline of symptom progression should be sought and the influence on the patient's daily life, as well as the impact on the family, should be assessed.

The physical exam should include a standardized evaluation of cognition. Many health care providers use the Folstein Mini-Mental Status Exam (MMSE). Although it is the best validated of the current tools, the Folstein suffers from reduced sensitivity and specificity early and late in the disease. It is also heavily affected by education level and by sensory or arthritic impairment. A recent study demonstrated that a new test, the seven-minute screen, is more sensitive and more specific in diagnosing early onset dementia; it may become more widely used in the future.[1]

Although not often the case, reversible causes of cognitive impairment should also be investigated. Tests include a complete blood count, electrolytes, renal and hepatic function, thyroid screening, erythrocyte sedimentation rate, laboratory evaluation for syphilis, and B_{12} and folate. Most clinicians obtain a chest X-ray and EKG, as well as a noncontrast CT brain scan. Occasionally, an EEG or lumbar puncture may be useful. AIDS dementia is an increasingly common cause of cognitive impairment, so HIV testing may be appropriate in some cases.

Because depression can present as dementia or coexist with it, the provider should screen for it. The Geriatric Depression Scale (GDS) is an effective and easily completed instrument. Scores of 6 or greater on a 15-point scale correlate well with depression. The scale is also useful documenting disease response to therapy. For a further description of the GDS, refer to the following chapter.

THE DEMENTIA–DELIRIUM SYNDROMES

Alzheimer's disease (AD) is the most common cause of progressive dementia. It produces a slow decline in cognitive function, usually beginning with short-term memory and gradually involving executive functions; eventually competence with less complex cognitive tasks declines. With loss of the ability to perform activities of daily living and to speak intelligibly, the patient enters the final stage of this devastating disease. The process often takes 8–10 years from diagnosis to death. AD usually begins after age 65; however, its onset may occur as early as age 40, appearing first as a memory decline, and, over several years, destroying cognition, personality, and the ability to function. Confusion and restlessness are common.[2]

Within the brain of the Alzheimer's patient, characteristic amyloid plaques and neurofibrillary tangles are the pathologic markers. These changes can be found in the brains of nondemented older adults, but they are more numerous in the tissues of AD patients. A decline in the neurotransmitter acetylcholine is also found. Although the entire brain decreases in size and weight, the frontal and temporal lobes as well as the hippocampus are specifically affected.

While the cause of the disease is not known, certain risk factors may predispose individuals to developing AD. These factors include female gender; aging; family history; head trauma; chromosomal mutations on chromosomes 1, 14, and 21; and possibly depression and hypothyroidism. Persons who inherit the homozygous ApoE 4 allele are known to be at much higher risk as they age. Also, they tend to become demented at an earlier age than those with heterozygous status or the ApoE 2 or 3 alleles. However, some persons with this genetic makeup do not develop any cognitive impairment, suggesting some other precipitating event or factor.

Behavior and personality changes are often the most difficult aspects of the disease for families to handle. Irritability and lack of initiative are early manifestations, and paranoia is a common symptom. Grief is intense as the patient withdraws and becomes unable to recognize loved ones as the disease progresses.

The course of AD can range from 5 to 20 years. On average, patients live for 8 years after they are diagnosed. It is estimated that 4.5 million Americans suffer from AD and that its prevalence will increase 27% by 2020, 70% by 2030, and nearly 300% by 2050.[3] The annual cost of care for AD ranges from $51 billion to $88 billion.[4] While aging remains the most significant risk factor for developing AD, the wise health professional should keep in mind that AD is not part of normal aging.

Symptoms or findings suggestive of **vascular dementia**, such as a history of stroke, hypertension, diabetes, or coronary artery disease, should be documented. Vascular dementia tends to progress at a more variable rate than AD, but in some patients it does respond to usual dementia therapy. Measures to reduce further stroke risk, such as antiplatelet agents, blood pressure control, lipid reduction, and glycemic control, may retard its progression.

Characterized by eosinophilic inclusion bodies in neuronal cytoplasm, **Lewy body disease** may coexist with or be mistaken for AD. Patients with this disease are demented but also appear Parkinsonian, with rigidity being a prominent feature. They often have visual hallucinations and become paradoxically agitated when treated with antipsychotics. If paranoia is severe enough to warrant treatment, that is, if it distresses the patient or others, quetiapine is thought to be the best agent and less likely to provoke the paradoxical response or increase rigidity. If sedation is necessary, benzodiazepines are considered the preferred drugs.

Delirium, also known as acute confusional state, may be misdiagnosed as dementia. It can be differentiated by its acute onset, disturbances of attention, and level of consciousness and by the presence of one or more precipitating factors. Hospitalized elders with dementia often develop delirium. Since medications are a common cause, a thorough review of prescription and nonprescription medication should be undertaken.

Mild cognitive impairment refers to the presence of cognitive dysfunction, usually mild memory problems, that is insufficient to produce difficulties in daily life. It is thought to be a prodromal state for AD. Investigators are attempting to determine if acetylcholinesterase inhibitors are effective in slowing the progression to full dementia. A 2005 study on donepezil suggests little or no effect.[5]

Returning to Zelda White, no abnormalities other than mild hypertension are found during evaluation. Her laboratory studies are unrevealing, and the CT scan is negative for subdural hematoma or stroke. Her Folstein Mini-Mental score is 20/30 (abnormal) and her GDS score is 3/15 (up to 5 is normal). The primary care clinician makes a diagnosis of AD.

- What pharmacological and nonpharmacological treatments would you suggest?
- What support systems would you put in place for Zelda's family?

THERAPY

Nonpharmacological Therapy of Dementia

Education is the mainstay of treatment. Family and patients need to know that this is a terminal disease, although life expectancy is 8–10 years at diagnosis. If the patient has decision-making capacity, advance directives, including resuscitation wishes, need to be discussed. Because nutrition and feeding are affected, use of a feeding tube may be considered; however, there is growing evidence that, in advanced dementia, artificial feeding tubes diminish quality of life and only marginally prolong life. Safety is also a concern, as patients may wander from their homes or may operate a motor vehicle in a reckless manner. Resources to assist patients and caregivers are readily available from the Alzheimer's Association.

Dealing with the behavioral complications of dementia is often the most difficult aspect for family and caregivers. Common problems include wandering, screaming, and misinterpretation of environmental stimuli, which can precipitate catastrophic aggression or agitated behavior. The best treatment for problem behaviors is to manipulate the environment, not the patient. Maintaining a standard routine helps dementia patients cope. The astute clinician should remain vigilant for behavior caused by pain or by undiagnosed or undertreated medical conditions, such as an infection.

Wandering is best managed by providing a safe place to wander and sufficient caloric supplementation to overcome increased nutritional demand. One should also attempt to find a reason for the pacing. Is there an unmet need? Possible causes should be sought. Sedation with drugs rarely is indicated and usually does not work well. Restraints often cause increased agitation and have been implicated in patient decline and even death.

Pharmacologic Treatment of Behavioral Disturbances

Many pharmacologic agents have been advocated for problem behaviors; however, a recent meta-analysis found that their efficacy is highly suspect.[6] The anticonvulsants valproate and carbamazepine have been used in low doses, as has the antidepressant trazodone. Valproate has been associated with hepatic abnormalities and carbamazepine has been associated with white cell abnormalities, although not usually with the low doses used for dementia-associated behavioral problems. Trazodone may cause orthostatic hypotension and priapism, but only infrequently when used in small amounts. It appears that low-dose, short-acting benzodiazepines may be the best agents for this purpose.[7]

Agitation can be a symptom of depression and may respond to antidepressants. Mirtazapine and the selective serotonin reuptake inhibitors (SSRIs) are the preferred agents. Mirtazapine frequently causes an increase in appetite and weight gain, which may be an advantage in these patients. Rarely, it can cause leukopenia or hepatic dysfunction. SSRIs may cause a syndrome of inappropriate antidiuretic hormone-like effect, resulting in hyponatremia, as well as the more common nausea and other side effects.

There is some evidence that the acetylcholinesterase inhibitors may be useful in decreasing the frequency of difficult behaviors and in lessening the caregiver burden related to them.

Pharmacologic Therapy for Memory Loss

Alzheimer's disease is associated with a decline in the neurotransmitter acetylcholine. Currently available therapy is designed to reduce the enzymatic degradation of this substance and thus increase the amount of acetylcholine available to the neurons. There are four agents on the market (in order of introduction): tacrine, donepezil, rivastigmine, and galantamine.

Tacrine is rarely used at this time because it requires multiple daily doses, often provokes cholinergic side effects such as nausea and diarrhea, and is associated with hepatocellular degradation in autopsy studies. Donepezil is given once daily, usually at bedtime, and requires only one dosage titration from 5 to 10 mg/day. Rivastigmine is dosed twice per day and requires slow escalation in dosage to avoid gastrointestinal side effects.[8] Some evidence suggests it may more selectively target the hippocampus, a portion of the brain important in memory that often is affected in AD. Galantamine also has nicotinic receptor activity, although the clinical significance of this activity is unknown. These agents have also been found to reduce neuron degeneration, primarily by blocking the formation of neurotoxic beta-amyloid protein and thus may also be disease-modifying.[9]

All of the cholinesterase inhibitors may slow the progression of cognitive decline sufficiently to delay nursing home placement, but none has been found to be effective in halting the neuronal death and brain atrophy associated with AD, Lewy body disease, and vascular dementia. There is some evidence that they may reduce behavioral complications of dementia.[10] If one agent is ineffective, a therapeutic trial of another is appropriate. However, withdrawal of the agent followed by reinstitution may produce loss of cognitive function that may never be regained.

These agents normally are well tolerated, but side effects, usually cholinergic in nature, can occur. Nausea, vomiting, and diarrhea are the most frequently cited, but cardiovascular effects such as bradycardia have been reported. Muscle cramps, tremor, weakness, insomnia, agitation, and nightmares also may result from these agents. Cholinesterase inhibitors may increase gastric acid secretion, so patients at risk for gastritis and peptic ulcers must be monitored closely.

There is no way to prevent or cure AD, but memantine (Namenda®), which is newly available in the United States, can help stop disease progression. Several current drugs that treat AD, drugs such as galantamine, do so by inhibiting an enzyme called acetylcholinesterase. This enzyme breaks down the brain neurotransmitter acetylcholine. It is acetylcholine that is badly affected in AD patients. But memantine works differently. It appears to protect the brain's nerve cells against glutamate, a messenger chemical involved in brain processing and in information storage and retrieval, that is released in excess amounts by cells damaged by AD or certain other neurological disorders. When glutamate binds to N-methyl-D-aspartate (NMDA) receptors, this attachment permits calcium to flow freely into the cell. Sustained elevation of glutamate leads to chronic overexposure to calcium, which in turn leads to cell degeneration. Memantine may prevent this destructive sequence by filling the NMDA receptor sites.

Memantine is indicated for moderate-to-severe dementia because of its ability to enhance vigilance, short-term memory, and concentration. It has few side effects, although agitation may occur.[11] One study found that it may be additive when used with a cholinesterase inhibitor.[12]

How should health care providers best counsel caregivers in the decision-making process of treatment for moderate-to-severe AD? In a recent study, four specific findings about how caregivers formulate treatment goals were presented:[13]

- Quality of life is a key factor in a caregiver's decision to pursue or not pursue specific treatments.
- The decision to forgo treatment is more likely as the dementia severity increases.
- The caregiver's mental health may influence the decision to forgo treatment.
- Specific patient and caregiver characteristics are associated with treatment decisions.

Does there come a point at which there is no value in slowing the progression of severe AD, given the disease's effect on the quality of life of the patient and the caregiver? Health care providers need to stay involved in the care of advanced dementia patients and the family. Support and education of the caregiver improve the overall care of the patient. When cognitive-enhancing drugs are discontinued, the possibility of a more rapid decline in the patient's condition needs to be understood by everyone involved in that patient's care.

Antipsychotic Therapy

Paranoia is a common manifestation of early dementia that may persist into later stages of the disease. Psychosis, hallucinations, and delusions are not uncommon in moderate-to-late stage dementia. Fortunately, these disturbing symptoms respond well to antipsychotic therapy. The hallucinations common to Lewy body dementia are the exception, as the patient may actually have an escalation of behavior. Usually, very low doses are adequate to control symptoms. Most clinicians prefer to use the newer agents risperidone, olanzapine, and quetiapine. While these have fewer extrapyramidal side effects, less hypotension, and a lower incidence of neuroleptic malignant syndrome than the older antipsychotic medications, they have been implicated in impaired glucose tolerance and excess cardiovascular mortality.[14] The drugs have been used for behavioral complications of dementia, but a recent meta-analysis questions their efficacy.[15] Thus, their use should be restricted to control of psychotic and paranoid symptoms.

Use of Complementary and Alternative Treatments

So, what happens when Zelda White's son walks into a pharmacy and while waiting for a prescription asks the pharmacist, "Is there nothing else that will help my Mom? I understand that vitamin E, estrogen, and aspirin have demonstrated some protective effect against AD-type dementia. What do you think?"

Attempts to arrest the cell death associated with dementing illnesses or to enhance memory have been made using various agents. Ginkgo biloba has been used for centuries. Many studies have failed to demonstrate its efficacy. Vitamin E has been touted for its antioxidant effects and therefore presumed neuroprotective effects. Early studies suggested it might be helpful, but more recent studies failed to demonstrate its usefulness. An increase in cardiovascular mortality associated with its use has led most clinicians to avoid recommending it. Estrogen showed promise in improving categorical reasoning, an ability lost early in dementia, but later research showed more harm than benefit.

Nonsteroidal anti-inflammatory agents have been associated with less risk of dementia, presumably by reducing inflammation in the neuronal plaques and tangles. The only study on their use in dementia had to be halted early because of excessive GI bleeding. This may have been related to the use of indomethacin; however, the newer COX 2 inhibitors also failed to show efficacy.[15]

The recent widespread use of the cholesterol-lowering class of medications known as reductase inhibitors or statins has provoked an intriguing possibility for their use in preventing or treating AD. Treatment seems to reduce the amount of beta-amyloid protein in brain tissues, which may retard progression of the disease. Although two agents, atorvastatin and simvastatin, have shown promise, larger studies are needed. Statins are not yet recommended for the prevention or treatment of dementia, except in those patients who also have a hyperlipidemic indication.

CARING FOR THE CAREGIVER

It is the obligation of health care providers to counsel caregivers in an unbiased approach to the treatment of AD as well as to the ethical, religious, and financial issues that arise during the decision-making process. One must take into account the unique characteristics and values of each individual patient/caregiver. The process should be approached with insight into interpersonal dimensions, qualities, and values. What are the fears, wishes, and bias of medical care? Is the patient/caregiver allowed to pursue all avenues of care? There is an endless list of questions to present, but the underlying theme is to step aside and allow patients to journey through their malady with the dignity of the true human spirit. Health professionals need only to offer the simple healing of providing comfort, care, and treatment while following the choices of each individual patient and to offer healing with the empathic care they themselves would want.

Oftentimes, caring for a patient with dementia requires a consideration of the caregiver as well. Caregivers can reliability predict the presence of dementia in the elderly they care for.[16] They are essential in monitoring the progression of the dementing illness and behavioral disruptions and in recognizing subtle changes that can herald an acute organic illness such as a urinary tract infection. Many patients with dementia would be unable to remain in a home setting if it were not for the hands-on care and supervision provided by caregivers. Situations that prompt institutionalization and warrant medical evaluation, including unwanted drug effects, are loss of function, development of incontinence, wandering, and behavioral disruptions.

Caregivers regularly disregard their own health, frequently skipping important preventive medicine modalities and ignoring minor symptoms. Reports of distress, anxiety, and depression among caregivers are higher than in the general population. Screening caregivers for their own needs and directing them to services such as respite care, home health care entities, support groups, and educational services can help ease this burden. Care of the caregiver benefits the patient and the whole family.

LATE-STAGE DISEASE AND END-OF-LIFE ISSUES

Alzheimer's disease and the other progressive dementias are terminal conditions. Factors associated with a rapid course of decline include male gender, earlier onset, lower education, advanced age, medical and mental health comorbidities, unstable environment, and poor caregiver status. As the patient's condition declines, continuing the conversation about family desires and needs for the individual is essential. Many medications can be discontinued, and an individualized careplan for symptom management should follow (Table 1). The issue of treating a new febrile illness and lower respiratory infections is difficult for caregivers and family. In late-stage dementia, aggressive antibiotic therapy has not been shown to improve survival or patient comfort more than symptom relief with antipyretics and analgesics. The identification of pain in dementia patients is extremely challenging; special skills combined with caregiver reports are essential (Table 2). Behavioral disruptions must be addressed with either medications or nonmedication approaches. Advice on communication and behavioral modalities should be consistent and clear.

Because of increasing numbers of patients with diseases that cause dementia, primary care physicians especially must be efficient in their assessment procedures. The advantages of early screening for dementia are:

- The patient's cognitive capacity to participate in his/her own medical care can be determined.
- An early diagnosis enables administration of medications that preserve cognitive functions.[17]

A focused questionnaire, completed by family caregivers about their family member who has signs of dementia, helps the clinician differentiate between patients with dementia with a variety of degenerative disorders and patients without dementia with other neurological disorders that often are mistaken for dementia. When a caregiver questionnaire is combined with a patient test (Mini-Mental Status Exam), an accurate prediction of whether the patient suffers from a true degenerative disease that causes dementia will likely ensue or cause the clinician to make a referral. The ultimate goal is to ensure that all patients who show signs of dementia receive appropriate medical management as early in the disease process as possible. A patient's careplan (Table 1) should include assessment of pain (Table 2), especially as the dementia moves into its later stages.

Table 1 Issues and suggestions for late-stage dementia patients' careplans

Functional decline	Ask the caregiver what is important.
	Don't see the patient as a "Passive Observer."
	Allow even minor participation in activities of daily living care.
	Break it down into simple steps.
	Remember that familiar, repetitive activities are comforting.
	Focus on familiar skills and activities.
	Provide cues and modeling.
	Strive for environmental consistency.
	Address pain and manage appropriately.
	Avoid sedation and plan the timing of medications.
	Avoid restraints.
	Provide prompted toileting and walking as able.
Prevent and treat comorbidities	Dehydration.
	Pressure ulcers.
	Falls and injury.
	Adverse drug reactions.
	Fecal impaction.
	UTIs.
	Contractures.
	Stratify conditions versus quality of life.
	Liberalize restrictions.
	Set new goals; for example, blood sugars.
	Careful medication review and elimination, such as:
	Calcium and alendronate in chairbound person.
	Anticoagulation in a frequent faller.
	Statin for mild-to-moderate dyslipidemia.
Recurrent infections	Hygiene and toileting.
	Immunization of patients, caregivers, and staff.
	Avoid overuse of antibiotics.
	Avoid dehydration.
	Nutritional support.
	Hand-washing and disinfectants.
	(*Clostridium difficile* is not controlled with hand sanitizer.)
Nutritional problems and weight loss	Weekly weights and monitoring.
	Increased lighting in environment.
	Address comorbidities and medications affecting appetite.
	Tailor foods to patient's likes.
	Liberalize medical diets as possible.
	Ease of feeding with adaptions, such as special utensils.
	Offer small, frequent amounts and courses.
	Swallowing evaluation for food consistency type.

Table 1 (continued)   Issues and suggestions for late-stage dementia patients' careplans

Pain evaluation and management	Change in symptoms and behavior, suspect source of pain.
	Use a dementia pain scale and caregiver cues to identify pain.
	Treat pain empirically.
	Watch for atypical medical causes of pain, such as ischemia or peptic ulcer disease.
	Predeath is painful and needs treating.

Table 2   Pain assessment in advanced dementia scale

Item	0	1	2
Breathing and vocalization	Normal	Occasional. Labored breath, short hyperventilations.	Noisy labored breath, long hyperventilation Cheyne–Stokes respirations.
Negative vocalization	None	Occasional. Moan, low and negative speech.	Repeated calling out, loud moaning, crying.
Facial expression	Smiling, inexpressive	Sad, frightened, frown.	Facial grimacing.
Body language	Relaxed	Tense, pacing, fidgeting.	Rigid, fists clenched, knees pulled up, striking.
Consolability	No need to console	Reassured or distracted by voice or touch.	Unable to console, distract, or reassure.

KEY POINTS

- The increasing prevalence of dementia mandates improved detection and treatment strategies.
- While progress has been made, much remains to be investigated.
- Clinicians must remain alert to current and developing therapies and be prepared to implement those that show efficacy.
- Since there is no cure for Alzheimer's disease, healing is through compassionate palliative care rather than curative medicine.
- With realistic expectations, a patient's function, verbalization, and behavior can be improved.
- Treatment must be individualized for each patient.
- Caregivers tend to wear down over time and neglect their own health. Support for caregivers is essential.
- Better education and better information about Alzheimer's disease and other dementias are needed.

REFERENCES

1. Meulen EF, Schmand B, van Campen JP, et al. The seven minute screen: a neurocognitive screening test highly sensitive to various types of dementia. *J Neurol Neurosurg Psychiatry.* 2004;75(5):700–5.
2. NINDS. Alzheimer's Disease Information Page. Bethesda, MD: National Institute of Neurological Disorders and Stroke.
3. Hebert LE, Scherr PA, Bienias JL, et al. Alzheimer disease in the US population: prevalence estimates using the 2000 census. *Arch Neurol.* 2003;60(8):1119–22.
4. Leon J, Cheng CK, Neumann PJ. Alzheimer's disease care: costs and potential savings. *Health Aff (Millwood).* 1998;17(6):206–16.
5. Lopez OL, Becker JT, Saxton J, et al. Alteration of a clinically meaningful outcome in the natural history of Alzheimer's disease by cholinesterase inhibition. *J Am Geriatr Soc.* 2005;53(1):83–7.
6. Standridge J. Current status and future promise of pharmacotherapeutic strategies for Alzheimer's disease. *J Am Med Dir Assoc.* 2005;6(3):194–9.
7. Sink KM, Holden KF, Yaffe K. Pharmacological treatment of neuropsychiatric symptoms of dementia: a review of the evidence. *JAMA.* 2005;293(5):596–608.
8. Farlow MR. Combination drug therapies for AD: progress is slow, but we must keep trying. *Geriatrics.* 2005;60(6):13–4.
9. Aupperle PM, Koumaras B, Chen M, et al. Long-term effects of rivastigmine treatment on neuropsychiatric and behavioral disturbances in nursing home residents with moderate to severe Alzheimer's disease: results of a 52-week open-label study. *Curr Med Res Opin.* 2004;20(10):1605–12.
10. Defillippi JL, Crisman ML, Clark WR. Alzheimer's disease. In: Dipiro JT, Talbert RL, Yee GC, et al., eds. *Pharmacotherapy: A Pathophysiologic Approach.* 5th ed. New York: McGraw-Hill; 2002:1174.
11. Livingston G, Katona C. The place of memantine in the treatment of Alzheimer's disease: a number needed to treat analysis. *Int J Geriatr Psychiatry.* 2004;19(10):919–25.
12. Reisberg B, Doody R, Stoffler A, et al. Memantine in moderate-to-severe Alzheimer's disease. *N Engl J Med.* 2003;348(14):1333–41.
13. Karlawish JH, Casarett DJ, James BD, et al. Why would caregivers not want to treat their relative's Alzheimer's disease? *J Am Geriatr Soc.* 2003;51(10):1391–7.
14. Wooltorton E. Olanzepine (Zyprexa): increased incidence of cerebrovascular events in dementia trials. *CMAJ.* 2004;170(9):1395.
15. Peskind E, Tangelos E, Grossberg G. A case-based approach to Alzheimer's disease. *The Clinical Advisor.* 2005;4(3):32–46.
16. Aisen PS, Schafer KA, Grundman M, et al. Effects of rofecoxib or naproxen vs placebo on Alzheimer disease progression: a randomized controlled trial. *JAMA.* 2003;289(21):2819–26.
17. Monnot M, Brosey M, Ross E. Screening for dementia: family caregiver questionnaires reliably predict dementia. *J Am Board Fam Pract.* 2005;18(4):240–56.

9

Diagnosis and Treatment of Depression in the Geriatric Population

DIPESH PATEL AND JOHN M. BOLTRI

Just as the French call the senior years the Third Age, we believe that the senior years do not need to be as dire and depressing as they are often made out to be. Every time in life has its ups and downs. Our senior years are no exception.

—**Editors, MedicineNet.com 2005**

OVERVIEW

Depression is very common in older adults, with one in six Americans 65 years of age or older suffering from some type of depression. Elderly patients are more likely to present with physical symptoms than psychological symptoms. It is important to have a high index of suspicion for depression in the elderly and to begin appropriate treatment at an early stage. The highest rate of depression occurs in the elderly, medically ill, hospitalized population, in which rates as high as 40% have been found. This chapter presents strategies for diagnosing depression in the elderly, followed by treatment recommendations for the most common causes of elder depression.

Mrs. Jane Smith, a 78-year-old widow whose husband died of cancer almost 1 year ago, is brought to the office by her younger sister. Jane has not been eating well and has lost some 15 pounds over the past 6 months. Jane also has trouble sleeping, which she attributes to her age. On further questioning, Jane says that though she knows she has no reason to get depressed, she misses her husband a lot. Then she begins to cry. Detailed physical exam is normal except for a flat affect. On the Geriatric Depression Scale (GDS), Jane scores 8 out of 15. Laboratory tests including CBC, liver profile, thyroid-stimulating hormone, and electrocardiogram are ordered. Jane is diagnosed with depression and started on a low dose of a selective serotonin reuptake inhibitor. At her follow-up visit 4 weeks later, her laboratory tests are all noted to be normal. She reports that she feels better and has gained about 2 pounds. Her sleep has improved, she now visits with the neighbors, and she has started socializing with friends again.

DEPRESSION BASICS

Depression is a common illness in all age groups, including the elderly. In spite of its prevalence, depression is underdiagnosed and undertreated in this group. The annual direct and indirect cost of depression in the United States is $43 billion.[1] Typically, elderly patients with depression do not report depressed mood but instead present with less specific symptoms such as insomnia, anorexia, and fatigue. Depression in the elderly has many serious consequences such as confusion, lethargy, dementia, and isolation. Depressed elderly are at particular risk for suicide. Fortunately, tools are available to accurately diagnose and treat most cases of elderly depression.[2]

As many as 5 million Americans (nearly 1 in 6) 65 years of age or older suffer from depression. The prevalence of depression in adults older than 65 years of age ranges from 7% to 36% in medical outpatient clinics, while for patients in long-term care facilities the prevalence ranges from 12% to 30%. However, the highest rate of depression, 40%, occurs in patients who are elderly, medically ill, and hospitalized.[1-5]

MAJOR DEPRESSION

Due to its association with suicide, major depression must be distinguished from other causes of depression such as dysthymia (chronic low-grade depression), mood disorders secondary to an underlying medical condition, grief reaction, and bipolar (manic depressive) disorder. With all forms of depression, it is important to rule out underlying causes of depression such as medications and chronic diseases.

According to the fourth edition of the *Diagnostic and Statistical Manual of Mental Disorders* of the American Psychiatric Association (DSM-IV),[6] the diagnosis of major depression requires the presence of at least five vegetative signs and symptoms. One of these must be either lowered mood or loss of interest and pleasure, and it must be present on a continuous basis for at least 2 weeks. The elements to ascertain a differential diagnosis are from the following DSM-IV criteria:

A—1. Depressed mood most of the day or nearly every day, as indicated by either subjective report (e.g., feels sad or empty) or observations made by others (e.g., appears tearful).
2. Markedly diminished interest or pleasure in all or almost all activities, most of the days or nearly every day (as indicated by either subjective report or observations made by others).
3. Significant weight loss when not dieting, weight gain (e.g., a change of more than 5% of body weight in a month), or decrease or increase in appetite nearly every day.
4. Insomnia or hypersomnia nearly every day. Psychomotor agitation or retardation nearly every day (observable by others, not merely subjective feeling of restlessness or being slowed down).
5. Feelings of worthlessness or excessive or inappropriate guilt (which may be delusional) nearly every day (not merely self-reproach or guilt about being sick).
6. Fatigue or loss of energy nearly every day.
7. Diminished ability to think or concentrate, or indecisiveness, nearly every day (either by subjective account or as observed by others).
8. Recurrent thoughts of death (not just fear of dying), recurrent suicidal ideation without a specific plan, or a suicide attempt or a specific plan for committing suicide.

B—The symptoms cause clinically significant distress or impairment in social, occupational, or other important areas of functioning.

C—The symptoms are not due to the direct physiological effects of a substance (e.g., a drug of abuse, a medication) or a general medical condition (e.g., hypothyroidism).

D—The symptoms are not better accounted for by bereavement (i.e., after the loss of a loved one). The symptoms persist for longer than 2 months or are characterized by marked functional impairment, morbid preoccupation with worthlessness, suicidal ideation, psychotic symptoms, or psychomotor retardation.

Many elderly patients with depression often initially seek medical attention for nonspecific problems. Most patients have decreased appetite and weight loss at the time of diagnosis. Sleep disturbances are common and are characterized by early awakening and inability to fall asleep. As a result, there is also often a feeling of tiredness and fatigue that may be expressed as a lack of energy. Many patients have inappropriate feelings of guilt and worthlessness. Occasionally patients may also have hallucinations, delusions, and suicidal thoughts. Some patients seek medical attention for nonspecific problems multiple times before a diagnosis is made. Major depression is treated with antidepressant medications and psychotherapy.

Patients with bipolar disorder (manic depressive disorder) often present to the office with symptoms of depression. Detailed history will reveal at least one prior episode of a manic event. It is important to distinguish bipolar disorder from other types of depression, as the treatment is both different and more complex. The diagnosis and treatment of this disorder is beyond the scope of this chapter. Most elderly patients with bipolar disorder should be managed with the help of a psychiatrist.

DYSTHYMIA

Dysthymia is a form of depression that is generally less severe but usually more chronic in nature. This condition has fewer than five of the nine symptoms required for the diagnosis of major depressive disorder (see DSM-IV criteria list). The symptoms have been present for at least 2 years. Dysthymia is treated with antidepressant medications and psychotherapy. In patients with dysthymia, as with all forms of depression, it is important to rule out underlying causes of depression such as medications or chronic diseases. Depression related to underlying chronic disease such as that due to hypo- or hyperthyroidism can be misdiagnosed as dysthymia. The depression will often resolve once the chronic disease is appropriately treated.

GRIEF REACTION

Grief comprises the myriad psychological, physiologic, and behavioral responses that accompany the human awareness of an irrevocable loss, such as a pending or actual loss of a close friend or relative. It is an extraordinarily powerful emotion that includes the following responses:

- **Psychological:** sense of loss, anguish, anger, apathy, dissociation, anxiety, guilt, fear, distractibility, and regressions.
- **Physiologic:** insomnia, agitation, anorexia, and autonomic symptoms.

There is great variability in the course of grief. Its length and intensity are related to closeness of the relationship between the survivor and the deceased.

Grief may last from a few weeks to several months. If grief persists beyond several months, the possibility of major depression needs to be ruled out. The DSM-IV lists several additional factors that should alert the clinician that major depression may be present in patients being treated for grief. These factors include:

- Preoccupation with death independent of the specific death of the loved one.
- Guilt unassociated with a death.
- Morbid preoccupation with worthlessness.
- Psychomotor retardation.
- Prolonged and marked functional impairment.
- Hallucinations not involving the deceased.

A benzodiazepine can be prescribed for a brief period of use to treat anxiety symptoms. Sleep disturbance can be treated with short-acting benzodiazepines or trazodone.[7-9]

SCREENING FOR DEPRESSION

Laboratory Testing

Patients presenting with signs and symptoms of depression should generally receive a laboratory evaluation for treatable causes of depression, as well as for abnormalities that may influence the choice of medication. Laboratory tests should include an electrocardiogram, urinalysis, general chemistry, complete blood count, B_{12}, rapid plasma reagin, folate level, medication levels if necessary, and thyroid-stimulating hormone. In special circumstances, other tests may also be indicated. These may include head computed axial

Table 1 Medications that cause depression[a]

Antibacterials	Ampicillin, dapsone, isoniazid, metronidazole, nitrofurantoin, sulfonamides, tetracycline
Anticonvulsants	Carbamazepine, ethosuximide, phenobarbital, phenytoin, primidone
Antihypertensives	Clonidine, guanethidine, methyldopa, propranolol
Antipsychotics	Fluphenazine, haloperidol
Cardiovascular medications	Digitalis, procainamide
Chemotherapeutics	Azathioprine, bleomycin, cisplatin, cyclophosphamide, doxorubicin, mithramycin, vinblastine, vincristine
Parkinsonian medications	Amantadine, bromocriptine, levodopa
Sedatives and anxiolytics	Barbiturates, benzodiazepines, chloral hydrate
Stimulants (depression usually from withdrawal)	Amphetamines, caffeine, methylphenidate
Hormones	Glucocorticoids, hormone replacement, oral contraceptives
Others	Cimetidine, disulfiram, metoclopramide, physostigmine, ranitidine

[a] Adapted from Reference 10.

tomography (CAT) scan, magnetic resonance imaging (MRI), and HIV testing.

Depression Scales and Screening Instruments

Risk factors for depression in elderly persons include a history of depression, chronic medical illness, certain medications (Table 1), female gender, being single or divorced, brain disease, and stressful life events. Up to 15% of widowed adults have potentially serious depression for a year or longer after the death of a spouse.[11]

Alcohol, certain medications (Table 1), and substance abuse are all associated with an increased risk for depression.

The most commonly used screening test for depression in the elderly is the 30-item Geriatric Depression Scale (GDS). Sensitivity is 80% and specificity is 100% if the score is above 13 out of 30.[12] The GDS is also available as a short form 15-item questionnaire. Sensitivity is 92% to 97% and specificity is from 55% to 81% if the score is above 5 out of 15.[13] A one-item screening question, "Do you often feel sad or depressed?" may screen as effectively as the GDS and also save time.[14]

It is important to note that the validity of most depression screening instruments is significantly decreased in patients with a Mini-Mental Status Examination (MMSE) score of 15 or less.[15] In patients who have cognitive deficits, interviewer-administered instruments such as the Cornell Scale for Depression in Dementia or the Hamilton Rating Scale for Depression are preferred.[16] Although these instruments require more time to administer, for cognitively impaired patients they are more appropriate than self-report instruments. The Cornell measure is designed to be administered by the patient's primary caregiver. The Cornell Scale for Depression in Dementia has 10 questions for patients and 20 questions for the caregiver. It has a sensitivity of 90% and a specificity of 75% if the score is above 12.[17] The Center for the Epidemiological Studies Depression Scale has 20 questions.[18]

Depression is not diagnosed using screening forms. Rather, it is diagnosed from history and a physical exam with laboratory testing to rule out organic causes of depression. In busy practices, screening forms and depression scales are useful for:

- Help in identifying individuals at risk for depression.
- Supporting a clinical diagnosis of depression.
- Assessing the effectiveness of treatment.

Depression scales are not a substitute for excellent clinical assessment. They should be used only as adjuncts to professional judgment, evaluation, and assessment.

PHYSICAL DISORDERS ASSOCIATED WITH DEPRESSION

There are a number of medical conditions in which depression is known to occur more commonly, often as a direct result of the illness. In many cases, once the illness resolves or is appropriately treated, the depression will resolve. In some cases, treatment for depression may need to continue long after the underlying illness has been addressed. The following illnesses have been associated with an increased incidence of depression: angina, myocardial infarction, cancer (pancreatic), stroke, intracranial tumors, multiple sclerosis, hypothyroidism, hyperthyroidism, AIDS, Addison's disease, Parkinson's disease, Cushing's disease, diabetes, chronic renal disease, hepatitis, syphilis, systemic lupus erythematosus, temporal arteritis, hypoglycemia, hypo- and hyperkalemia, hypo-and hypernatremia, vitamin deficiencies, dementia, and pernicious anemia.

TREATMENT OF DEPRESSION

Depression is treatable in the vast majority of elderly patients, with up to 75% of elderly patients responding to treatment.[2] Effective management requires a biopsychosocial approach combining pharmacotherapy and psychotherapy.[19,20] The goals of therapy include:

- Improved quality of life.
- Enhanced functional capacity.
- Improvement in medical health status (when possible).
- Increased longevity.
- Lower health care costs.

Studies show that older patients with depression benefit most from aggressive, persistent treatment.[20] Therapy for older patients should generally be continued for longer periods than are typically applied in treating younger patients.[21]

Antidepressant medication is appropriate not only for primary depression but also for depression associated with medical conditions such as cancer, heart and pulmonary diseases, arthritis, stroke, and Parkinson's disease. Elderly patients with depression secondary to a chronic disease often require long-term treatment. In situations such as depression due to a chronic illness that improves with treatment (such as hypothyroidism), a trial period off the antidepressant medication is warranted once the chronic illness is in remission.

Most experts recommend continuing treatment for 1 year for the first episode of major depression in the elderly. For patients who have had three episodes of major depression, therapy should be continued for life. For those who have had two episodes, the recommendation is less clear. The patient's progress as well as clinical factors should guide the therapy. Prior to discontinuing therapy, patients should be free of symptoms of depression. Upon discontinuation of therapy, patients should notify the physician of recurrence of the symptoms. In order to ensure that the patient remains in remission, he or she should be seen every 1–2 months during the first 6–12 months after discontinuing therapy and then about every 3 months after the first year.[22]

Selective Serotonin Reuptake Inhibitors

Selective serotonin reuptake inhibitors (SSRIs) are the drugs of choice for treating most types of depression. SSRIs are comparatively safe and work just as well as tricyclic antidepressants, but without many of the undesirable cholinergic side effects such as somnolence, orthostatic hypotension, and cardiac dysrhythmias. In addition, SSRIs have a much lower potential for toxicity in overdose. Common side effects of SSRIs include weight loss, agitation, insomnia, fatigue, dry mouth, constipation, nausea, diarrhea, headache, anxiety, and sexual dysfunction.

The pure SSRIs are fluoxetine (Prozac®), paroxetine (Paxil®), sertraline (Zoloft®), escitalopram (Lexapro®), citalopram (Celexa®), and duloxetine (Cymbalta®).

Fluoxetine

The dosage of fluoxetine is 10–40 mg/day. Its half-life is 2–3 days. Its metabolite norfluoxetine has a half-life of 7–9 days. Fluoxetine and its metabolite inhibit CYP450-2D6. Common side effects include weight loss, agitation, insomnia, and sexual dysfunction. The main concern with use in the elderly is the long half-life.

Paroxetine

The dosage of paroxetine is 10–40 mg. The half-life is 21 hours, and it inhibits CYP450-2D6. Paroxetine is more helpful with anxiety symptoms. Common side effects include nausea, gastrointestinal upset, constipation, and hyponatremia. The main concern for use in the elderly is higher anticholinergic effects. It also has the potential for interaction with monoamine oxidase inhibitors (MAOIs) and tricyclic antidepressants.

Sertraline

The dosage of sertraline is 25–200 mg/day. Its half-life is 26 hours. The initial pathway of metabolism for sertraline is N-demethylation. N-Desmethylsertraline has a plasma terminal elimination half-life of 62–104 hours. Common side effects include sexual dysfunction, fatigue, insomnia, and dry mouth.

Escitalopram

The dosage of escitalopram is 10–20 mg once a day. The mean terminal half-life is about 27–32 hours. CYP3A4 and CYP2C19 are the primary isozymes involved in the N-demethylation of escitalopram. Escitalopram's area under curve (AUC) and half-life are increased by approximately 50% in elderly subjects. Common side effects include dry mouth, constipation, nausea, somnolence, insomnia, sexual dysfunction, and hyponatremia.

Duloxetine

The dosage of duloxetine is 20–60 mg/day. It has an elimination half-life of 12 hours (range 8–17 hours) and inhibits both CYP1A2 and CYP2D6. Common side effects include nausea, dry mouth, constipation, fatigue, decreased appetite, and somnolence. The concerns with this drug are to avoid use in end-stage renal disease, hepatic insufficiency, and uncontrolled narrow-angle glaucoma. Blood pressure should be monitored prior to initiating treatment and periodically during treatment.

Citalopram

The usual starting dose of citalopram is 20 mg/day. It has an elimination half-life ($t_{1/2}$) of 33 hours and reaches a peak plasma concentration in 2–4 hours. This drug is 80% protein bound and is greater than 80% bioavailable from an oral dose, but plasma concentrations of this drug and all SSRIs are greater in the elderly than in young patients. Note that SSRIs are extensively distributed in the tissues and, with the exception of citalopram, may have a nonlinear pattern of drug accumulation when given over long periods. Citalopram has few to no anticholinergic effects and produces little sedation, but like other SSRIs, seizures, as an ADR, are something to watch out for. Other side effects, which are generally mild and short-lived, are nausea, vomiting, and diarrhea; sexual dysfunction in both males and females; headache; insomnia; and fatigue.

Tricyclic Antidepressants

Tricyclic antidepressants have a nonspecific mechanism of action. This category includes the tertiary amines amitriptyline, imipramine, trimipramine, and doxepin, and the secondary tricyclic antidepressants nortriptyline, bupropion, venlafaxine, mirtazapine, and trazodone.

Tricyclic antidepressants inhibit presynaptic serotonin and norepinephrine reuptake, have high anticholinergic effects, inhibit alpha-1-adrenergic receptors (orthostatic hypotension), and inhibit histamine-1 receptor action (sedation). They also prolong cardiac repolarization, leading to lengthening of the QT interval.[23] Caution is required in geriatric patients with cardiovascular disease, narrow-angle glaucoma, benign prostatic hyperplasia, urinary retention, or a history of seizures. Anticholinergic effects can cause confusion. These agents should be administered at bedtime to help decrease the impact of their anticholinergic side effects. Due to the potential for the development of the serotonergic syndrome, extreme caution should be used when combining SSRIs with tricyclic antidepressants.

Amitriptyline (Tertiary)

The dosage of amitriptyline is 25–300 mg. Side effects include strong anticholinergic effects, sedation, cardiac effects, weight gain, lower seizure threshold, and orthostatic hypotension. Generally, it should not be used with antiarrhythmics and MAOIs. Other tricyclic antidepressants, such as clomipramine, doxepin (Sinequan®), trimipramine, and imipramine (Tofranil®), have similar side effects. This class of drugs should be avoided in the elderly.

Nortriptyline (Secondary)

The dosage of nortriptyline is 25–250 mg. It generally should not be used with antiarrhythmics and MAOIs. Side effects include hypotension, confusion, dry mouth, and urinary retention. Some other secondary tricyclics are protriptyline (15–60 mg) and desipramine (25–300 mg). They should all be used with caution in patients with coronary artery disease, arrhythmias, narrow-angle glaucoma, benign prostatic hyperplasia, seizures, and urinary retention.

Bupropion (Wellbutrin®) (Secondary)

Bupropion is a relatively weak inhibitor of the neuronal uptake of norepinephrine, serotonin, and dopamine and does not inhibit MAO. It is presumed that this action is mediated by noradrenergic and/or dopaminergic mechanisms. The dosage is 100–300 mg/day in divided doses three times a day. Side effects include neuropsychiatric disturbances, primarily agitation and abnormalities in mental status; gastrointestinal disturbances, primarily nausea and vomiting; neurological disturbances, primarily seizures, headaches, and sleep disturbances; and dermatologic problems such as rash, hypotension, and hypertension. Bupropion should be avoided in patients with seizures.

Venlafaxine (Effexor®) (Secondary)

This drug is a potent inhibitor of neuronal serotonin and norepinephrine reuptake and a weak inhibitor of dopamine reuptake. The dosage is 75–375 mg/day in divided doses.

Side effects include weight change, appetite change, hyponatremia, seizures, mydriasis, increased cholesterol, and, at higher doses, increased blood pressure.

Mirtazapine (Remeron®) (Secondary)

Mirtazapine acts as an antagonist at the central presynaptic α_2-adrenergic inhibitory autoreceptors and heteroreceptors. This action is postulated to result in an increase in central noradrenergic and serotonergic activity. Mirtazapine is a potent antagonist of 5-HT_2 and 5-HT_3 receptors. Mirtazapine is also a potent antagonist of histamine (H_1) receptors, a property that may explain its prominent sedative effects. It is a moderate peripheral α_1-adrenergic antagonist, a property that may explain the occasional orthostatic hypotension reported in association with its use. Mirtazapine is a moderate antagonist at muscarinic receptors, a property that may explain the relatively low incidence of anticholinergic side effects associated with its use. The dosage is 15–45 mg/day.

It has a half-life of about 20–40 hours. Side effects include somnolence, dizziness, increased appetite, weight gain, cholesterol/triglycerides elevation, transaminase elevation, and seizures.

Mirtazapine is excreted mainly through the renal system. Therefore, it should be used cautiously in the geriatric population since many elderly have impaired renal function in spite of having a normal creatinine.

Trazodone (Secondary)

The mechanism of trazodone antidepressant action in humans is not fully understood. In animals, trazodone selectively inhibits serotonin uptake by brain synaptosomes and thus potentiates the behavioral changes induced by the serotonin precursor 5-hydroxytryptophan. The half-life of trazodone is 6–9 hours. The dosage is 50–300 mg at bedtime. Side effects include priapism, blurred vision, constipation, confusion, and nausea.

PSYCHOSOCIAL INTERVENTIONS

Findings from several randomized clinical trials suggest that the combination of pharmacological and psychosocial interventions is more effective than either intervention alone in preventing recurrence of major depression.[22,24] Expert consensus findings recommend the combined use of antidepressant treatment and psychotherapy for treating late-life depression, especially for episodes in which there is a clearly identified psychosocial stressor.[2,22]

Interventions likely to be efficacious in older adults include problem-solving therapy, interpersonal therapy, brief psychodynamic therapy, and reminiscence therapy. Cognitive therapy, behavioral therapy, and cognitive–behavioral therapy have the greatest empirical support for effectiveness in the treatment of geriatric depression.[25,26]

In **electroconvulsive therapy (ECT),** an electrical current is passed through the cerebral hemispheres. Treatment is given under anesthesia and with muscle relaxants. It is mostly indicated for severe depression that has not responded to the other treatments. ECT is also indicated when speedy response is necessary, such as in severely depressed patients with suicidal ideation or serious risk of self-neglect.

ECT is a very effective treatment for a major depressive disorder with or without psychotic features. Unfortunately, ECT is often overlooked as a potential treatment for the elderly. ECT is a very safe method of treating depression in elderly patients.[27] It can often be life-saving in situations where antidepressants have been ineffective and in cases in which the patients are suicidal and more rapid treatment is needed.

ECT typically consists of between 6 to 10 treatments that are given two or three times per week.

The benefits are that ECT acts speedily in major depression and is generally safe, especially with unilateral ECT. Although modern procedures for ECT are very safe, some patients may find the prospect of ECT frightening. ECT is also associated with transient short-term memory loss.

ECT is often combined with medications that require monitoring. Patients should be evaluated for any evidence of confusion. If confusion or memory disturbance is present more than 2 weeks after the end of ECT treatment, reevaluation should be performed and the ECT deferred. Rarely, maintenance ECT may be continued over an indefinite period.

Relative contraindications to ECT include any condition that renders the patient unfit for anesthesia, current use of MAOIs (should be discontinued 2 weeks before ECT), and any condition associated with increased intracranial pressure.

A systematic review of ECT in younger and older adults with moderate-to-severe depression found that real ECT was more effective than simulated

ECT (control group), and that ECT was more effective than antidepressant medication for the short-term treatment of depression.[28] In another systematic review of ECT in the elderly, no firm conclusions could be drawn about whether ECT is more effective than antidepressant therapy alone.[29] ECT was found to be a faster and more effective treatment for patients with medication-resistant depression.

KEY POINTS

- Depression is a common problem in the elderly population that is associated with significant morbidity and mortality.
- Depression is often underdiagnosed and undertreated.
- Patients presenting with depressive symptoms should be evaluated with a thorough history and focused laboratory testing, and underlying causes should be identified and treated.
- Chronic illnesses often complicate depression evaluation and treatment.
- Depression surveys such as the Geriatric Depression Scale are helpful adjuncts for the evaluation of depression.
- Although elders with depression may present with atypical symptoms, they benefit from treatment with SSRIs and often require prolonged periods of treatment.
- ECT is a safe, effective, and underutilized depression treatment for the elderly.

REFERENCES

1. Hirschfeld RM, Keller MB, Panico S, et al. The National Depressive and Manic-Depressive Association consensus statement on the undertreatment of depression. *JAMA*. 1997;277(4):333–40.
2. Alexopoulos GS, Katz IR, Reynolds CF 3rd, et al. The expert consensus guideline series: pharmacotherapy of depressive disorders in older patients. *Postgraduate Medicine Special Report*. Minneapolis: The McGraw-Hill Companies, Inc.; 2001:1–86.
3. Koenig HG, Blazer DG. Minor depression in late life. *Am J Geriatr Psychiatry*. 1996; 4(4):S14–S21.
4. Koenig HG, Blazer DG. Epidemiology of geriatric affective disorders. *Clin Geriatr Med*. 1992;8(2):235–51.
5. Butler RN, Lewis MI. Late-life depression: when and how to intervene. *Geriatrics*. 1995;50(8):44–55.
6. American Psychiatric Association. *Diagnostic and Statistical Manual of Mental Disorders*. 4th ed, Text Revision. Washington, DC: American Psychiatric Association; 2000.
7. Jacobson JL, Jacobson AM. *Psychiatric Secrets*. 2nd ed. Philadelphia: Hanley and Belfus; 2000:163–5.

8. Grief and bereavement. *Psychiatr Clin North Am.* 1987;10(3):329–515.

9. Burnell GM, Burnell AL, eds. *Clinical Management of Bereavement: A Handbook for Healthcare Professionals.* New York: Human Sciences Press; 1989.

10. Birrer RB, Vemuri SP. Depression in later life: a diagnostic and therapeutic challenge. *Am Fam Physician.* 2004;69(10):2375–82.

11. Boswell EB, Stoudemire A. Major depression in the primary care setting. *Am J Med.* 1996;101(6A):3S–9S.

12. Yesavage JA, Brink TL, Rose TL, et al. Development and validation of a geriatric depression screening scale: a preliminary report. *J Psychiatr Res.* 1982-83;17(1):37–49.

13. Sheikh JI, Yesavage JA. Geriatric depression scale (GDS): recent evidence and development of a shorter version. In: Brink TL, ed. *Clinical Gerontology: A Guide to Assessment and Intervention.* New York: Haworth; 1986:165–73.

14. Mahoney J, Drinka TJ, Abler R, et al. Screening for depression: single question versus GDS. *J Am Geriatr Soc.* 1994;42(9):1006–8.

15. McGivney SA, Mulvihill M, Taylor B. Validating the GDS depression screen in the nursing home. *J Am Geriatr Soc.* 1994;42(5):490–2.

16. Hamilton M. A rating scale for depression. *J Neurol Neurosurg Psychiatry.* 1960 Feb; 23:56–62.

17. Alexopoulos GS, Abrams RC, Young RC, et al. Cornell Scale for Depression in Dementia. *Biol Psychiatry.* 1988;23(3):271–84.

18. Radloff LS. The CES-D scale: a self-report depression scale for research in the general population. *Applied Psychological Measurement.* 1977;1:385–401.

19. Dunner DL. Therapeutic considerations in treating depression in the elderly. *J Clin Psychiatry.* 1994;55(Suppl):48–58.

20. Charney DS, Miller HL, Licinio J, et al. Treatment of depression. In: Schatzberg AF, Nemeroff CB, eds. *The American Psychiatric Press Textbook of Psychopharmacology.* 2nd ed. Washington, DC: American Psychiatric Press; 1998:575–601.

21. Alexopoulos G. *Pharmacotherapy of Depressive Disorders in Older Patients.* Minneapolis: McGraw-Hill Healthcare Information; 2001.

22. Reynolds CF 3rd, Frank E, Perel JM, et al. Nortriptyline and interpersonal psychotherapy as maintenance therapies for recurrent major depression: a randomized controlled trial in patients older than 59 years. *JAMA.* 1999;281(1):39–45.

23. Preskorn SH. Recent pharmacologic advances in antidepressant therapy for the elderly. *Am J Med.* 1993;94(Suppl 5A):2S–12S.

24. Lenze EJ, Dew MA, Mazumdar S, et al. Combined pharmacotherapy and psychotherapy as maintenance treatment for late-life depression: effects on social adjustment. *Am J Psychiatry.* 2002;159(3):466–8.

25. Laidlaw K. An empirical review of cognitive therapy for late life depression: does research evidence suggest adaptations are necessary for cognitive therapy with older adults. *Clin Psychol Psychother.* 2001;8(1):1–14.

26. Gatz M, Fiske A, Fox LS, et al. Empirically validated psychological treatments for older adults. *J Ment Health Aging.* 1998;4(1):9–46.

27. Tomac TA, Rummans TA, Pileggi TS, et al. Safety and efficacy of electroconvulsive therapy in patients over age 85. *Am J Geriatr Psychiatry.* 1997;5(2):126–30.

28. UK ECT Review Group. Efficacy and safety of electroconvulsive therapy in depressive disorders: a systematic review and meta-analysis. *Lancet.* 2003;361(9360):799–808. Reviewed in: *Clinical Evidence.* 2004;12:1389–434 Level A.

29. Van der Wurff FB, Stek ML, Hoogendijk WL, et al. Electroconvulsive therapy for the depressed elderly. *Cochrane Database Syst Rev.* 2003,2:CD003593. Reviewed in: *Clinical Evidence.* 2004; 12:1389–434 Level A.

10

Pharmacotherapy Issues of Managing Chronic Pain in the Geriatric Population

PHILIP S. WHITECAR

Pain is temporary. It may last an hour or a day, or a year but eventually it will subside and something else will take its place. If I quit, however, it lasts forever.

—Lance Armstrong, American cyclist

OVERVIEW

This chapter looks at issues surrounding the decades of pain that many elderly have to contend with. Many health care providers do not deal with their patients' pain needs in an effective and team-based approach, especially when the elderly may be unwilling or unable to express themselves. This chapter provides insights into the use of opioids, non-opioids, and other adjuvants to therapy that help control various types of pain. The importance of preventing side effects and choosing correct medications for special needs is stressed. Barriers and assessment techniques are covered in order to help a clinician understand how the undertreatment of pain in the elderly has become so prevalent. The chapter also describes for clinicians a key tool: a stepwise approach for the selection of pain medication. All in all, this chapter underscores the complexities of diagnosing (assessing) and treating chronic pain in the elderly in alignment with best practices recommended by relevant professional organizations.

Nancy Melville is a 75-year-old woman who suffers from chronic pain in her lower back as a result of an accident about 5 years ago in a car in which she was a passenger. Her husband died in that car accident. Her medical records do not indicate if she suffered a herniated disk or a ruptured disk but she was placed on oxycodone–aspirin medication shortly after the accident and has been using it ever since because she complains of constant pain. Nancy now shares a house with two other widows, both of whom consider her to be quite sedentary, as she spends a lot of time in bed and watching TV. To her physician and pharmacist Nancy is always saying, "You know I have this constant pain in my back and from time to time my legs just tingle. Can't I take more of my pain medication?" Besides her oxycodone–aspirin tabs 2 q6h, she is taking metoprolol 50 mg BID, digoxin 0.125 mg OD, fluoxetine 75 mg HS, and hydrochlorothiazide 25 mg OD.

- What do you think may be at issue with Nancy's constant pain 5 years after the car accident?
- What nondrug therapy might be suggested for her?
- In order to enhance compliance, ensure that her therapy is successful, and prevent adverse effects, what information should Nancy be given?
- What can you suggest to optimize Nancy's medication regimen?
- What do you think about the fact that tricyclic antidepressants are sometimes considered as first-line therapy for neuropathic pain?

EPIDEMIOLOGY AND PREVALENCE OF PAIN IN THE ELDERLY

Chronic pain is an issue for up to 40%–60%[1] of community-dwelling elderly, and 40%–80% of institutionalized elderly patients also complain of pain. But what is pain? It has been defined as an unpleasant sensory and emotional experience associated with actual or potential tissue damage, or it is described in terms of such damage.[2] Additionally, chronic pain is often described as pain that has lasted for at least 3 months, but a more useful definition is pain that extends beyond the expected time of healing.[3]

Elderly patients often suffer from acute, recurrent, chronic, and end-of-life pain. Pain from cancer, neurological illnesses, skin ulcers, diabetic neuropathy, and postsurgery are common among elderly individuals, as are arthritis and other bone and joint problems.[4]

Radiographic severity of osteoarthritis of the knee correlates well with increased pain, impaired function, and psychological dysfunction. Data from a national survey indicate that the prevalence of musculoskeletal pain affecting the neck, back, hip, and knee is greater in older persons (mean age 75) than in younger persons (mean age 40). Of interest in this study, even when the prevalence of pain in a particular location was similar in the two groups, the effect of the pain on impairing activities of daily living and in disturbing the quality of life was greater in the older group.[5]

In addition to the common complaint of joint pain, one research study noted that nocturnal leg pain or cramps and leg pain while walking are also common in the elderly.[6] A majority of patients with pain also reported interference with sleep, activities of daily living, or movement. Interestingly, those more than 85 years of age were less likely to complain of pain.

With so much pain in the community and in institutions, it is amazing to discover that chronic pain is undertreated in the general population and that it remains a significant public health issue. This problem is common in older adults in long-term care settings, with recent studies demonstrating that up to 80% of nursing home residents who experience substantial pain are undertreated.[7] In a study of pain in the hospital, elderly patients had lower pain intensity levels and higher satisfaction with pain control, yet overall they received worse pain management.[8] Given the resources most hospitals and nursing homes have today, including frequent evaluations by nursing personnel, the problem of untreated pain should be an issue amenable to marked improvement.

Pain of moderate-to-severe intensity is undertreated in almost 50% of cancer patients, and a higher percentage often have poorly controlled end-of-life pain.[9] A significant gap appears when these percentages are compared to estimates by pain specialists, who note that almost 90% of patients with pain could obtain very good pain relief with proper therapy.[9] A recent study of patients with metastatic cancer revealed that 67% reported daily pain, and in 62% it was severe enough to limit their function. Only 42% of these patients were prescribed appropriate analgesics.[10]

Inadequate management of pain in the elderly who choose to work results in increased health care costs and absenteeism, as well as diminished quality of life. Chronic pain has been associated with depression, sleep disturbance, emotional and psychosocial stress, functional loss, impaired cognition, anxiety, and social withdrawal.[11] Pain has also been found to negatively affect sleep, social activities, ambulation, and activities of daily living, and it is associated with anxiety and depression in spite of the fact that guidelines have been established for the treatment of chronic pain in the elderly and that newer therapies and safer approaches to using pain medications are available. Thus, the undertreatment of chronic pain in the elderly persists,[12] despite the work of several professional organizations to generate clinical and prescribing guidelines.

The following guidelines to aid in managing pain in the elderly are available:

- The American Geriatrics Society clinical practice guidelines.[12]
- The American Medical Directors Association guidelines for the management of pain in the long-term care setting.[13]
- The American Pain Society guidelines for the management of pain in osteoarthritis, rheumatoid arthritis, and juvenile arthritis.[14]
- The World Health Organization analgesic ladder approach to pain management.[15]

Barriers to Appropriate Pain Management for the Elderly

Due to its subjective nature, the severity of pain is often difficult to measure, especially among the elderly, who often are unable to talk about their pain in terms that make sense to a clinician. Also, many clinicians view pain as a symptom rather than a disease, and since it is not the central focus of the medical or treatment encounter, the result is often undertreatment of pain. In addition, pain is often viewed by many clinicians as being either purely physical or psychological, and thus they ignore the evidence that most patients with pain have both a physical and psychological component to their pain.

It is not uncommon for clinicians to fear criminal prosecution[16] or professional sanctions for "overprescribing" pain-relieving medications. Other provider-related barriers include nurses' and physicians' lack of knowledge about pain and its treatment, especially matters related to addiction, tolerance, and side effects of opioids, and their lack of skill in assessing and managing pain effectively.[17] Failure to routinely assess and document pain[18] and inappropriate concerns about the safety of opioids compared with nonopioid analgesics has been labeled opiophobia.

But not all undertreatment of pain is the fault of the clinician; patient and social barriers play a role as well. Barriers include society's perceptions of aging as well as the belief by many that pain is simply a part of aging. In fact, one study of nonhospitalized patients found that many elderly believe their pain is part of the aging process, thus justifying their not wanting to "bother" their physician about it out of fear that complaining may cause problems.[19] Elderly patients are more likely to fear some pain medications, thus reinforcing their physicians' beliefs. They may also be more likely to suffer the side effects of pain medications and therefore be reluctant to ask about improving their pain control.

Barriers to effective pain control also occur at the health system level. They include:[20]

- A lack of institutional commitment to pain management.
- A failure to standardize pain assessment.
- A lack of a team approach to pain management.
- A lack of accountability for pain management practices.

Cultural and gender differences in attitudes toward pain and in reporting it to physicians have led to a large body of literature that documents disparities in pain management among racial and ethnic minorities for diverse pain conditions in many kinds of treatment settings. For example, African American and Hispanic patients are more likely to receive inadequate analgesia or be denied opioids.[21]

The Physiology of Pain and Types of Pain

Acute pain can be caused by pressure, heat, cold, injury, or chemical agents that stimulate a variety of receptors in the skin and underlying tissues. Once stimulated, receptors then activate primary afferent fibers, which transmit the sensation of pain and its characteristics and other associated nonpain-related information up the spinal cord, where the brain interprets the sensation. At the spinal level, the process becomes more complicated and less well understood. What is known is that the transmission of pain-related information from primary afferent nerves to secondary afferent nerves is done via ascending up several pathways in the spinal column to multiple locations in the midbrain, cerebellum, and cerebrum. There N-methyl-D-aspartate (NMDA) receptors are critical to acute pain transmission and to the creation of an eventual chronic pain syndrome. Transmitters released from stimulation by primary afferents cause the blockade of NMDA receptors to be lifted. This action amplifies impulse transmission in the acute pain situation, but it can lead to amplification of pain in the chronic situation. This process is the principal reason why treating neuropathic pain successfully is so difficult.[22]

Once pain information reaches the brain, it is conveyed to cognitive, emotional, and autonomic centers where it is processed, experienced, and integrated with previous pain experiences. Each of these centers will then send an outgoing transmission down the spinal column to the dorsal horn to either augment or diminish the incoming transmission. The multiple routes of transmissions and processing centers coupled with the patient's previous pain experiences explain at least some of the difficulty in treating pain.

There is no apparent age-related difference in pain by sensory/affective descriptors or in the presence of associated depressed mood.

PAIN CLASSIFICATION

Most clinicians prefer to describe pain in terms of either its etiology or its severity: mild (1–3 on a 10-point scale), moderate (4–6), or severe (7–10). The "faces" scale is often used for children, but it can be appropriate for the elderly as well.

Pain may also be classified according to its etiology; however, in many disease states, several etiologies of pain are simultaneously present, for example, cancer or vascular disease. Most chronic pain has components of both physical and psychogenic etiologies (Table 1).

Today, most clinicians use quality-of-life indicators to measure a patient's ability to return to work, dance, sleep, get out of bed unassisted, play sports, or take up hobbies again as better measures of coping with pain. Such assessments are more compelling because they help the clinician work with what is most important to the patient. Finally, many elderly patients are impaired cognitively and thus the clinician must rely on other sources of information such as home visits and direct observation to assess the patient's pain. This assessment process is critical if the elderly patient is to be prescribed an agent that provides relief with few adverse effects and that fits in with the other concerns relevant to a geriatric patient.

Table 1   Etiology of pain and associated symptoms

Types of Pain		Symptoms and Signs
Somatic	Myofascial	Well localized, achy, throbbing or dull, worse with movement, tender to palpation.
	Bone	Intermittent or constant, achy or throbbing, well localized, tender to palpation, not always worse with movement or better with rest.
	Rheumatic	Tender, inflamed or warm joints, decreased range of motion, achy.
Psychogenic		Various presentations, may be associated with unusual presentations, may have minimal to no peripheral findings.
Visceral		Poorly localized, cramping, colicky or achy
Neuropathic	Peripheral	Sharp, tingling, burning, deep pain, may radiate, possible allodynia or hyperalgesia.
	Central	Various presentations, may have minimal to no peripheral findings, though often historical evidence of injury/illness.
	Sympathetic	Inconsistent, hot/cold sensations, sharp and shooting or numb, possible allodynia or hyperalgesia.

Assessment of Pain

A broad approach to pain assessment in the elderly, including those with cognitive or functional impairments, is critical to arriving at an appropriate therapy. The starting point is to gather from the patient an explanation of the pain and its severity. There are no objective markers for pain, so the patient's story is assumed to be accurate. Pain in the elderly may be assessed using standard pain assessment tools, including numeric rating scales, verbal descriptor scales, the faces pain scales, and visual analogue scales. More comprehensive tools include the Wisconsin Brief Pain Inventory and the McGill Pain Questionnaire. At the minimum, one should assess the severity, locations, aggravating and alleviating factors, and qualities of the pain. Critical elements of the assessment include noting related psychosocial factors, especially psychiatric illness and addiction history. Physical examination and diagnostic studies should be used to confirm the history and pinpoint the cause(s) of the pain and to aid in choosing a treatment.

Another important element in assessing pain in the elderly is to ask how it affects function. Assess pain during movement and at rest, remembering that severe limitations in activities may be extremely burdensome. Finally, one should assess the elderly for additional diseases, organ dysfunctions, and current medication use, since medications can cause limitations as well as complicate treatment regimens. Concern about the possibility of addiction should not outweigh the assessment for pain. Several screening tools (e.g., SOAPP[23]) have been developed to help assess the risks of using opioids.

Cognitively impaired patients tend to underreport pain, but when questioned directly, they can be capable of giving valid responses.[24] Several tools have been tested and found helpful in assessing pain in dementia patients.[25]

Steps to take when assessing pain in the cognitively impaired are:[25]

- Ask the patient.
- Ask family and caregivers.
- Note facial expression.
- Note body posture.
- Note vocalizations.
- Assess appetite.
- Assess patient's ability to interact.

Treatment of Pain in the Elderly

Guidelines for management of pain in the elderly by using pharmaceuticals are based on the World Health Organization three-step analgesic ladder,[15] in which selection of a medication and its dosage depends on the severity and type of pain the patient is experiencing. Patients with mild pain are started on acetaminophen or a nonsteroidal anti-inflammatory drug (NSAID) with or without the addition of adjuvant medications. Pain that is moderate in intensity often requires opioids in addition to starting or maximizing step 1 therapies. Patients with severe pain or pain unresponsive to step 2 therapy usually require treatment with opioids.[26]

In addition to assessing the correct level of pain, the clinician can take several other steps to achieve good overall pain control in the elderly:

- Identify the goals the patient has regarding pain control. Improved pain relief or sleep or mood or function while minimizing side effects are all reasonable goals. Patients in acute pain may choose pain relief over all other goals, whereas patients with chronic pain may choose to focus on improving function.
- Individualize treatment, as certain types of pain respond well to the addition of adjuvant medications along with using analgesics (e.g., neuropathic or visceral pain). No single analgesic is appropriate for every patient with pain.

- Try to maintain or maximize the functional ability of the patient. Improved function may improve the patient's sense of well-being, which often improves his/her perceived level of pain.
- Minimize side effects of analgesics by choosing those with fewer drug interactions and side effects or those the patient is known to already tolerate. Certain medications have almost unavoidable side effects. One example is the use of opioids resulting in constipation. Therefore, when choosing this type of medication, try to prevent these anticipated consequences.
- Ensure that treatment is comprehensive, with the use of physical, psychological, or integrative approaches almost always an appropriate complement to analgesic use.
- Use the least invasive route of administration.
- Reassess the patient frequently. Older patients reported more pain relief post-op while receiving the same dose of medication as younger patients.[27] Therefore, a general rule in the elderly is to start with a low dose of analgesic and gradually increase it.[12]

Each one of the preceding steps should be undertaken in a systematic way, while addressing each of the patient's concerns. If care is being provided in a nonurgent setting and if the physician is convinced that opioids are appropriate, an opioid use trial should be proposed. The results of the trial should include patient self-assessments about the changes in their pain; in addition, changes in function should be assessed by both the patient and the physician. The patient should demonstrate proper use of the opioid medication. The patient should be informed of both the potential risks and the benefits of opioid therapy.

While treatment for acute perioperative pain uses combinations of opioids, NSAIDs, and local and general anesthetics to address all aspects of pain, treatment for chronic or end-of-life pain needs to be even broader in its application to address the complex underlying physiology coupled with the additional cognitive and emotional aspects. A successful approach used by pain centers combines targeting multiple sites simultaneously in the pain transmission pathway with antidepressants, opioids, anticonvulsants, and anti-inflammatory agents and using cognitive behavioral therapy and physical modalities. It has been noted that an older person on six medications is 14 times more likely to have a drug reaction than a younger person on six medications.[28] This situation seems to argue against using multiple medications to adequately address pain. However, carefully assessing the patient for medication interactions and starting with low dosages can maximize pain relief and minimize side effects and interactions.

USING ANALGESICS IN THE ELDERLY

Nonopioid analgesics, including acetaminophen and NSAIDs, are commonly used to treat pain in the elderly. Since the acetaminophen half-life is not related to age, the dose does not have to be adjusted for age.[29] Acetaminophen causes significant liver toxicity at high doses or with chronic use at usual doses; therefore, it is generally recommended to restrict acetaminophen use to 3000 mg/day in the elderly.[12] In addition, it has been noted that an increased risk of renal failure exists in those with long-term or high-dose use of acetaminophen.[30] Although nonsteroidal analgesics are often used for pain in the elderly, their side effect profile is such that they require close monitoring. Unfortunately, there is a relative infrequency of inclusion of the aged in NSAID trials, so the true incidence of side effects of these agents may not be fully understood.[31] One study discovered a three- to eight-fold increase in peptic ulcer disease with the use of NSAIDS in aged patients.[32]

NSAIDs often worsen hypertension, as they block prostaglandins, which stimulate renin and/or act as vasodilators.[33] NSAIDs can cause significant renal adverse effects (fluid retention, hyperkalemia, decreased renal blood flow, acute renal failure). In addition, the use of high-dose COX-2 inhibitors has now been associated with cardiovascular side effects, including vasoconstriction and increased platelet aggregation. Two of the three COX-2 inhibitors on the market have been withdrawn and use of the third has been curtailed.

Higher doses of NSAIDs are not necessarily associated with better pain relief. Therefore, to limit the potential for NSAID-induced adverse effects the lowest effective dose and shortest duration of therapy should be used.[12] The use of aspirin in the elderly at analgesic dosages has been associated with similar gastrointestinal, renal, and hepatic side effects. Choline magnesium salicylate may be safer than NSAIDs and it is as effective.

Here are some principals of opioid use in the elderly.[34] Once a patient is no longer opioid naive, titration upward can be done using immediate or sustained-release opioids. When titrating opioids, the key is to increase the dose by a percentage of the current dose, with increases ranging from 25% to 50% based on pain rating and the patient's clinical condition. Opioid dosage may be increased 50% to 100% in a 24-hour period for severe pain. However, in debilitated patients or those with decreased renal or hepatic function, smaller increases over longer time periods may be more beneficial in preventing severe side effects. Although smaller increases will be effective for moderate pain, increases of less than 25% are usually ineffective.

Short-acting agents can be titrated every 2–4 hours until either adequate analgesia is reached (usually defined as > 50% reduction in pain) or side effects such as sedation are encountered. Sustained-release products can be escalated every 24–48 hours, whereas transdermal fentanyl and methadone should not be increased more frequently than every 3–6 days. Longer periods of time should be reserved for debilitated patients. Once a patient is stable, sustained-release opioids are more convenient and provide a steady level of drug to prevent the highs and lows associated with short-acting agents, which should minimize side effects and maximize pain control, although there is no evidence that these long-acting agents are better tolerated by the elderly.

When using sustained-release opioids, it may be important to provide "breakthrough" pain medication. This medication is a short-acting opioid, which can be used prior to predictable pain-inducing activities or for sudden onset of severe pain. Ten percent of the total daily dose of the sustained-release opioid should be available every 4 hours for breakthrough pain. For those individuals who are on high-dose opioids and who have severe breakthrough pain, transmucosal fentanyl may be used. It is important to remember to increase the "rescue" or breakthrough short-acting dose as the baseline dose increases.

Patients may respond to certain opioids unpredictably, even if they respond very well to others. Therefore, if a patient has a poor response to one opioid or has intolerable side effects, switching to another opioid should be attempted rather than avoiding use of this whole class of drugs.

Switching between opioids requires calculating the equianalgesic dose and then decreasing by 25% for severe pain or up to 50% in moderate pain. The decrease in dosage is due to the combined effects of the previous opioid and the new one (Table 2). Follow-up should be at short intervals until improved pain control and function have been achieved with minimal or controlled side effects. The correct dose of analgesic that achieves these goals is often unique for each patient and may need to be arrived at by a trial over time; therefore, analgesic doses should be titrated until pain relief is achieved or intractable side effects occur. Failure of a specific analgesic drug cannot be determined unless the dose is increased to treatment-limiting toxicity. There is no maximal or "correct" opioid dose. Patients at high risk or in severe pain may need to be seen frequently, using the pain management follow-up guidelines in Table 3.

Table 2 Opioid conversions

Medication	Single Dose Equivalent		Daily Dose Equivalent		Usual Starting Dose	
	Parenteral	Oral	Parenteral	Oral	Parenteral	Oral
Morphine	5 mg	15 mg	30 mg (5 mg q4h)	90 mg (15 mg q4h)	2 mg q4h	5 mg q4h
Morphine SR (MS Contin®)	na	na	na	90 mg (45 mg q12h)	na	15 mg q12h
Oxycodone (Percocet®)	na	10 mg	na	60 mg (10 mg q4h)	na	5 mg q4h
Oxycodone SR (Oxycontin®)	na	na	na	60 mg (30 mg q12h)	na	10 mg q12h
Methadone	1.5 mg	5 mg	See below	See below	5 mg q8h	5 mg q8h
Hydromorphone (Dilaudid®)	0.75 mg	3.75 mg	1.5 mg q8h	20 mg (4 mg q5h)	0.75 mg q4h	1.5 mg q4h
Hydrocodone (Vicodin®)	na	15 mg	na	90 mg (15 mg q4h)	na	5 mg q6h
Codeine (Tylenol #3)	na	90 mg	na	540 mg (NR)	na	5 mg q4h
Tramadol (Ultram®)	na	100 mg	na	600 mg (NR)	na	50 mg q8h
Meperidine (Demerol®)	50 mg	150 mg (NR)	300 mg (50 mg q4h)	900 mg (NR)	25 mg q4h	50 mg q4h (NR)
Fentanyl (Duragesic®)	na	na	25 mcg/hr patch		25 mcg/hr patch	

NR = not recommended

Methadone Conversion Chart

Morphine Daily Equivalent (mg)	Morphine to Methadone Ratio
<30	2 to 1
30–99	4 to 1
100–299	8 to 1
300–499	12 to 1
500–999	15 to 1
>1000	20 to 1

Table 3 Keys to quality pain management follow-up care[35]

Analgesia	Assess effectiveness of pain relief.
Activities of daily living	Monitor functional improvement.
Adverse reactions	Prevent, diagnose, and treat side effects.
Aberrant drug-taking behaviors	Make note of and address behaviors of concern.
Affect	Note change in affect and its relation to medication or overall improvement.
Adherence to treatment plan	Assess whether patient is compliant and making progress toward improvement.
Appropriateness of opioids	Make note of your assessment that opioids are helpful in this individual.

DEALING WITH TOLERANCE, ADDICTION, DIVERSION, AND MISUSE OF ANALGESICS IN THE ELDERLY

Defining Terms

The American Society of Addiction Medicine, American Pain Society, and American Academy of Pain Medicine have issued consensus statements on the definitions of tolerance, addiction, and dependence in an effort to clear up confusion among addiction and pain specialists on the meanings of these terms.[36]

Tolerance is defined as "an adaptive process in which exposure to a drug induces physiologic changes that result in a diminution of one or more of the drug's effects over time."

Addiction is "a primary, chronic, neurobiologic disease, with genetic, psychosocial, and environmental factors influencing its development and manifestations characterized by behaviors that include one or more of the following: impaired control over drug use, compulsive use, cravings, and continued use despite harm."

Physical dependence is a state of physiologic adaptation to an opioid that is manifested by a drug-class-specific withdrawal syndrome that can be precipitated by abrupt cessation, rapid dose reduction, decreasing blood level of the drug, and/or administration of an antagonist.

While tolerance has been studied and documented, it may be uncommon from a clinical perspective. When tolerance occurs, it usually is easily addressed by making minor changes in opioid dosing. Persons requiring

Table 4 Patient behaviors requiring physician attention[38]

Yellow Flags	Red Flags
Lost prescriptions	Prescription forgery
Drug hoarding	Injecting oral formulations
Early refills	Buying prescription drugs
Poor compliance with treatment plan	Abuse of illicit drugs
Many drug "allergies"	Unauthorized dose escalations
Sharing pain medications	Selling prescription drugs
Refusing long-acting opioids	Using drug for another purpose
Requesting frequent drug escalations	Reporting psychic effects
Refusing generics	Doctor shopping
Aggressive complaining	Scams
	Requesting several controlled substances

substantial changes in opioid dosing should be evaluated for worsening disease or improper medication use before tolerance to the drug is assumed to be the reason for such a request.

Physical dependence is not characterized by the behaviors of addiction, and withdrawal symptoms will reverse promptly with resumption of the opioid. Pseudoaddiction is the development of behaviors typical of addiction in a patient whose pain is undertreated. The differentiating factor from addiction is that the concerning behaviors cease once the pain is treated appropriately.[37] Diversion is the illicit obtaining and distribution of controlled medications by patients or health care professionals. Drug diversion is usually associated with patient behaviors similar to those of addicts.

Table 4 identifies patient behaviors related to addiction, tolerance, and diversion that clinicians need to watch for and pay attention to; Table 5 suggests ways to minimize diversion and inappropriate use.

Clinical Pearls for Treating Neuropathic Pain in the Elderly

Neuropathic pain may be peripheral due to direct nerve injury, often from trauma or cancer growth. Neuropathic pain may also be of central origin, due to remodeling of the sensory pathway from chronic undertreated pain or from direct injury to spinal nerves. Neuropathic pain is poorly tolerated by most people and is poorly responsive to opioid therapy alone. However, several medications have been found to be helpful for neuropathic pain, individually and collectively.[39] Tricyclic antidepressants have long been known to help with diabetic neuropathy, postherpetic neuralgia (PHN), and other

Table 5 Strategies to minimize diversion or inappropriate use

Maintain control of prescription pads.

Consider using duplicate, numbered, or tamper-resistant prescription pads.

Communicate regularly with pharmacists.

Obtain photo ID of all new opioid patients.

Avoid phone refills unless a long history of controlled pain and appropriate behavior exists.

Minimize requests to change medication dose over the phone; evaluate in person.

Avoid refills on schedule III opioids or multiple prescriptions for schedule II opioid.

Have the patient choose a pharmacy, and write the pharmacy name on the prescription.

neuropathies.[40] In a study of PHN, amitriptyline reduced pain prevalence by more than one-half upon follow-up at 6 months.[41] The effectiveness of the tricyclic antidepressants is dose-dependent, so titration is necessary to minimize side effects. Amitriptyline, nortriptyline, and desipramine have been found to be very successful in treating PHN, but the latter two drugs may be safer in the elderly due to fewer anticholinergic side effects.

The serotonin–norepinephrine reuptake inhibitors (SNRIs) venlafaxine and duloxetine are effective for neuropathic pain and may cause fewer side effects than the tricyclic antidepressants in the elderly.[42] Selective serotonin reuptake inhibitors (SSRIs) have not been found to relieve neuropathic pain. Anticonvulsants are effective treatments for all types of neuropathic pain.[43] Due to the need for titration up to an effective dosage, they are often used in combination with analgesics. It should be noted that anticonvulsants may interfere with vitamin D metabolism, which can be problematic in elderly homebound patients.[44] Gabapentin is commonly used for central neuropathic pain, since its side effect profile is minimal if the dose is gradually increased. Gabapentin is not metabolized and should be used with caution in patients with renal impairment. Gabapentin is also excreted unchanged in the urine and can accumulate with decreased renal function.[45]

Topiramate has several mechanisms of action, but for pain it does not seem to be any more effective than older anticonvulsants. With topiramate, no age-related differences in pharmacokinetics are seen in elderly patients versus younger adults; however, the possibility of age-associated renal functional abnormalities should be considered. The clearance of topiramate is reduced by roughly 42% to 52% in renal dysfunction. Hydrochlorothiazide and estrogens are among its few drug interactions.[45]

Although the evidence for use of lamotrigine, valproic acid, pregabalin, and zonisamide is not as strong as for gabapentin, they are worth considering if the patient cannot tolerate gabapentin. The elderly exhibit a lower clearance and longer lamotrigine half-life when compared to young adults. Lamotrigine should be used with caution in patients with hepatic disease or impairment because the drug is extensively metabolized by the liver. Lamotrigine should be used with caution in patients with severe renal impairment or renal failure, including patients on dialysis. Valproic acid should not be used in patients with liver disease or decreased liver function due to its hepatotoxicity. Haloperidol and bupropion are among its few drug interactions.[45] Pregabalin has few drug interactions and does not induce the P450 system, so it may represent a safer choice in the elderly.[45] Zonisamide is primarily excreted renally, so its dose must be decreased in patients with decreasing renal function. It has few drug interactions.[45]

The older anticonvulsants are as effective for neuropathic pain and less expensive than newer anticonvulsants, although the old ones tend to have more side effects. Phenytoin has several contraindications, including arrhythmias, bone marrow suppression, and jaundice. Also, it has a multitude of drug interactions, including antiarrhythmics, warfarin, fluoxetine, antiretroviral drugs, cimetidine, methotrexate, and several of the newer antipsychotics. Phenytoin must be used with caution in the presence of liver disease, due to decreased metabolism.[45]

For postherpetic neuralgia, the cyclovirs have been found to decrease pain prevalence at 6 months.[46] The lidocaine patch is effective for relieving all types of peripheral neuropathic pain and has minimal side effects.[47] Capsaicin was found to be minimally beneficial for PHN, but it is poorly tolerated.[48]

Bone pain is a distinct type of pain that is neurochemically different from inflammatory and neuropathic pain. Bone pain can be intermittent, although it often becomes chronic. It can be exacerbated by normally non-painful activities. It is common (up to 70%) in breast and prostate cancer. NSAIDs, due to their antiprostaglandin activity, are especially useful in bone pain. Corticosteroids are also helpful for this type of pain, especially when the pain is acute. Opioids alone can be effective for relieving bone pain, but combination therapy often is required. Bisphosphonates are effective in about 50% of patients with bone cancer.[49]

PAIN, THE ELDERLY, AND DRUG SIDE EFFECTS
The pharmacological treatment of pain in the elderly must be balanced by minimizing side effects. The elderly may metabolize certain medicines more

slowly than a younger patient would. Thus, individualization of therapy is the best way to ensure that patients maintain a balance between symptom management and side effects. Some patients value comfort and function equally, requesting relief of pain and other symptoms with as little impact on their cognitive abilities and physical functioning as possible. Other patients are often willing to compromise their functionality in order to gain greater comfort. The therapeutic window between effectiveness and toxicity is much narrower in elderly patients, and those over 60 years of age have up to a 20% risk of adverse drug reactions (ADRs), which is significantly higher than for younger patients.[50] This increased risk is also related to the greater prevalence of polypharmacy and comorbidities in the elderly, as well as to the physiologic changes that occur with aging. For this reason, the American Geriatrics Society recommends starting with a lower dose of analgesic medication and carefully titrating upward in older patients.[12]

One of the most important aspects of medication side effects is prevention. Beers has noted several medications that are generally inappropriate in the elderly. These include meperidine, pentazocine, propoxyphene, indomethacin, cyclobenzaprine, amitriptyline, and doxepin.[28]

Issues of Renal Failure, Medications, and the Elderly

In elderly patients with decreased renal function, use of all NSAIDs, morphine, meperidine, and gabapentin requires great caution.[13] Morphine metabolites are excreted renally, so it is possible for iatrogenic overdose to occur in patients with renal failure. The renal clearance of normeperidine, a metabolite of meperidine, was significantly slower in older individuals and correlated with creatinine clearance.[51] Since NSAIDs will worsen renal failure, their use should be severely curtailed.

Issues with the Use of Opioids in the Elderly

Opiate analgesics have clearly emerged as an acceptable treatment for end-of-life pain as well as chronic pain in the elderly. Pure opiates do not have a ceiling effect with respect to organ toxicity and should be considered in the management of pain in the elderly. A review of randomized controlled studies revealed no evidence that one sustained-release opioid was better than another, nor were there any drugs with better safety profiles. Comparisons of long-acting and short-acting oxycodone demonstrated equal effectiveness.[52]

Opioid side effects are more common in older patients, especially those more than 60 years of age, than in younger patients.[53] Elderly patients may have alterations in pharmacokinetic or pharmacodynamic parameters when compared to younger populations. One of the most common concerns is related to the relative decrease in renal elimination that is seen with increasing age. Calculation of an elderly patient's creatinine clearance will give an estimation of renal function and help with selecting or adjusting medication doses. While clearance of opioids is decreased with age, the bioavailability of morphine and hydromorphone is unaffected.[54,55]

Assessment of side effects is a vital first management step. Symptoms attributable to opioid pain medications, especially in older patients and patients with advanced illness, may in fact be related to concurrent medical problems, other drugs, metabolic disturbances, or underlying disease progression. In addition, the occurrence and intensity of opioid-related side effects may not remain constant; patients' responses to opioids can change over time. Therefore, monitoring and assessment of side effects must be ongoing. The most common opioid side effects include constipation, nausea, respiratory depression, sedation, and urinary retention. Development of constipation is always a concern for elderly patients on chronic opioid therapy. Prophylactic bowel regimens should be started whenever opioids are begun.[12] In general, a stimulant-type laxative (e.g., senna), with or without a stool softener (e.g., docusate sodium), is often advisable,[14] whereas bulk-forming agents (e.g., psyllium) should be avoided in opioid-induced constipation.

Transdermal fentanyl has usual opioid side effects, though some studies have found it to be better tolerated than other opioids.[56] One must remember to provide short-acting opioids for 12–18 hours when starting transdermal fentanyl, which is metabolized by the CYP3A4 system and has drug interactions with some common medications, including calcium channel blockers and phenothiazine. Dosage must be reduced in both liver and renal failure. In general, elderly patients should not be prescribed transdermal fentanyl if they are opioid naïve and should be closely monitored for any signs of opioid toxicities when using this agent. Malnourished or infected patients may have too much free drug or release the drug from reservoir too rapidly. Fentanyl is also available in a transmucosal "lollipop" for rapid relief of severe breakthrough pain. Due to its strength, it should not be used in opioid-naïve patients. Generally, it is reserved for use in severe end-of-life pain in patients on large doses of opioids.[45]

Hydromorphone is available only in a short-acting formulation without acetaminophen. It has few drug interactions and the typical opioid side effects. Dosage must be decreased as renal function decreases.[45]

Oxycodone is available in a short-acting formulation with and without acetaminophen. It is also available in a controlled-release formulation. It has few drug interactions and its side effects are typical of opioids. Dosage must be decreased in renal failure.[45]

Morphine use is contraindicated in ileus, respiratory depression, shock, and status asthmaticus. Morphine use in patients with renal failure is associated with a greater incidence of side effects in the elderly. A metabolite of morphine, morphine-6-glucuronide, can cause cognitive dysfunction if it accumulates, which is much more likely in patients with decreased renal function.[45] Spinal administration of morphine is not associated with fewer side effects than oral or intramuscular morphine,[57] so this route should be considered only if intramuscular or oral routes are not available or successful.

Hydrocodone comes in formulations with acetaminophen, and so its daily dosage is limited by this addition. Hydrocodone has few drug interactions among those agents used by the elderly.[45]

Propoxyphene has not been shown to be any more effective than acetaminophen, and it causes significant problems in the elderly. Elimination of propoxyphene is prolonged in the elderly, mostly from decreasing renal function. Its active metabolite has a long half-life of more than 30 hours and has antiarrhythmic effects. There are numerous drug interactions, including beta-blockers, tricyclic antidepressants, barbiturates, and older anticonvulsants.[45]

Codeine is metabolized to morphine by the CYP2D6 system in the liver; therefore, the dosage should be decreased in patients with liver disease. Also, because of this conversion to morphine, the dosage should be reduced in patients with renal dysfunction. Acetaminophen limits this combination product to low dosages. The drug interactions of codeine are similar to those of morphine.[45]

The partial agonists butorphanol, buprenorphine, and nalbuphine generally are not to be used long term for pain. However, because of their limited side effects and drug interactions, they are excellent choices for acute transient pain. Elderly patients are at somewhat higher risk of the CNS side effects from these drugs.

Pentazocine can cause delirium and confusion in the elderly, so it should not be used in this population.[58] Though all of these drugs can accumulate with renal impairment, this is probably of little practical importance since they are not supposed to be used chronically. Use of these agents in opioid-tolerant patients may precipitate withdrawal reactions.

Meperidine can cause delirium, seizures, dysphoria, and myoclonus secondary to accumulations of normeperidine, which is more common in those with poor renal function, such as the elderly.[28]

The following simple four-step plan addresses the issue of opioid side effects in the elderly:[59]

1. Decrease the opioid dose by 25%–50% if the patient is sedated.
2. Treat side effects such as nausea, vomiting, constipation, sedation, altered cognition, and pruritus.
3. Rotate the opioids if nausea, vomiting, altered cognition, myoclonus, or pruritus occurs.
4. Switch the route of administration if side effects persist.

Adjuvant Therapies for Pain in the Elderly

Several physical, environmental, psychological, and invasive techniques are available as either primary treatments or secondary options for those patients whose pain is unresponsive to medical treatment. Physical modalities, especially manual medicine (osteopathic, chiropractic, and physical therapy), acupuncture, and exercise all have some evidence of improvement in pain and function,[60] even in cancer pain. The evidence for TENS and ultrasound is not as strong.[60] Hypnosis can be useful in patients with event-specific pain. Relaxation techniques and guided imagery have been shown to improve patients' sense of control and decrease pain.[61] Invasive procedures such as neuromodulation, dorsal root entry zone lesioning, cordotomy, radiofrequency lesioning, intrathecal delivery systems, and implantable pumps may be used for those rare cases of unrelieved severe pain that is expected to last at least a few months.[62-65]

Issues Surrounding Concomitant Psychiatric Illness in the Elderly with Pain

Between 33% and 50% of patients requiring palliative care meet diagnostic criteria for a psychiatric disorder, yet up to half remain undiagnosed. The most common disorders are the dementias, anxiety, and depression.[66] Asking the patient "are you depressed" was found to be an adequate screening tool for depression.[67] Venlafaxine (Effexor®) may have fewer side effects than the tricyclic antidepressants while still providing effective treatment for depression and as an adjunct for pain management[42] or in palliative care.

KEY POINTS

- The elderly have pharmacological and nonpharmacological treatments available to them to adequately address the vast majority of their pain.
- Persistent pain is unlike acute pain in that acute pain is caused by a disease whereas chronic pain can become a disease.
- The key to successful control of pain in the elderly is to listen to the patient and to his/her caregivers, and then to help with ensuring that the therapeutic options used are safe.
- To control pain, ensure that therapy begins at low doses.
- Short-acting, less potent opioids are often good starting drugs.
- If short-acting opioids are effective, the guidelines recommend switching patients to long-acting opioids, reserving the short-acting opioids for breakthrough pain.
- Adjuvant drugs are useful in treating neuropathic pain. Such drugs as tricyclic antidepressants and anticonvulsants such as gabapentin (Neurontin®) and topiramate (Topamax®) are useful, assuming the patient can tolerate their anticholinergic and cardiovascular side effects.
- Remember that pain management is as frustrating for the elderly as it is for the clinician, especially when polypharmacy is involved.
- Anticipate side effects and keep channels of communication open with patients and their caregivers.
- Pain management in the elderly is a team effort and requires the active involvement of physicians, pharmacists, and nurses in both community and institutional settings.
- All patients have a fundamental right to adequate relief of pain.
- Nurses, physicians, pharmacists, and lay caregivers all have a role in ensuring a better quality of life for the elderly in pain.
- Pharmacists especially have a role in educating patients and their loved ones and caregivers, as well as community and institutional professionals, about the medications being used.
- Pharmacists are especially suited to recommend dosage forms and adjunct medications and to talk with patients about the outcomes of therapy.

REFERENCES

1. Herr KA, Garand L. Assessment and measurement of pain in older adults. *Clin Geriatr Med.* 2001;17(3):457–78.
2. Pain terms: a current list with definitions and notes on usage. Recommended by the IASP Subcommittee on Taxonomy. *Pain.* 1979;6(3):249–52.
3. Turk DC, Okifuji A. Pain terms and taxonomies of pain. In: Loeser JD, Butler SH, Chapman CR, et al., eds. *Bonica's Management of Pain.* 3rd ed. Philadelphia: Lippincott, Williams and Wilkins; 2001:17–25.
4. O'Brien T, Welsh J, Dunn FG. ABC of palliative care. Non-malignant conditions. *BMJ.* 1998;316(7127):286–9.
5. Davis MA, Ettinger WH, Neuhaus JM, et al. Knee osteoarthritis and physical functioning: evidence from the NHANES I epidemiologic followup study. *J Rheumatol.* 1991;18:591–8.
6. Mobily PR, Herr KA, Clark MK, et al. An epidemiologic analysis of pain in the elderly: The Iowa 65+ Rural Health Study. *J Aging Health.* 1994;6(2):139–54.
7. Bernabei R, Gambassi G, Lapane K, et al. Management of pain in elderly patients with cancer. SAGE Study Group. Systematic Assessment of Geriatric Drug Use via Epidemiology. *JAMA.* 1998;279(23):1877–82. Erratum in: *JAMA.* 1999;281(2):136.
8. McNeill JA, Sherwood GD, Starck PL. The hidden error of mismanaged pain: a systems approach. *J Pain Symptom Manage.* 2004;28(1):47–58.
9. Levy MH. Pain management in advanced cancer. *Semin Oncol.* 1985;12(4):394–410.
10. McCaffery M. Helping patients who deny pain. *Nursing.* 1999;29(10):14.
11. Ferrell BA. Pain management. *Clin Geriatr Med.* 2000;16(4):853–74.
12. Guidelines for Treatment of Pain in the Elderly. *J Am Geriatr Soc.* 2002;50(6 Suppl):S205–24.
13. American Medical Directors Association. *Chronic Pain Management in the Long-Term Care Setting.* Columbia, MD: American Medical Directors Association; 1999.
14. Simon LS, Lipman AG, Jacox AK, et al. *Pain in Osteoarthritis, Rheumatoid Arthritis, and Juvenile Chronic Arthritis.* Glenview, IL: American Pain Society (APS); 2002.
15. World Health Organization, Cancer Pain Relief and Palliative Care, Report of WHO Expert Committee. WHO Technical Report Series, Geneva: WHO; 1990.
16. Glajchen M. Chronic pain: treatment barriers and strategies for clinical practice. *J Am Board Fam Pract.* 2001;14(3):211–8.
17. Oneschuk D, Fainsinger R, Hanson J, et al. Assessment and knowledge in palliative care in second year family medicine residents. *J Pain Symptom Manage.* 1997;14(5):265–73.
18. Brunelli C, Costantini M, Di Giulo P, et al. Quality of life evaluation: when do terminal cancer patients and health-care providers agree? *J Pain Symptom Manage.* 1998;15(3):151–8.
19. Ferrell BR, Ferrell BA. Easing the pain. *Geriatr Nurs.* 1990;11(4):175–8.
20. Berry PH, Chapman CR, Covington EC, et al. *Pain: Current Understanding of Assessment, Management, and Treatments.* Reston, VA: National Pharmaceutical Council; 2001.
21. Green CR, Anderson KO, Baker TA, et al. The unequal burden of pain: confronting racial and ethnic disparities in pain. *Pain Med.* 2003;4(3):277–94.
22. Besson JM. The neurobiology of pain. *Lancet.* 1999;353(9164):1610–5.

23. Butler SF, Budman SH, Fernandez K, et al. Validation of a screener and opioid assessment measure for patients with chronic pain. *Pain.* 2004;112(1-2):65–75.
24. Parmelee PA. Pain in cognitively impaired older persons. *Clin Geriatr Med.* 1996; 12(3):473–87.
25. Closs SJ, Barr B, Briggs M, et al. A comparison of five pain assessment scales for nursing home residents with varying degrees of cognitive impairment. *J Pain Symptom Manage.* 2004;27(3):196–205.
26. Ahmedzai S. Current strategies for pain control. *Ann Oncol.* 1997;8(Suppl. 3): S21–S24.
27. Bellville JW, Forrest WH, Miller E, et al. Influence of age on pain relief from analgesics. A study of postoperative patients. *JAMA.* 1971;217(13):1835–41.
28. Beers MH. Explicit criteria for determining potentially inappropriate medication use by the elderly: an update. *Arch Intern Med.* 1997;157(14):1531–6.
29. Divoll M, Abernethy DR, Ameer B, et al. Acetaminophen kinetics in the elderly. *Clin Pharmacol Ther.* 1982;31(2):151–6.
30. Perneger TV, Whelton PK, Klag MJ. Risk of kidney failure associated with the use of acetaminophen, aspirin, and nonsteroidal anti-inflammatory drugs. *N Engl J Med.* 1994;331(25):1675–9.
31. Rochon PA, Fortin PR, Dear KB, et al. Reporting of age data in clinical trials of arthritis. Deficiencies and solutions. *Arch Intern Med.* 1993;153(2):243–8.
32. Griffin MR. Epidemiology of nonsteroidal anti-inflammatory drug-associated gastrointestinal injury. *Am J Med.* 1998;104(3A):23S–29S.
33. Ruoff GE. The impact of nonsteroidal anti-inflammatory drugs on hypertension: alternative analgesics for patients at risk. *Clin Ther.* 1998;20(3):376–87.
34. Doyle D, Hanks GWC, MacDonald N, eds. *Oxford Textbook of Palliative Medicine.* New York: Oxford University Press; 1993.
35. Passik SD, Kirsh KL. Probing the paradox of patients' satisfaction with inadequate pain management. *J Pain Symptom Manage.* 2002;24(4):361–3.
36. Savage S, Covington EC, Heit HA, et al. *Definitions Related to the Use of Opioids for the Treatment of Pain: A consensus document from the American Academy of Pain Medicine,* the American Pain Society and the American Society of Addiction Medicine. Glenview, IL: American Academy of Pain Medicine, the American Pain Society, and the American Society of Addiction Medicine; 2001.
37. Weissman DE, Haddox JD. Opioid pseudoaddiction—an iatrogenic syndrome. *Pain.* 1989;36(3):363–6.
38. Passik SD, Kirsh KL, Whitcomb L, et al. Pain clinicians' rankings of aberrant drug-taking behaviors. *J Pain Palliat Care Pharmacother.* 2002;16(4):39–49.
39. Waller A, Caroline NL. *Handbook of Palliative Care in Cancer.* 2nd ed. Boston: Butterworth-Heinemann; 2000:31.
40. Gill D, Hatcher S. Antidepressants for depression in medical illness. *Cochrane Database Syst Rev.* 2000;(4):CD001312.
41. Bowsher D. Postherpetic neuralgia and its treatment: a retrospective survey of 191 patients. *J Pain Symptom Manage.* 1996;12(5):290–9.
42. Mattia C, Paoletti F, Coluzzi F, et al. New antidepressants in the treatment of neuropathic pain. A review. *Minerva Anestesiol.* 2002;68(3):105–14.
43. McQuay HJ, Moore RA, Eccleston C, et al. Systematic review of outpatient services for chronic pain control. *Health Technol Assess.* 1997;1(6):i–iv, 1–135.

44. Gloth FM 3rd, Gundberg CM, Hollis BW, et al. Vitamin D deficiency in homebound elderly persons. *JAMA*. 1995;274(21):1683–6.

45. Clinical Pharmacology Drug Database, Gold Standard, 2005.

46. Alper BS, Lewis PR. Does treatment of acute herpes zoster prevent or shorten postherpetic neuralgia? *J Fam Pract*. 2000; 49(3):255–64.

47. Galer BS, Jensen MP, Ma T, et al. The lidocaine patch 5% effectively treats all neuropathic pain qualities: results of a randomized, double-blind, vehicle-controlled, 3-week efficacy study with use of the neuropathic pain scale. *Clin J Pain*. 2002;18(5): 297–301.

48. Dworkin RH, Schmader KE. Treatment and prevention of postherpetic neuralgia. *Clin Infect Dis*. 2003;36(7):877–82.

49. Goudas L, Carr DB, Bloch R, et al. *Management of Cancer Pain. Evidence Report/ Technology Assessment No. 35*. Rockville, MD: Agency for Healthcare Research and Quality; 2001:102. AHRQ Publication No. 02-E002.

50. Seidl LG, Thorton GF, Smith JW, et al. Studies on the epidemiology of adverse drug reactions: III. Reactions in patients on a general medical service. *Bulletin of The Johns Hopkins Hospital*. 1966;119:299–315.

51. Boreus L, Odar-Cederlof I, Bondesson U, et al. Elimination of meperidine and its metabolites in old patients compared to young patients. In: Foley K, Inturrisi C. *Opioid Analgesics in the Management of Cancer Pain, Advances in Pain Research & Therapy*, Vol. 8. New York: Raven Press; 1986:167–9.

52. Chou R, Clark E, Helfand M. Comparative efficacy and safety of long-acting oral opioids for chronic non-cancer pain: a systematic review. *J Pain Symptom Manage*. 2003;26(5):1026–48.

53. Forman WB. Opioid analgesic drugs in the elderly. *Clin Geriatr Med*. 1996;12(3): 489–500.

54. Baillie SP, Bateman DN, Coates PE, et al. Age and the pharmacokinetics of morphine. *Age Ageing*. 1989;18(4):258–62.

55. Hays H, Hagen N, Thirlwell M, et al. Comparative clinical efficacy and safety of immediate release and controlled release hydromorphone for chronic severe cancer pain. *Cancer*. 1994;74(6):1808–16.

56. Payne R, Mathias SD, Pasta DJ, et al. Quality of life and cancer pain: satisfaction and side effects with transdermal fentanyl versus oral morphine. *J Clin Oncol*. 1998;16(4): 1588–93.

57. Klinck JR, Lindop MJ. Epidural morphine in the elderly. A controlled trial after upper abdominal surgery. *Anaesthesia*. 1982;37(9):907–12.

58. Hanks GW. The clinical usefulness of agonist-antagonistic opioid analgesics in chronic pain. *Drug Alcohol Depend*. 1987;20(4):339–46.

59. Cherny N, Ripamonti C, Pereira J, et al. Strategies to manage the adverse effects of oral morphine: an evidence-based report. *J Clin Oncol*. 2001;19(9):2542–54.

60. Wright A, Sluka K. Nonpharmacological treatments for musculoskeletal pain. *Clin J Pain*. 2001;17(1):33–46.

61. Syrjala KL, Donaldson GW, Davis MW, et al. Relaxation and imagery and cognitive-behavioral training reduce pain during cancer treatment: a controlled clinical trial. *Pain*. 1995;63(2):189–98.

62. Falci S, Best L, Bayles R, et al. Dorsal root entry zone microcoagulation for spinal cord injury-related central pain: operative intramedullary electrophysiological guidance and clinical outcome. *J Neurosurg*. 2002;97(2 Suppl):193–200.

63. Jones B, Finlay I, Ray A, et al. Is there still a role for open cordotomy in cancer pain management? *J Pain Symptom Manage.* 2003;25(2):179–84.
64. Shah RV, Ericksen JJ, Lacerte M. Interventions in chronic pain management. 2. New frontiers: invasive nonsurgical interventions. *Arch Phys Med Rehabil.* 2003;84(3 Suppl 1):S39–44.
65. Wallace MS. Treatment options for refractory pain; the role of intrathecal therapy. *Neurology.* 2002;59(5 Suppl 2):S18–S24.
66. Ita D, Keorney M, O'Slorain L. Psychiatric disorder in a palliative care unit. *Palliat Med.* 2003;17(2):212–8.
67. Massie MJ, Holland JC. The cancer patient with pain: psychiatric complications and their management. *J Pain Symptom Manage.* 1992;7(2):99–109.

11

Nutrition and Exercise in the Elderly

Y. MONIQUE DAVIS-SMITH AND JOHN M. BOLTRI

All parts of the body if used in moderation and exercised in labors to which each are accustomed, become thereby healthy and well developed, and age slowly; but if unused and left idle, they become liable to disease, defective in growth, and age quickly.

—Hippocrates

OVERVIEW

Aging and good nutrition are presented as inseparable elements of a long life. Also covered in this chapter is how medications interact with food to affect the usefulness of the medication. Respiratory, musculoskeletal, cardiovascular, and central nervous system changes that occur with normal aging are discussed relative to their effect on chronic disease. Additionally, the demographic profiles of those who regularly exercise are discussed. Exercise itself is an investment in helping keep the body healthy so it is better able to stave off disease and to prevent any decline in the ability to defend against disease as a person ages or becomes inactive. The authors present several "prescriptions" to help the elderly patient live a healthier and longer life through appropriate exercise and attention to appropriate nutrition.

Ruth Smith is an 80-year-old widow with osteoarthritis and hypertension. During a follow-up visit for hypertension, she expresses concern about how her osteoarthritis affects her ability to maintain her activities of daily living. Specifically, she has trouble opening jars and turning door knobs due to pain and weakness in her hands. Further questioning discloses that she is also having some difficulty with gait and balance. Her blood pressure is controlled, and her fasting lipid profile, glucose, and cardiac function are normal. You prescribe an exercise program specifically designed to decrease her arthritic pain and fall risk, strengthen her muscles, and improve her gait and balance. In addition, you recommend the use of kitchen utensils designed to aid arthritic patients and suggest that she take calcium and vitamin D.

- What other steps could you suggest?
- What things might Ruth do for herself?

AGING AND NUTRITION

Longevity and quality of life are dependent on adequate nutrition. The elderly have special nutritional needs due to age and disease processes. Their lean body mass diminishes and body fat increases, leading to a decrease in energy needs.[1] The usual caloric needs for the elderly range from 1900 to 2400 calories a day, depending on the individual's level of activity. The daily protein requirement necessary for maintaining muscle mass for healthy elders is 0.8 to 1.0 g/kg. Fat consumption should remain at 30% of total caloric intake, fiber intake should be 25–30 g per day, and water intake should be six to eight glasses a day (Table 1).[2] The elderly food pyramid includes vitamin and mineral supplements due to a lower caloric need and a proportionally higher requirement for various vitamins and minerals. The Nutrition Screening Initiative (NSI) developed these recommendations based upon the food pyramid concept.[3]

Proper nutrition in the elderly increases disease resistance, hastens recovery from an acute illness, and improves outcome after surgical and medical interventions and trauma.[4] Aging is associated with physiological changes that impact nutrition. Many elderly experience an age-related decline in their perception of taste and smell, and many have difficulty with chewing and swallowing. It is essential for physicians to evaluate the nutritional

Table 1   Daily nutrition guide for older adults

Liquids	6–8 glasses
Grains	4–8 or more servings
Fruits	2–4 servings
Vegetables	2–5 servings
Meat	2–3 servings
Dairy	2–4 servings
Fats	1–3 servings
Dietary supplements:	calcium 1200 mg
	vitamin D 400 IU

status of their elderly patients. This evaluation should include a review of dietary habits, medication use, chronic illness, and social history.[5]

Social isolation is a common problem for seniors that negatively impacts nutritional status. At least 10% to 20% of widows and widowers have clinically significant depression during the first years of bereavement. This can significantly affect the elder's nutritional status.[6] The special diets required by chronic conditions (e.g., hypertension, diabetes, and renal disease) may take extra effort to prepare and may cost more. The elderly with conditions like these who lack motivation, knowledge, adequate income, or skill are more likely to make poor dietary choices.[7] Also, some of the medications taken by elderly patients may alter taste, cause gastrointestinal discomfort, or interfere with nutrient absorption (Table 2).

The physician should assess, diagnose, and treat conditions associated with or contributing to poor nutritional status, making recommendations or referring the patient to a registered dietitian when necessary. Body mass index (BMI) is a validated measure of over/under/normal weight. The recommended BMI range in the elderly is 22–27. Serum albumin is a nonspecific indicator of poor nutritional status and is associated with increased morbidity and mortality when less than 3.5 g/dL. Another indicator of poor nutritional status is a sharp decline in the cholesterol level. It is also beneficial for the physician to use a Functional Health Status Assessment Tool and Activities of Daily Living measurement when evaluating the nutritional status of the elderly patient.[8]

DEMOGRAPHICS

By 2030, approximately 70 million Americans will be more than 65 years of age.[9] This age group will represent 20% of the population, a majority of

Table 2   Chronic illness medications and their effects on nutrition[a]

Chronic Obstructive Pulmonary Disease
  Theophylline derivatives: anorexia, nausea
  Cromolyn: anorexia, nausea
  Corticosteroids: increased appetite, bone demineralization, wasting of lean muscle mass
Congestive Heart Failure
  Diuretics: electrolyte abnormalities
  Digitalis: anorexia, nausea
Coronary Heart Disease
  Statins: elevated liver enzymes
  Niacin: gastrointestinal distress
Dementia
  Cholinesterase inhibitors: nausea, diarrhea, anorexia
  Anticholinergics: dry mouth, delayed gastric emptying, constipation
  Antidepressants: alteration of appetite
Diabetes Mellitus
  Insulin: hypoglycemia
  Sulfonylureas: epigastric fullness, heartburn, nausea
  Biguanides: anorexia, diarrhea
  Alpha glucose inhibitors: flatulence, diarrhea

[a] From Reference 3.

whom will be women. Although there is often a decrease in physical activity associated with aging, the concept of a decrease in habitual activity being a normal part of the aging process is debatable. There is, however, cultural reinforcement to the idea that physical activity should diminish with aging.[10] In both developed and undeveloped societies, senior citizens are encouraged to "take it easy," retire, or pass responsibility on to younger adults. For a variety of reasons, organized sporting activities infrequently include the senior population.

Physical inactivity is one of the leading causes of premature death in the United States.[11] Physical fitness is directly related to physical activity, with the more physically active elders being more physically fit. Fitness appears to be a better predictor of longevity than body weight, with the lowest death rates observed in people with the highest fitness levels.[12] Even among frail and very old adults, physical activity improves mobility and functioning.[13] Older people who exercise daily have better balance and are less likely to fall than those who do not exercise.[14] The CDC and American College of Sports Medicine recommend that adults engage in a moderate intensity

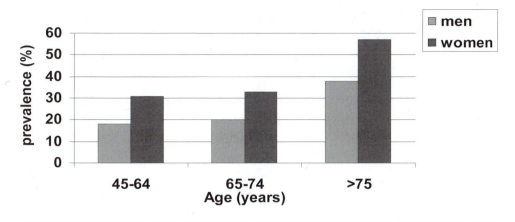

Figure 1   Prevalence of physical inactivity among the elderly. (Data from the Third National Health and Nutrition Examination Survey, 1988 to 1994. Adapted from Reference 19.)

activity (e.g., walking 3–4 mph) for at least 30 minutes per day on most, preferably all, days.[15] Regular physical activity in the elderly is associated with improved health, reduced disease-specific risk, reduced age-related morbidity, increased functional capacity, increased independence, and increased quality of life.[16,17] Even when initiated late in life, physical activity can reverse the age-related declines in maximal aerobic capacity (VO_2max) and reduce both disease-specific morbidity and all-cause mortality.[18]

The prevalence of physical inactivity, defined as less than 30 minutes of moderate exercise on most days, increases with age. In all age groups, women are less active than men (Figure 1).[19] For senior citizens, age, ethnicity, income, fear of crime, and chronic disease can impact confidence and ability to exercise.[20] Four out of five individuals older than age 65 have at least one chronic health condition, and 20% have a chronic disability.[21] Even though increased physical activity carries some risk, the benefits of exercise outweigh the risk of inactivity in most elderly.

Regular exercise, a minimum of 30 minutes of moderate activity on most days, can reduce mortality as well as facilitate opportunities for social interactions and enhance one's sense of well-being.[22] Exercise programs may also lead to social interactions that provide the emotional and physical support that helps seniors remain active in the community and reduces the need for formal health care services.[23] Among older adults who engage in regular physical activity, 42% exercise both for the enjoyment and for the physical benefits of the activity.[24] Walking and gardening are the most prevalent forms of physical activity among adults 65 years or older in the United States.

Table 3 Physiologic changes associated with aging that affect physical activity[a]

System	Effect of Aging	Physiologic Outcome	Effect of Exercise
Cardiovascular	↓ cardiac output ↑ blood pressure ↓ maximal heart rate ↓ oxygen-carrying capacity	↓ aerobic capacity (VO_2max) ↑ cardiovascular risk ↓ maximal work capacity	Weight control; reduced blood pressure; reduced risk of developing diabetes.
Respiratory	↓ vital capacity	↓ respiratory efficiency	Enhanced work performance capabilities.
Musculoskeletal	↓ muscle mass and strength ↓ bone density ↓ synovial fluid viscosity ↓ in height	↓ ability to perform independent activities of daily living ↑ fracture risk ↑ risk of musculoskeletal injury	Promotion of bone, muscle, and joint health.
Central nervous system	↓ number of motor neurons ↑ reaction time	↓ neuromuscular efficiency ↑ risk of injury	Improved self-esteem; reduced risk of falling; reduced depression and anxiety.

[a] Adapted from Reference 25.

PHYSIOLOGIC CHANGES ASSOCIATED WITH AGING

Although there are normal physiological changes associated with aging, "healthy old age" is not an oxymoron. In the absence of disease, the normal decline of the physical condition associated with aging generally imposes few restrictions on activities of daily living regardless of age. However, as individuals age, they are more likely to suffer from disabilities, diseases, and the side effects of medications. Aging is typically characterized by a progressive loss of muscle and bone mass, strength, cardiovascular capacity, and flexibility (Table 3).[25] Between the ages of 65 and 85 there is an annual loss of 1% to 2% in muscle strength and 3% to 4% in power.[26] These changes are attributed to sarcopenia, or muscle wasting. Exercise levels commonly decline with age because of chronic medical conditions and physical activity–limiting illnesses.[27] Therefore, there is a wide range of physical capabilities and limitations in the elderly. When considering physical activity, it is useful to categorize senior adults into two groups, those who are apparently healthy

Table 4 Physical capabilities of the elderly[a]

Apparently Healthy	Has Chronic Illness
No significant limitations on physical activity	Has at least one underlying medical condition that influences physical capabilities
Requires no assistance performing activities of daily living	Changes in activity level require special consideration

[a] Available at http://www.sgcard.org/pp/elderly.html (accessed April 25, 2005).

and those who have chronic illness (Table 4). An exercise prescription for a healthy elder will be markedly different from one for an elder with a chronic illness. Physicians should evaluate the effects of specific chronic illnesses on the elder's ability to exercise.

Cardiovascular

It is difficult to distinguish between normal aging and the pathology that develops with inactivity. Autopsy studies show that as many as 60%–70% of older subjects have some evidence of coronary vascular disease.[28] Although the maximal heart rate decreases with age, stroke volume is generally well maintained. Due to an increase in afterload (decreased compliance of the great vessels), the elderly do not increase their cardiac output with exercise as well as younger people. A reduction in exercise capacity can occur due to reduced arterial O_2 content. The reduction in arterial O_2 content may occur due to anemia (poor diet, B_{12} deficiency, gastrointestinal bleeding), altered peripheral distribution of the available cardiac output, and chronic chest diseases that lead to a decrease in pulmonary diffusing capacity. With aging, there is an increased prevalence of episodic orthostatic hypotension and a progressive increase in systolic pressures at rest as well as during exercise. These factors should be considered when developing an exercise plan.

Respiratory

Respiratory function in the elderly is often altered by kyphosis, ankylosis of the joints in the rib cage, and weakness of abdominal wall muscles. There is a progressive decline in the ciliary function of the bronchial tree and an increased risk for aspiration, thereby increasing the risk of pulmonary infection in the aging population. Pulmonary compliance increases slightly, decreasing the PaO_2, as elastic tissue is progressively lost. In spite of this, respiratory function appears to remain adequate for the needs of exercise in most elderly.[29]

Musculoskeletal

Rheumatic complaints in one or more joints are common in the elderly. In almost one-fourth of the senior population with rheumatic complaints, there is moderate-to-severe limitation of daily activities.[30] Osteoarthritis is the most common form of arthritis, with more than 80% of 60-year-olds having some form of this disease. Genetics, previous acute joint disease, and metabolic disorders may accelerate the rate of joint degeneration. Much of the disability associated with osteoarthritis is probably secondary to deconditioning, muscle weakness, and joint degeneration. Several studies have demonstrated the value of physical therapy and specific exercise programs, particularly aquatic therapy, for treatment of persons with established arthritis.[31,32] In addition to overuse and trauma, important contributing factors to osteoarthritis and the effects on the musculoskeletal system are being overweight and obesity.

Some of the functional consequences of aging are:

- Decreased range of motion.
- Stiffening or "gelling" of the arthritic joint after a period of immobility.
- Loss of stability, particularly at the knee joint.

Aging is also associated with a progressive decrease in standing height, principally as a result of a change in structure of the intervertebral disks. With aging, the nucleus pulposus of the disks is compressed or collapses. Osteoporosis, weakening of the muscles of the back, and osteoarthritis of the vertebral joints are other factors that increase kyphosis in the elderly. Senescence is associated with a progressive loss of both minerals and matrix from the bones. Predisposition to hip fractures in older individuals is due to a progressive loss of both trabecular and compact bone. Strains, sprains, and tendon rupture can occur as a result of loss of resilience in collagen and bone.

Sarcopenia, muscle wasting that impedes the frail elder's ability to undertake activities of daily living, is a major factor leading to deterioration in the quality of life for affected individuals. Muscle atrophy is associated with a decrease in lean muscle mass. There is a decrease in muscle fiber size and number. Decreased habitual physical activity and aging contribute to the total loss of muscle tissue. Conversely, regular sustained physical activity can help decrease muscle and bone wasting.

Central Nervous System

Many aspects of memory, cognition, and information processing deteriorate with age.[33] Factors contributing to poor cerebral performance include depression, poor literacy, Alzheimer's disease, medications, and cardiovascular disease. Sleep patterns are also altered with the aging process, with deep, slow-wave sleep being replaced by shallow, stage 2 sleep. Several reports have suggested that regular exercise can enhance cerebral function in the elderly, but the explanation for this phenomenon is uncertain.[34,35] It is known that regular sustained exercise increases endorphins, dopamine, and catecholamine. As a result, regular physical activity may lessen anxiety and depression, increase self-esteem, and increase one's attention span.

ADVANTAGES OF EXERCISE FOR THE ELDERLY

Regularly active elderly persons have a 20% higher functional level than their sedentary counterparts.[36] The elderly who exercise also appear to have an improved quality of life due to improved physical functioning and enhanced psychological well-being. Exercise is one of the few interventions that can restore loss of physiologic capacity.[37] Regular exercise contributes to both mobility and independence by preserving skeletal muscle strength, aerobic capacity, and bone density. Aerobic exercise training improves the ability of aging skeletal tissue to resist injury.[38] Exercise also enhances balance, reaction time, and coordination.

EXERCISE, DISEASE MANAGEMENT, AND DISEASE PREVENTION

For Diabetes

Regular exercise can lead to improved glucose tolerance in persons of any age who have diabetes or impaired glucose tolerance. Although glucose tolerance decreases with age, moderate-intensity aerobic training has a favorable effect on glucose tolerance and may lead to an improvement in diabetes control and a decreased requirement for medications. Regular exercise may also help delay or prevent the onset of diabetes in persons with prediabetes. This effect can reduce the development of diabetes and help to control blood glucose levels.[39] Physicians should keep in mind that, to prevent a hypoglycemic event, patients medicated with insulin and oral hypoglycemic agents may need to decrease their medication doses based on the amount of exercise.

For Cardiovascular Disease

Regular exercise decreases obesity risk and therefore cardiovascular risk as well as decreasing circulating triglycerides and increasing high-density lipoprotein cholesterol. Low-intensity aerobic training significantly reduces blood pressure in the elderly who take medication for hypertension. Blood pressure decreases significantly after 3 months of regular physical activity and stabilizes at a lower level by the end of 9 months of sustained training.[40] Persons taking beta-blockers cannot be monitored by the target heart rate method for endurance intensity because of the tendency of this medication to reduce the heart rate. Such patients can be monitored using the talk test described in the section *Guidelines for Activity Prescriptions*. Medications that cause orthostatic hypotension should be used with caution in order to avoid exacerbation of orthostasis caused by fluid loss during exercise. Patients taking blood pressure medications who begin a sustained exercise program may need a reduction in their medication to prevent hypotension; such patients should be monitored carefully.

For Musculoskeletal Changes

An exercise program with weight-bearing exercise at moderate intensity and gait training is highly effective in offsetting the decline in bone mineral density and has a positive effect on postural stability.[41,42] Exercise, combined with home hazard modifications and vision correction, reduces the number of at-home falls among the elderly.[43] The impact of exercise on falls in the elderly is primarily due to improved balance.[44]

PREEXERCISE EVALUATION

Primary care physicians are cognizant of the ramifications of physical inactivity. Diabetes, hypertension, coronary artery disease, hyperlipidemia, obesity, and depression are linked with physical inactivity. Most primary care physicians would like to incorporate counseling about physical activity into their daily practice; however, time constraints, lack of skills, and inadequate reimbursement limit the ability to do so consistently and effectively. There are, however, physician office visits that offer the opportunity for a physical activity assessment:

- During the annual physical.
- At the time of diagnosis or management of a chronic disease (hypertension, diabetes).
- During the evaluation for a fall or fracture.

Brief written questionnaires can also effectively assess physical activity. The authors use the following question as part of an annual health assessment of adults; "On average, how many days per week do you exercise for at least 30 minutes?" Answer choices are: none, 1 or 2 days, 3 or 4 days, 5 or 6 days, or daily.

During a physical activity assessment, the patient should be asked about any physical activity during the past week. The provider should identify if the patient performs 30 minutes of moderate activity on most days of the week and whether the patient engages in lifestyle activities such as taking the stairs instead of the elevator or choosing a parking space distant from the entrance of a building. The patient's sedentary time (watching TV, talking on the phone, using the computer) should be described. Physicians should take time to evaluate the patient's level of knowledge about the risk and benefits of exercise and explore any perceived barriers to exercise.

In individuals with unstable cardiac disease, the risk of exercise may outweigh the potential benefits. For this reason, an accurate history and physical examination are necessary to make the clinical decision to have the patient undergo exercise stress testing or additional cardiac evaluation prior to initiating a program of regular physical activity. Indications and contraindications for clinical exercise testing are noted in Table 5. Some patients may be appropriately referred to a cardiac or pulmonary rehabilitation program. Rehabilitation programs may be beneficial for the frail elder and for those who have recently experienced a newly diagnosed or an exacerbation of a chronic pulmonary or cardiac illness.

Regardless of their health status, all elderly individuals should have medical clearance from a physician prior to initiating a new program of physical activity. This evaluation should focus on cardiovascular risk factors, physical and mental limitations, and other signs and symptoms that may be worsened by exercise or inactivity (Figure 2). Based on the patient's medical history, physical exam, and the type of exercise program the patient is planning to begin, an exercise stress test may be a necessary step in the evaluation. However, most healthy elderly patients can initiate a moderate activity program without a stress test. Moderate physical activity is described in Table 6. Elderly patients should be counseled to seek medical attention if they experience any chest pain, palpitations, undue dyspnea, fatigue, or lightheadedness during exercise.[45] Patients with pulmonary disease should be counseled on the use of their peak flow meter and have their pulmonary disease maximally controlled with appropriate medical therapy prior to initiating an exercise program.

Table 5   Clinical exercise testing indications and contraindications[a]

Indications

Evaluation of patients with suspected coronary artery disease.
   Typical angina pectoris.
   Atypical angina pectoris.

Evaluation of patients with known coronary artery disease.
   Following myocardial infarction.
   Following therapeutic intervention.

Screening of healthy, asymptomatic patients.
   Individuals in high-risk occupations (e.g., pilots, law enforcement officers).
   Men older than 40 and women older than 50 who are sedentary and plan to initiate a vigorous
      exercise program.
   Individuals who are identified as being at risk based on multiple cardiac risk factors or
      concurrent chronic diseases.

Evaluation of exercise capacity in patients with valvular heart disease (excluding severe aortic
   stenosis).
Evaluation of patients with cardiac rhythm disorders.
Evaluation of exercise-induced arrhythmia and response to treatment.
Evaluation of rate-adaptive pacemaker setting.

Contraindications
Absolute contraindications

Recent myocardial infarction.
Unstable angina.
Acute myocarditis/pericarditis.
Acute systemic infection.
Symptomatic heart failure.
Symptomatic aortic stenosis.

Relative contraindications

Severe hypertension (uncontrolled).
Persistent arrhythmias (poorly controlled).
Obstructive cardiomyopathy.
Uncontrolled diabetes or thyroid disease.
Systemic neuromuscular, musculoskeletal, or rheumatologic disease that limits the patient's
   ability to exercise.
Heart block (2nd or 3rd degree atrioventricular block).
Stenotic valvular heart disease.
Undifferentiated electrolyte abnormalities (e.g., hypokalemia, hypomagnesemia).

---

[a]   From American College of Sports Medicine; Franklin BA, Whaley MH, Howley ET, et al., eds. *ACSM's Guidelines for Exercise Testing and Prescription.* 6th ed. Philadelphia, Pa: Lippincott Williams & Wilkins; 2000; and Gibbons RJ, Balady GJ, Beasley JW, et al. ACC/AHA guidelines for exercise testing. A report of the American College of Cardiology/ American Heart Association Task Force on Practice Guidelines [Committee on Exercise Testing]. *JACC.* 1997:260–315.

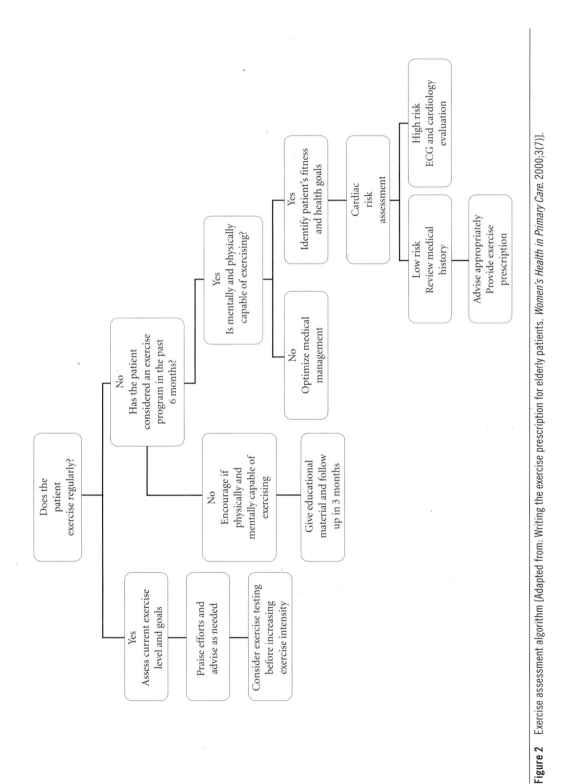

Figure 2 Exercise assessment algorithm [Adapted from: Writing the exercise prescription for elderly patients. *Women's Health in Primary Care.* 2000;3(7)].

Table 6 Activity level [a]

Light-Intensity Activities
Less than 3.0 metabolic equivalents (METS)
Less than 3.5 kcal/minute
60 minutes
    Walking slowly
    Golf, powered cart
    Swimming, slow treading
    Gardening or pruning
    Bicycling, very light effort
    Dusting or vacuuming
    Conditioning exercise, light stretching or warm-up

Moderate-Intensity Activities
3.0–6.0 METS
3.5–7 kcal/minute
30 minutes
    Walking slowly
    Aerobics (water aerobics and aerobic dancing)
    Dancing
    Team sports (softball, basketball, etc.)
    Putting groceries away
    Golf, pulling or carrying clubs
    Swimming, recreational
    Mowing a lawn, power motor
    Tennis, doubles
    Bicycling 5–9 mph, level terrain, or with a few hills
    Scrubbing floors or washing windows
    Weight lifting, Nautilus machines or free weights

Vigorous Activities
Greater than 6.0 METS
More than 7 kcal/minute
20 minutes
    Racewalking, jogging, or running
    Swimming laps
    Mowing lawn, hand mower
    Tennis, singles
    Bicycling more than 10 mph, or on steep uphill terrain
    Moving or pushing furniture
    Very competitive sports (football, soccer, etc.)
    Circuit training
    Backpacking

[a] From Reference 48.

ACTIVITY PRESCRIPTIONS FOR ELDERLY PATIENTS

Many primary care physicians admit that they rarely discuss exercise regimens with their patients.[46] Most health care providers receive minimal formal training in strategies for discussing the benefits of exercise, tailoring exercise programs to meet individual needs, or facilitating adherence to an exercise regimen.

Exercise History

Assess the patient's life-history of physical activity and interest. Elderly persons who have previously been active are more likely to maintain an exercise program than are those who have never been active. During this visit, the provider might also evaluate the person's musculoskeletal injury history as well as the amount of time the patient is sedentary. The discussion should be tailored to the patient's medical conditions.

Current Activity Level

Assessment of the patient's past 2 months of activity will aid in tailoring the initial exercise program to the patient's current level of fitness. The patient's concerns about exercise should be discussed, including perceived barriers to exercise, fear, and lack of time. The physician should help the patient learn to incorporate exercise into daily living.

Level of Interest and Social Preferences

Patients involved in the development of their own exercise regimen will be more likely to adhere to that regimen. Some patients prefer to exercise in a group or in a club setting, whereas others prefer to exercise alone or at home. Many elderly people lead very lonely lives. Group exercise programs may offer an opportunity to increase the social contacts for an elderly patient. The literature does support an interaction between physical activity and social functioning. The regular exerciser can anticipate an increase in the social contacts that are often lacking in a senior's life.

Guidelines for Activity Prescriptions

The three main components of an activity regimen for elderly patients are:[47]

- Cardiovascular conditioning.
- Muscular conditioning.
- Balance and flexibility training.

Elderly patients generally prefer moderate intensity activity.[48] Target heart rates can be utilized to determine the appropriate intensity of activity (maximum heart rate = 220 – patient age). The talk test is easier for elderly patients to use because it does not require the heart rate to be monitored. It is also useful for individuals who are beginning an activity program or are fearful of excessive exertion.[49] Advise patients to exercise to a level where they are able to have a conversation without experiencing undue breathlessness. Some patients who use the talk test may fail to achieve the level of intensity required to improve cardiovascular fitness. Such patients can use the talk-sing test, exercising at a level where he or she can comfortably talk but would be unable to sing. Another way to monitor exercise intensity is the Borg scale of perceived exertion. It is based on a linear relationship between heart rate and the level of perceived physical exertion.[50]

KEY POINTS

- Helping the elderly understand that nutrition and exercise contribute to their health and well-being is a responsibility of all their caregivers and health professionals.
- The nutritional and exercise status of the elderly can be ascertained easily during a routine conversation with a caring health professional.
- Nutritional status can be adversely affected by social isolation, declining sense of taste, and medication side effects.
- Age-related decline in exercise can be addressed by exploring the patient's medical problems, past history of exercise, and motivation.
- The clinician can provide specific nutrition and exercise advice, tailored to the situation, that can help elders live longer and have a better quality of life.

REFERENCES

1. Lorefalt B, Wissing U, Unosson M. Smaller but energy and protein-enriched meals improve energy and nutrient intakes in elderly patients. *J Nutr Health Aging.* 2005; 9(4):243–7.
2. Bidlack WR, Smith CH. Nutritional requirements of the aged. *Crit Rev Food Sci Nutr.* 1988;27(3):189–218.
3. A physician's guide to nutrition in chronic disease management for older adults. Available at: http://www.aafp.org/nsi (accessed May 5, 2005).
4. Position of the American Dietetic Association: cost-effectiveness of medical nutrition therapy. *J Am Diet Assoc.* 1995;95(1):88–91.

5. Evans WJ. Exercise and nutritional needs of elderly people: effects on muscle and bone. *Gerontology.* 1998;15(1):15–24.
6. Ferry M, Sidobre B, Lambertin A, et al. The SOLINUT study: analysis of the interaction between nutrition and loneliness in persons aged over 70 years. *J Nutr Health Aging.* 2005;9(4):261–8.
7. Callen BL, Wells TJ. Screening for nutritional risk in community-dwelling old. *Public Health Nurs.* 2005;22(2):138–46.
8. Berner YN. Assessment tools for nutritional status in the elderly. *Isr Med Assoc J.* 2003;5(5):365–7.
9. AARP. National Blueprint. *Increasing Physical Activity among Adults Age 50 and Older.* Princeton, NJ: Robert Wood Johnson Foundation; 2001.
10. Shephard RJ, Rode A. *The Health Consequences of "Modernization": Evidence from Circumpolar Peoples.* New York: Cambridge University Press; 1996.
11. McGinnis JM, Foege WH. Actual causes of death in the United States. *JAMA.* 1993; 270(18):207–12.
12. Talbot LA, Morrell CH, Metter J, et al. Comparison of cardiorespiratory fitness versus leisure time physical activity as predictors of coronary events in men aged < or = 65 years and > 65 years. *Am J Cardiol.* 2002;89(10):1187–92.
13. van der Bij AK, Laurant MG, Wensing M. Effectiveness of physical activity interventions for older adults: a review. *Am J Prev Med.* 2002;22(2):120–33.
14. Gillespie LD, Gillespie WJ, Robertson MC, et al. Interventions for preventing falls in elderly people. *Cochrane Database Syst Rev.* 2003;(4):CD000340.
15. Increasing physical activity: A report on recommendations of the Task Force on Community Preventive Services. *MMWR Recomm Rep.* 2001;50(RR-18)1–14. Available at: http://www.cdc.gov/mmwr/preview/mmwrhtml/rr5018a1.htm.
16. Kahn EB, Ramsey LT, Brownson RC, et al. The effectiveness of interventions to increase physical activity. A systematic review. *Am J Prev Med.* 2002;22(4 Suppl):73–107.
17. Physical Activity and Older Americans: Benefits and Strategies. June 2002. Agency for Healthcare Research and Quality and the Centers for Disease Control and Prevention. Available at: http://www.ahrq.gov/ppip/activity.htm (accessed May 5, 2005).
18. Fiatarone MA, Marks EC, Ryan ND, et al. High-intensity strength training in nonagenarians. Effects on skeletal muscle. *JAMA.* 1990;263(22):3029–34.
19. Christmas C, Andersen RA. Exercise and older patients: guidelines for the clinician. *J Am Geriatr Soc.* 2000;48(3):318–24.
20. Clark DO, Nothwehr F. Exercise self-efficacy and its correlates among socioeconomically disadvantaged older adults. *Health Educ Behav.* 1999;26(4):535–46.
21. Singh MA. Exercise and aging. *Clin Geriatr Med.* 2004;20(2):201–21.
22. Bean JF, Vora A, Frontera WR. Benefits of exercise for community-dwelling older adults. *Arch Phys Med Rehabil.* 2004;85(7 Suppl 3):S31–42; quiz S43–4.
23. Schechtman KB, Ory MG. The effects of exercise on the quality of life of frail older adults: a preplanned meta-analysis of the FICSIT trials. *Ann Behav Med.* 2001;23(3), 186–97.
24. National Center for Health Statistics. *Health, United States, 1999.* Data from the National Health Interview Survey.
25. Barry HC, Eathorne SW. Exercise and aging. Issues for the practitioner. *Med Clin North Am.* 1994;78(2):357–76.
26. Kirkendall DT, Garrett WE Jr. The effects of aging and training on skeletal muscle. *Am J Sports Med.* 1998;26(4):598–602.

27. Evans WJ. What is sarcopenia? *J Gerontol A Biol Sci Med Sci.* 1995 Nov;50 Spec No: 5–8.
28. Elveback L, Lie JT. Continued high incidence of coronary artery disease at autopsy in Olmsted County, Minnesota, 1950 to 1979. *Circulation.* 1984;70(3):345–9.
29. Babcock MA; Paterson DH, Cunningham DA, et al. Exercise on-transient gas exchange kinetics are slowed as a function of age. *Med Sci Sports Exerc.* 1994;26(4):440–6.
30. Pullar T, Wright V. Disease of the joints. In: Pathy MSJ, ed. *Principles and Practices of Geriatric Medicine.* 2nd ed. New York: John Wiley and Sons; 1991:1237–74.
31. Misner JE, Massey BH, Bemben MG, et al. Long-term effects of exercise on the range of motion of aging women. *J Orthop Sports Phys Ther.* 1992;16(1):37–42.
32. Hopkins DR, Murrah B, Hoeger WW, et al. Effect of low impact aerobic dance on the functional fitness of elderly women. *Gerontologist.* 1990;30(2):189–92.
33. Spirduso WW. *Physical Dimensions of Aging.* Champaign, IL: Human Kinetics; 1995.
34. Dustman RE, Emmerson R, Shearer D. Physical activity, age, and cognitive neuro-psychological function. *J Aging Phys Act.* 1994;2:143–81.
35. Whitehurst M. Reaction time unchanged in older women following aerobic training. *Percept Mot Skills.* 1991;72(1):251–6.
36. Shephard RJ. Fitness and aging. In: Blais C, ed. *Aging into the Twenty First Century.* Downsview, ON: Captus University Publications; 1991:22–35.
37. Westerterp KR. Daily physical activity and aging. *Curr Opin Clin Nutr Metab Care.* 2000;3(6):485–8.
38. Elward K, Larson EB. Benefits of exercise for older adults. A review of existing evidence and current recommendations for the general population. *Clin Geriatr Med.* 1992;8(1):35–50.
39. DiPietro L, Seeman TE, Stachenfeld NS, et al. Moderate-intensity aerobic training improves glucose tolerance in aging independent of abdominal adiposity. *J Am Geriatr Soc.* 1998;46(7):875–9.
40. Motoyama M, Sunami Y, Kinoshita F, et al. Blood pressure lowering effect of low intensity aerobic training in elderly hypertensive patients. *Med Sci Sports Exerc.* 1998;30(6):818–23.
41. Snow CM, Shaw JM, Winters KM, et al. Long-term exercise using weighted vest prevents hip bone loss in postmenopausal women. *J Gerontol A Biol Sci Med Sci.* 2000; 55(9):M489–91.
42. Welsh L, Rutherford OM. Hip bone mineral density is improved by high-impact aerobic exercise in postmenopausal women and men over 50 years. *Eur J Appl Physiol Occup Physiol.* 1996;74(6):511–7.
43. Province MA, Hadley EC, Hombrook MC, et al. The effects of exercise on falls in elderly patients. A preplanned meta-analysis of the FICSIT Trials. Frailty and Injuries: Cooperative Studies of Intervention Techniques. *JAMA.* 1995;273(17):1341–7.
44. Li F, Fisher KJ, Harmer P, et al. Delineating the impact of Tai Chi training on physical function among the elderly. *Am J Prev Med.* 2002;23(2 Suppl):92–7.
45. American College of Sports Medicine Position Stand. Exercise and physical activity for older adults. *Med Sci Sports Exerc.* 1998;30(6):992–1008.
46. Wee CC, McCarthy EP, Davis RB, et al. Physician counseling about exercise. *JAMA.* 1999;282(16):1583–8.
47. Mazzeo RS, Tanaka H. Exercise prescription for the elderly: current recommendations. *Sports Med.* 2001;31(11)809–18.

48. U.S. Department of Health and Human Services. Physical Activity and Health: A Report of the Surgeon General. Atlanta, GA: U.S. Department of Health and Human Services, Centers for Disease Control and Prevention, National Center for Chronic Disease Prevention and Health Promotion; 1996.

49. Persinger R, Foster C, Gibson M, et al. Consistency of the talk test for exercise prescription. *Med Sci Sports Exerc.* 2004;36(9):1632–6.

50. Dawes HN, Barker KL, Cockburn, J, et al. Borg's rating of perceived exertion scales: Do the verbal anchors mean the same for different clinical groups? *Arch Phys Med Rehabil.* 2005;86(5):912–6.

12

Natural Medicines Used by the Elderly: A Common Sense Dose of Reality

ALAN C. MCKELVEY

A person should not be making decisions about what dose of herbal supplements to take any more than he or she should decide what dose of penicillin to take.

—**Kathy Golden**

OVERVIEW

This chapter offers a comprehensive introduction to the most common natural products used by the elderly and the significance of these products in the armamentarium of their health care. To help health professionals better understand the need for increased patient–practitioner dialogue on these products, which are often deemed harmless or innocuous, 20 of the most popular natural products are presented in some detail. The demographics relative to users of these products are also presented in order to help focus the health professional's attention on the cultural influences, beliefs and attitudes, and use of natural products in those over 65 years of age. The goal of this chapter is to help health professionals realize that most elderly patients will never talk about their use of herbal medications until the health professionals they see become proactive and initiate such dialogue.

Steven McNeal, RPh, lives in a small suburb of a large, urban metropolis in the Midwest, where he took over a community pharmacy from its owner of 22 years. He has now been at this pharmacy for 4 years and has slowly won the acceptance of the locals. One morning, John Abbott comes into the pharmacy to pick up his refills and talk to Pharmacist McNeal. John suffered a mild stroke (transient ischemic attack, or TIA) several months ago and has since had a stent placed in his heart. Because he is an at-risk patient, John is taking ticlopidine 250 mg BID, and the calcium channel blocker verapamil, 40 mg TID, for control of his blood pressure and slightly irregular heartbeat.

Now, as he's picking up his prescriptions, John tells Pharmacist McNeal that he'd had some memory loss after the stroke but has been taking ginkgo biloba for 2 months and believes it has helped his memory. In addition, he has been making a concerted effort to eat healthier and has been drinking two glasses of grapefruit juice daily, one in the morning and one in the evening. Concerned at this revelation, the pharmacist next asks if he had told his doctor that he was taking ginkgo and drinking grapefruit juice regularly. John replies that he hasn't told his doctor, that issues of memory loss and trying to have a healthy lifestyle were not things he'd talked to a doctor about. He just had to take control of his own health.

This scenario raises a number of concerns and questions, such as:

- When older patients are at risk for stroke, what medical readings or kinds of education about natural products do they receive or are they directed to?
- What is the likelihood that the elderly are spending their money on natural products that are not indicated for their conditions or that could be dangerous?
- Is the use of natural products more prevalent among individuals who come from societies where natural products are primarily used?
- What are the principal medical conditions for which older patients use natural products?
- How can members of the health care team best obtain from their patients information about their use of natural product and nonprescription drugs?
- How does the Internet affect an older American's ability to acquire relevant, correct, and applicable information about nonprescription drugs and natural products?

- Since elderly patients tend to look for relief from symptoms and not necessarily a cure from disease, what can a clinician expect to find regarding the taking of nonprescription or natural products by seniors?

REGULATORY ISSUES

Many people are familiar with the Norman Rockwell painting of an elderly depression-era pharmacist compounding a liquid cough medicine for a sick child. In those days, it would have been difficult to find any compounding recipe that did not call for at least one natural product. With the introduction of "modern pharmaceuticals" throughout the 1940s, 1950s, and 1960s, the use of natural products was largely abandoned in the United States, as were the regulatory controls over natural products that were in place due to the *National Formulary* (NF) and the joint public–private sector regulatory body, the *United States Pharmacopeia* (USP). Thus, as the 21st century proceeds, it is not the NF or USP that people turn to, but rather to Internet sites, dubious healers, lay magazines, and other sources touting natural products as superior to, safer than, or equal in efficacy to modern medicines. Figures from 1997 indicate that, in the United States, among those persons taking prescription medicines, one in five is also taking at least one herbal preparation, at a total cost of $5.1 billion per year. This higher usage requires that all health professionals be familiar with these products and at a level higher than what the general public knows.[1] Although most "studies" of herbal medicines present claims that they work as indicated, these studies:

- Tend to be nothing more than testimonials.
- Are conducted in foreign countries.
- Are done without standardized products.
- Are done without regard to standardized dosing and, as such, present flawed results having limited usefulness, application, and interpretation.[2]

Furthermore, some risks in the use of natural products in the United States occur because these products are regulated as dietary supplements under the Dietary Supplement Health and Education Act of 1994 (DSHEA). Thus, supplements without proven safety or efficacy studies can be marketed without any intervention by the Food and Drug Administration (FDA) until a well-documented problem occurs.

A FAILURE TO COMMUNICATE

In the movie *Cool Hand Luke*, great attention is paid to the phrase, "what we have here is a failure to communicate," and so it is with natural products. In one recent study of the medication follow-up of patients at least 55 years of age who were admitted to a hospital, it was found there was at least one discrepancy or failure to continue the current medications in 65% of the patients.[3] Thus, it is likely that elderly people get admitted to a hospital minus at least one medication they are taking and this discrepancy is either dismissed or the medication is discontinued without appropriate discussion with the patient. In this same study, 12% of the medication discrepancies resulted from herbal products being withheld upon admission to the hospital. The message to patients is a strong one: these products are not useful and helpful even though there may be evidence that some herbal supplements actually do have therapeutic benefit.

Such problems are compounded in community settings, as another study indicates that physicians inquire about nonprescription medications in only about one-third of their patient encounters.[4] Yet consumers spent more than $2 billion on nonprescription analgesics, vitamin preparations, and cold, allergy, and sinus products in 2004 alone.[5] Thus, it is likely that many elderly patients take nonprescription products or dietary supplements or natural products without their physician's knowledge. Furthermore, it is also likely that elderly patients will not accurately communicate what they are taking and the dosages of the products they are taking, which is why caring professionals should ask to see the bottles for all medications rather than a list of medications.

The failure to discuss nonprescription drugs, natural products, and other dietary supplements can and does lead to unnecessary hospitalizations. For instance, results from a study looking at the use of nonprescription non-steroidal anti-inflammatory drugs (NSAIDs) found that patients had an adjusted odds ratio of being admitted to a hospital for upper gastrointestinal bleeding five times greater than a control group because they knowingly used NSAIDs in greater than recommended doses during the index week of the study.[6]

NATURAL PRODUCT USE AMONG THE ELDERLY: A DEMOGRAPHIC PROFILE

One authoritative resource that examined why people take natural medicines and what they do take is the 2002 National Health Interview Survey.[7]

This study, which was conducted among 31,044 adult Americans over the age of 18, examined 27 different categories of complementary and alternative medicine (CAM) use, including the use of natural products. It was found that the greatest complementary therapy used was prayer, at a rate of 43% among adults. The second most used CAM category was natural products, with 18.9% of Americans over the age of 18 having used at least one natural product in the last 12 months. CAM, including massage therapy, is used by more than 62% of Americans each year.[7]

Women are more likely than men to use CAM. Also, CAM use is more prevalent among older Americans than among younger adults, since older Americans have more medical conditions and disease states to cope with than younger Americans do.[7]

The survey also found that the use of CAM was related to ethnic and cultural factors. For example, Asian adults, with a 43.1% usage rate, are more likely to use CAM than are Caucasian adults, at 35.9%, or African American adults at 26.2%. Further, this survey revealed that the higher the education level of an individual, the more likely was use of CAM therapy. In the age range of 65 and older, individuals with public health insurance were more likely to use CAM than were individuals with private health insurance. Where one comes from also affects the use of CAM; for those who come from countries with access to plants and other botanical products, the use of CAM is higher. Former smokers are also more likely to use CAM, which explains why a high percentage of patients completing smoking cessation courses use some sort of alternative therapy in their attempt to quit smoking.

Interestingly, 26% of Americans who start CAM do so at the behest of a conventional medical professional, which somewhat belies the notion that CAM therapy is almost solely initiated by the patient without medical supervision.[7] CAM therapy is not necessarily limited to easy or simple medical conditions. High cholesterol, asthma, and hypertension were the three disease states for which CAM was found to be used most often.

The 2002 Survey of Complementary and Alternate Medicines included questions on 27 types of CAM therapy used in the United States. Ten of those therapies were provider-based; the remaining, which included natural products, vitamins, and diets, could be used by the patient without provider assistance. About 19% of the population surveyed had used at least one natural product in the past year to self-treat the following prevalent conditions:

- Back pain or back problems
- Head or chest cold
- Neck pain or problems
- Joint pain or stiffness
- Anxiety/depression
- Arthritis, gout, lupus, or fibromyalgia
- Stomach or intestinal illness
- Severe headache or migraine
- Recurring pain
- Insomnia or trouble sleeping

There are hundreds of natural products purported to be helpful in these conditions. However, no matter how good the advertising claims are, the truth is that only about 60 have any merit.[8] It is known with certainty that the majority of U.S. citizens who take natural products never mention that they do so to their personal physician or pharmacist. Unfortunately, unknown numbers of physicians and pharmacists fail to ask patients whether they routinely take natural products. As a consequence, the elderly spend vast sums on the purchase of natural products, many of which are ineffective or not indicated as effective for the patient's condition. Pharmacists can provide an invaluable service by screening patients for natural product use and preventing adverse drug reactions (ADRs) or drug interactions that these products may cause. It would be beneficial, in the team approach to patient care, to have community pharmacists regularly, as part of patient assessment, inquire about natural product use. This step could be especially helpful, since the most common source of information about natural products seems to be the Internet, a medium that was never expected to be a truthful and accurate supplier of information. Although the Internet does supply information, discovering its truthfulness usually is left to those who capture and apply information, not those who supply it.

A PRIMER ON THE MOST COMMONLY PURCHASED NATURAL PRODUCTS

Although there are hundreds, if not thousands, of natural products sold in this country to the American consumer, many consumers are dismayed to learn that there are only about 60 products proven to be at least somewhat effective. The three resources that provide health professionals with extensive information on natural products are:

- *Natural Medicines Comprehensive Database*[8]
- *The Review of Natural Products*[9]
- *Tyler's Honest Herbal*[10]

The following brief discussion covers the 20 top selling herbal and dietary supplements of those 50+ natural products that have some efficacy. Those discussed here represent a significant percentage of the natural products purchased in a community pharmacy. As a reminder to the reader, many pharmacies keep on their shelves at least one of the natural product resource books mentioned above or have other natural product information in computer databases. The pharmacist has always been, and will remain, a significant source of information on natural products, not only for patients but also for local health care practitioners.

Echinacea

In 2004, the second most purchased natural product in the United States was echinacea.[11] Although echinacea is widely used and researched, its active ingredients remain somewhat of a mystery. Traditionally, this product was used as a wound-healing agent and an immunostimulant.[9] Echinacea is rated as possibly effective for the common cold.[8] The average dose of this natural product varies according to which species is being used; the evidence for its effectiveness in treating the common cold is best for *E. purpurea* and *E. pallida*.

Ginseng

Ginseng was the seventh most widely sold natural product in this country during 2002.[11] The term ginseng is generic, as different subspecies are prevalent around the world; examples include American ginseng, Siberian ginseng, Panax ginseng, as well as Asian, Chinese, Korean, Oriental, Japanese, Chikusetsu, Chu Je, Western, Five Fingers, San-Chi, Tien-Chan, Himalayan, Canadian, Vietnamese, and Zhuzishen ginseng.[9] Ginseng root should contain at least 1.5% ginsenosides, as that is how preparations are standardized. The typical extract contains 4%–7% ginsenosides.[9] Ginseng is rated as possibly effective for cognitive function in otherwise healthy, middle-aged people.[8] As with most natural products, evidence shows that ginsenoside content varies with the species of the root, the age of the root, its geographical location, the season, and even the curing method.[9] One study that analyzed various chemical ginseng products from 11 different countries found that among 14 of the purest preparations, the ginsenoside content ranged from 1.9% to 8.1% (wt/wt). When 17 different ginseng products were analyzed from Sweden, it was found total ginsenoside content varied from 2.1 to 13.3 mg per capsule or tablet.[9] American ginseng has two indications for which it is possibly effective. It is listed as possibly effective in reducing the number of colds and reducing postprandial glucose levels.[8] A significant drug interaction with ginseng is its lowering effect on the INR in patients taking warfarin.[8]

Ginkgo Biloba

One of the more popular natural products used in those over 55 is ginkgo biloba, which is considered to be the last living specimen of an ancient tree species. Also considered to be the oldest living plant in the world, ginkgo survived the last Ice Age in the mountains of central China. In the 1700s, ginkgo was brought from China to other parts of the world, particularly Europe and France, for cultivation. Ginkgo is one natural product that has been extensively studied over the last 10 years. Books such as *The Complete German Commission E Monographs*[12] or *Tyler's Honest Herbal*[10] provide some basics, but they are more than 6 years old and lack the tremendous changes in the last 5 years in the thinking about ginkgo. Areas of research on ginkgo center on its role in age-related memory impairment, altitude sickness, cold intolerance, cognitive function, dementia, diabetic retinopathy, glaucoma, intermittent claudication, premenstrual syndrome, and vertigo; the *Natural Medicines Comprehensive Database* lists ginko use as possibly effective for all these indications.[8] Also, fairly decent data show that ginkgo may also have a cerebrovascular effect by improving circulation.[10] The daily dose of ginkgo ranges from 60 to 360 mg of dried leaf extract two or three times a day, depending on the indication. In Germany, millions of prescriptions have been written for gingko biloba extract, and it is also available as a non-prescription drug.[10] The standards in Germany are much higher, of course, and the herbal market is regulated in a manner similar to that for prescription medications in the United States.

Garlic

A second product that is popular in the American marketplace is garlic. In 2004, it was the most popular natural product sold in the United States.[11] In *The Complete German Commission E Monographs*, last updated in 1994, garlic is listed as having two official uses.[12] However, in the 2005 edition of the *Natural Medicines Comprehensive Database*, garlic had nine entries in its "possibly effective" category.[8] Some conditions for which garlic may be effective are atherosclerosis, hyperlipidemia, hypertension, prostate cancer, decreased tick bites, and tinea infections. The dosing of garlic extract for hyperlipidemia and hypertension is 600–1200 mg divided daily into three doses.[8] For tinea infections, studies have used the ajoene constituent as a 0.4% cream, a 0.6% gel, and a 1% gel applied twice daily for 1 week.[8] The only drug interaction of importance is that with saquinavir where the area-under-the-curve has been reduced by approximately one-half. Thus, garlic should be avoided in these patients as well as in patients taking other protease inhibitors.

Glucosamine/Chondroitin

One of the more widely sold natural products in the United States is the combination product of glucosamine and chondroitin, although each is available separately. Glucosamine is considered likely to be effective in osteoarthritis, as is chondroitin.[8] The most recent trial in patients with moderate-to-severe pain at baseline found that the group taking the combination of glucosamine 1500 mg per day and chondroitin 1200 mg per day had significantly less pain and better function than the placebo group, the glucosamine-only group, the chondroitin-only group, and the celecoxib group, although these results were not highlighted.[13] Furthermore, a recent meta-analysis suggests that glucosamine may be effective in delaying the progression of and improving the symptoms of osteoarthritis of the knee.[14]

There are 13 different names for glucosamine sulfate.[8] Glucosamine is found in natural mucopolysaccharides, mucoproteins, and chitin. Of these three, chitin is the most important source. Chemically, chitin is a biopolymer that is cellulose-like. Glucosamine has proven to be one of the safest and least troublesome of all natural products. While there are a number of concerns, most of them seem to be theoretical rather than actual. Dosing of glucosamine to treat osteoarthritis has been 1.5 g per day, either as a single or divided dose. Higher doses have been used and marketed; however, documentation for these doses is lacking. For chondroitin, the dosage is usually 200–400 mg three times daily or 1000–1200 mg as a single daily dose.

Fish Oils

Fish oil is commonly referred to as omega-3 fatty acid. The two fatty acids that are used interchangeably with the term omega-3 are eicosapentaenoic (EPA) and docosahexaenoic (DHA). Marine sources containing the highest content of omega-3 fatty acids are fatty fish such as mackerel, halibut, salmon, blue fish, mullet, sable fish, menhaden, anchovy, herring, lake trout, cohoe, and sardines.[9] Omega-3 fatty acids are metabolized into a class of biologically active, 20-carbon compounds called eicosanoids. These eicosanoids are potent regulators of blood pressure, blood clotting, childbirth contractions, and gastric secretions, as well as immune and inflammatory responses.[9]

The original research that pointed to the value of omega-3 acids in the prevention of cardiovascular diseases was the result of the observation that Greenland Eskimos, despite consuming more than 40% of their calories as fat, exhibited a very low incidence of coronary heart disease. Since then the benefit of consuming fish oil to reduce cardiovascular events has been demonstrated in at least four well-known, large studies, one being the 1989 Diet and Reinfarction Trial (DART).[15] This study found almost a 30% decrease over 2 years in overall mortality in men who ate fatty fish twice a week over those who did not. Worldwide, tens of thousands of people have been enrolled in studies to evaluate the effect of fish oil on cardiovascular mortality and there is a growing body of evidence that strongly suggests a cardioprotective effect from fish oil.

The mechanism of action of fish oil is thought to be an antiarrhythmic effect. Fish oil has been used after coronary artery bypass surgery to successfully reduce the number of patients experiencing atrial fibrillation.[16] Fish oils can lower blood pressure and decrease triglycerides, and they have been approved in other countries for use after a myocardial infarction to reduce the incidence of sudden cardiac death. In the United States, a prescription fish oil by the trade name of Omacor® has recently been marketed and approved for use to lower triglycerides. The capsules contain approximately 1 g of esterified EPA and DHA, and the dosage is two capsules twice daily.

Fish oil has also been used as an adjunct in treating depression; a better response to the antidepressant has been obtained in five of seven studies.[17] The mechanism of action is thought to be the promotion of neuronal growth in the dentate gyrus of the hippocampus. Sales of fish oil constitute a large proportion of the dietary supplement sales in this country. Given the uses and the overall safety profile, telling a patient who has had an infarction to stop taking fish oil may well constitute malpractice. Taking it may be a case of intelligent compliance on the part of patients and fruitful discussion is called for rather than stopping the fish oil on admission to the hospital, as is routinely done.

Saw Palmetto

It is estimated that 95% of the men who reach age 90 will have some sort of prostate disorder. An enlarged prostate is the number one self-treated condition among men. Many men treat this condition with saw palmetto, a natural product that has been around for several centuries. Early in the 20th century, saw palmetto was used as mild diuretic therapy for chronic cystitis and enlarged prostate.[4] When routinely used in the treatment of enlarged prostate, saw palmetto is considered likely to be effective.[1-4]

Saw palmetto's mechanism of action has been thoroughly studied. It has antiandrogenic, antiproliferative, and anti-inflammatory properties that seem to be responsible for improving the symptoms of benign prostatic hyperplasia.[1] Although saw palmetto does not seem to reduce the size of the prostate, it does relieve the symptoms of urgency. Saw palmetto berries contain large amounts of beta phytosterol and other plant sterols.[2] The beta phytosterol seems to be the predominant product.[4] In addition, saw palmetto contains numerous other chemicals; considerable research is ongoing to determine the pharmacological effects of saw palmetto and its constituents. Saw palmetto's pharmacological effects are possible because of the numerous chemical compounds within the product.

Saw palmetto's drug interactions are considered theoretical and not proven. It does not have any known side effects other than GI upset. Saw palmetto does not have any contraindications.[3] The normal dose is 320 mg of active ingredient that has been extracted with a lipophilic solvent.

Ginger

Ginger was originally grown in countries with warm climates, such as India, Jamaica, and China, where it has been used medicinally since 500 BC. It has been used worldwide as a flavoring agent, and its reputation in Asian medicine for reducing motion sickness is currently the subject of much research. As anybody who has gone on a cruise knows, there's not a lot to be said for a case of motion sickness. The mainstay of motion sickness treatment is either scopolamine patches or nonprescription antihistamines (Dramamine®), which can be quite sedating to some people.

In the last 15–20 years, there have been seven double-blind studies conducted on volunteers comparing 940 mg of powdered ginger, 100 mg of the antihistamine dimenhydrinate, and a placebo; each was consumed 25 minutes prior to tests conducted in a tilted, rotating chair. The initial study, done almost 20 years ago with 36 college students, has been repeated six times. In four out of the six subsequent studies, the initial findings that ginger helps in preventing motion sickness have been borne out. In the initial study, 36 subjects were given the ginger preparation, or dimenhydrinate, or placebo and placed blindfolded in a rotating chair. Subjects who received ginger root remained in the chair an average of 5.5 minutes, compared to 3.5 minutes for the antihistamine group, and 1.5 minutes for the placebo group. It is believed that the pharmacological action of ginger is related to the diterpenoid constituent gulonolactone, which has been shown to produce activity as a $5HT_3$-antagonist. This same mechanism of action is shown by ondansetron (Zofran®), another antiemetic drug used in treating chemotherapy-induced nausea and vomiting.

At this time, there are no reports of any toxicity associated with ginger. In theory, however, large doses of ginger could depress the central nervous system and cause cardiac arrhythmias. Ginger also might tend to exacerbate bleeding tendencies in susceptible individuals in certain disease states, although this is a hypothesized, not a documented, reaction. The use of ginger in pregnancy is controversial. The German Commission E has taken a conservative stance and is advising women not to use ginger during pregnancy for morning sickness. There is some concern, although most feel it is unfounded, that ginger could cause spontaneous abortion.

Soy

Among the top 10 natural products sold in the United States are soy products. The first recorded mention of soy was during the reign of the Chinese emperor Chung Nang in 2838 BC. At that time it was considered to be China's most important crop.[2] Soy is indicated as likely to be effective in treating hyperlipidemia. Soy products reduce total serum cholesterol by 9%, low-density lipoprotein cholesterol by 13%, and triglycerides by 11% after 1–2 months of therapy.[1] Soy also is possibly effective in reducing the risk of osteoporosis, lowering fasting blood sugar levels in diabetics, and reducing diarrhea symptoms, and it seems to work on mental symptoms, hypertension, kidney disease, osteoporosis, and prostate cancer. Research is being done on all of these possibly effective indications, with much new data likely to come out in the next 5 years. The estrogenic effect of soy derives from the isoflavinones. Soy products seem to help approximately 30% of the women who take them for postmenopausal symptoms, making the failure rate 70%.[1] However, another report shows that menopausal symptoms of hot flashes are reduced by 45%.[2] Soy should also have a positive effect on osteoporosis by retarding it. This is one of the hottest areas of soy research, with data coming out almost monthly. Soy is considered safe during pregnancy and lactation. Drug–drug interactions are minimal.

Melatonin

One of the most common questions health professionals are asked by the elderly is, "What can I do to get a good night's sleep?" When responding to such a question, community pharmacists usually find that it has not been posed to the person's family physician. Among the countless articles and folklore and urban legends about products that will ensure a good night's sleep, the one natural product that has received a fair amount of press over the last 12–14 years is melatonin. During this time, its exact indications and its niche in the insomniac market have varied considerably. Melatonin is a natural hormone produced by the pineal gland and extrapineal tissue. Considered effective in treating circadian rhythm disorders and sensory disturbances,[1] melatonin is also believed to be possibly effective in treating narcotic pain withdrawal, delayed sleep phase syndrome, and simple insomnia.

In the human body, tryptophan is converted to serotonin, which is the immediate precursor of melatonin. This final step in the synthesis of melatonin is inhibited by light and stimulated by darkness. For instance, winter polar nights affect the natural sleep/wake cycle. In the early 1990s, it was thought that melatonin was the panacea pharmacologists and pharmaceutical researchers had been looking for to help insomniacs. Unfortunately, the effectiveness of melatonin is limited. It is metabolized by the liver and has a half-life of less than 1 hour.[1] Since hormones in the human body generally do not have just one receptor site, but many (for example, estrogen has effects on skin, blood vessels, and bone density), it is likely that in the next few years, melatonin will have other indications.

There are not a lot of documented medical condition interactions with melatonin, but there are three drug interactions of note:

- Caffeine, which can elevate melatonin levels.
- Acetaminophen, which may have its effectiveness reduced by melatonin.
- Fluvoxamine, which may elevate melatonin levels, increasing drowsiness.[2]

There are other theoretical drug interactions, but none has been proven.

One commonsense caution with melatonin is that it does cause drowsiness. Thus, if any other medication, such as a tricyclic antidepressant for pain,

Ambien® for sleep, or Neurontin® for neurological pain, is being taken by the patient, it can potentiate the drowsiness of melatonin and delay waking up in the morning. The typical oral dose of melatonin for insomnia is 0.3–5 mg at bedtime.[1] Specific recommendations for travelers are:

- For eastbound travel, patients take a preflight early morning treatment of melatonin, followed by a treatment at bedtime for 4 days after arrival.
- For westbound travel, patients should take melatonin for 4 days at bedtime when in a new time zone.

Milk Thistle

Milk thistle is a product that was used extensively during the Middle Ages, fell out of use early in the 20th century, and now has regained popularity.[4] The use of milk thistle as a liver protectant goes back to the time of the Greeks and Pliny the Elder, the great Roman physician.[2] Milk thistle consists of several active ingredients, the most active being silymarin. Silymarin itself consists of several constituents, the three most active chemicals being silibinin, silydianin, and silychrintin.[3]

In the American natural product literature, milk thistle has five uses for which its effectiveness has been proven insufficient. However, four of its five indications are for treating/preventing conditions affecting the liver, alcohol-related liver damage, mushroom poisoning, hepatitis B or C, and toxin-induced liver damage. Milk thistle is also considered possibly effective for diabetes, which also is mediated through the liver.[1] Unfortunately there are, as yet, no good independent clinical data to support this. One reason milk thistle may be potentially effective is that after its ingestion and subsequent metabolism in the liver, it undergoes enteropathic recirculation, with a much higher concentration in the liver than in any other part of the body. It is a potent tumor necrosis factor inhibitor.[1] Silymarin alters cell membranes and prevents toxin penetration of the liver. One constituent of milk thistle's silymarin is silibinin, which decreases synthesis of cholesterol in the liver. With regard to viral hepatitis, silymarin may inhibit the antifibrotic and anti-inflammatory effects in viral infections.

An explanation for milk thistle's hepatoprotective effects may be its actions which either alter the liver cell membrane structure or block the absorption of toxins into the cells. Hepatoprotection by silymarin also can be attributed to its ability to increase the intracellular concentration of glutathione, a substance required for detoxifying reactions in liver cells. Milk thistle is also an antioxidant that is more potent than vitamins C and E. Even though milk thistle's hepatoprotection has not been conclusively established with good, well-organized, scientific, reproducible studies, it is believed by some that milk thistle protects the liver by stimulating RNA and DNA synthesis, resulting in regeneration of the liver.[2]

Milk thistle has no known interactions with other drugs. Principal side effects include chills, high fever, headaches, angina, orthostatic circulatory disturbances, and allergic reaction.[3] Milk thistle, which is marketed in this country as a dietary supplement in the form of capsules containing 140 mg of silymarin,[4] is normally given as a total daily dosage of 420 mg or one capsule of 140 mg three times a day.[1]

Black Cohosh

One of the more common questions health professionals get is what products, besides estrogens, are available to treat hot flashes and other menopausal symptoms. One such product is black cohosh. Black cohosh has been used for more than 200 years, originally by Native Americans, somewhat generically, in the treatment of "diseases of women." During the last century, it became one of the principal ingredients in the well-known product Lydia Pinkham's vegetable compound.[4] Black cohosh has had many proposed medical uses, but in the last 50 years the only indication that has received serious research has been the treatment of hot flashes and other symptoms of menopause. By 1962, at least 14 clinical reports, although not controlled clinical trials in the modern sense, involving 1500 patients had been published in Germany. German practitioners from the 1950s and early 1960s reported the efficacy of black cohosh in premenopausal and menopausal symptoms, including reduction of hot flashes and improvement of depressive moods.[4]

The three major pharmacological actions of black cohosh root are:

- Estrogen-like action,
- Leuteinizing hormone suppression, and
- Binding to estrogen receptors.[3]

The only significant ADR of black cohosh root appears to be GI upset.[1,3] The only two drug interactions involving black cohosh root are increasing blood levels and possible toxicities of docetaxel and doxorubicin, both chemotherapy drugs. There is also some preliminary supposition that black cohosh root could increase the risk of metastatic breast cancer.

The dosing of black cohosh root to manage symptoms of menopause is two to four 20-mg tablets twice a day. Therapeutic effects usually begin after 2 weeks, with maximum effect seen in 8 weeks.[2]

Zinc Lozenges

One of the more interesting natural products is the element zinc. Although used for many medical conditions, zinc is medically proven in the treatment of sore throats and wound healing.[2] Other conditions for which zinc is possibly effective are age-related macular degeneration, certain cases of ADHD, gingivitis, herpes simplex, muscle cramps, pneumonia, and venous leg ulcers. Zinc comes in eight salt forms. As is true with iron and calcium, patients need to look at the number of milligrams of zinc that each product contains. As one of the five micronutrients important in healing, zinc has been studied extensively in this area and is fairly universally acclaimed to promote the healing of wounds and shorten the duration of healing. Zinc is contained in more than 300 enzymes in the body, including the ones for wound healing.

Zinc has also been touted for the prevention of the common cold and the treatment of sore throat. Most data show that zinc is ineffective in the prevention of the common cold. But other research shows that in higher doses zinc is probably effective in the treatment of sore throat.

Out of more than 300 biological functions, zinc is important for the formation of neutrophils, natural killer T-cells, and lymphocyte feeding, which are necessary for the destruction of cold viruses.[1,2] Zinc has not been shown to be effective on mature cold viruses,[2] which explains why almost all reports indicate that zinc must be started within the first 3 days of cold symptoms in order for it to be effective. One mechanism of action for zinc is blocking the adhesion of mature rhino viruses to receptors in human tissue, thus blocking the progression of the cold. Most of the recent studies in sore throat treatment have used lozenges that contain 23 mg of zinc. The lozenges, which are to be taken every 2 hours, should not be used for more than 14 days. Most studies show that lozenges with a zinc content of less than 10 mg are ineffective. Furthermore, lozenges with the free zinc ion, rather than zinc gluconate or zinc sulfate, have been shown to be the most effective. Drug interactions involving zinc include tetracyclines, quinolones, thiazide diuretics (hydrochlorothiazide), and captopril.

Camphor

Another natural product that has been around since the time of the Romans and Greeks is camphor, which comes from the wood of the tree *Cinnamomum camphora*. Camphor is approved in Europe and by the FDA, but there are differences between European camphor and products sold in the United States. In Europe, manufacturers use commercial concentrations of up to 20% camphor, whereas the highest concentration used in the United States is 11%. Also, in Europe they tend to use camphor for a longer duration of therapy. In the United States it is used for short-term therapy only, that is, no more than 14 days. The FDA has indicated camphor for nonprescription use for three medical conditions: cough, pain, and pruritus. Camphor-containing products are not approved for children, nor are they approved for women who are pregnant or breastfeeding.

As a counterirritant, camphor works on reducing pain and pruritus. In the body, there are short and long nerve fibers that carry pain signals to the brain. Camphor acts on the long nerve fibers. A person's brain normally can concentrate on only one signal from an area of the body, whether the signal is pain or itching. When camphor is applied to the skin, the nerves that it irritates block the brain's reception of an unpleasant stimulus from the original area, hence the term counterirritant. There are other counterirritants on the market, but camphor is considered the preferred product in this country.[1]

Several generations ago, camphor was used internally. Due to the toxicity of oral camphor products, particularly in causing death in young children, all oral preparations of camphor were taken off the U.S. market about a generation ago. The only documented ADR of topical camphor is an occasional rise of liver enzymes.[1] Topical camphor has no known interactions with drugs or foods. For topical use on the skin for itching, cold sores, and hemorrhoids, a 1%–3% ointment is usually used three or four times a day. As a counterirritant for pain, the concentration of camphor-containing products is 3%–11%. Camphor-containing products for pain are applied one to four times a day. For an antitussive (Vicks® chest rub), a layer of 4.7% to 5.3% is applied to the throat and chest areas; the area can be covered to increase absorption.

Selenium

Some good preliminary data indicate that selenium can reduce the risk of prostate cancer. Selenium is frequently given with vitamin E and is purported to be useful for a wide variety of disease states. People take selenium to treat HIV, hypothyroidism, and Osgood-Schlatter disease and to prevent certain cancers. It has been studied in the prevention of colon, prostate, and, most recently, breast cancer. It has been shown to be effective in reducing the risks of prostate cancer, particularly in those individuals whose selenium levels have been shown to be low. At this point, the use of selenium in treating breast cancer is too preliminary to draw any conclusions. Selenium has been shown not to have any effect on the rates of colon cancer.

Selenium's mechanism of action remains unknown, but it is thought to be due to its antioxidant activity. If selenium levels are below 1000 micromoles/L, selenium activates glutathione peroxidase, which reduces oxidative stress by handling free radicals and hydrogen peroxide. At plasma concentrations above 2000 micromoles/L, selenium paradoxically increases cellular oxidation. It should be noted that selenium can cause acute toxicity, which can include the symptoms of nausea, vomiting, fatigue, irritability, and weight loss. Patients taking selenium should absolutely not take any more than the recommended daily amount. The only known interaction with other herbs or dietary supplements is with dietary iron, which can significantly decrease the absorption of the selenium. Patients taking a statin drug (Crestor®, Lescol®, Lipitor®, Pravachol®, Zocor®) need to check with their prescriber, as selenium can lower the absorption of these drugs.

The human body needs about 70 mcg/day, which can usually be obtained from food sources, such as lobster, clams, crabs, oysters, and nuts, but most people get their selenium from supplements. Whether it is taken for cancer prevention or as a supplement, patients should be cautioned against taking any more than 200 mcg of selenium per day, as it may lead to fragile, thickened nails, diarrhea, reduced sensation in hands and feet, fatigue, and irritability. Doses above 800 mcg/day can lead to tissue damage. Most standalone supplements contain 80–200 mcg/tablet or capsule.[1] Selenium sources do differ in content amounts, as some multivitamins contain only 20 mcg. An NIH-supported, 10-year cancer prevention trial using a tablet containing 200 mcg of selenium as brewer's yeast suggests that dietary supplements of the trace element selenium may significantly lower the incidence of prostate, colorectal, and lung cancers in persons with a history of skin cancer, but the study was too preliminary for a public health recommendation.

Witch Hazel

Witch hazel, a product that was on the market 100 years ago and is still on the market today, has a number of purported uses. However, the only one for which there is good documentation is in the treatment of hemorrhoids. Witch hazel, which is used alone or topically in products such as Tucks® pads, contains about 7%–10% tannins, although there is some dispute about the actual percentage. It is these tannins and their ability to tighten distended veins and restore vessel tone that explain the use of witch hazel in varicose vein treatment (hemorrhoids are essentially varicose veins that protrude from the skin). Tannins applied topically to broken skin or mucous membranes induce protein precipitation,[1] which tightens up superficial cell layers and shrinks colloidal structures, thereby causing capillaries to constrict. The decreasing vascular permeability approximates an anti-inflammatory agent. The astringent activity of tannins also causes an indirect antibacterial effect. Given that it is a topical application, it does not have any particular interactions with drugs, food, or laboratory tests. For topical hemorrhoid treatment, witch hazel liquid can be applied up to six times a day or after each bowel movement.

Emu Oil

From Australia, a relatively new natural product, emu oil, has been brought to the American market. This product was originally used by the Aboriginal people of Australia for a wide variety of conditions. The Emu Producers International Cooperative Oil Refineries produce 5000 pounds of oil daily for commercial use in cosmetics such as eye cream, moisturizers, and hair products.[1] People use emu oil for:[1]

- Improving cholesterol levels, as a source of polyunsaturated and monounsaturated fatty acids.
- Weight loss.
- As a cough syrup for colds and coughs.
- Sore muscles, aching joints, pain, or inflammation.
- Carpal tunnel syndrome, sciatica, shin splints, and gout relief.

However, nearly all clinical and scientific studies focus on the anti-inflammatory properties of emu oil.[2] Probably the best definitive clinical study to date was when five different preparations of emu oil were examined in Wistar rats. The oils came from emu birds raised in five different habitats. Three of the five groups of rats were given injections of emu oil, and two others had topical application. All five groups showed clinical benefit in the treatment of arthritis. The topical use of emu oil was roughly equivalent to the administration of oral ibuprofen in rats. In a very small study of 10 men, emu oil was used for approximately 6 months on surgical scars to reduce scarring. When compared to the placebo group, emu oil did show a significantly greater reduction in scarring.[2]

Emu oil contains a number of chemicals including, but not limited to, myristic, palmitic, palmitoleic, stearic, oleic, linolic, and linolenic fatty acids.[1] Linolic acid is the agent believed to ease muscle aches and joint pain. Oleic acid is considered to have local anti-inflammatory effect. Emu oil appears to have the ability to penetrate the skin, perhaps in part because it does not contain phospholipids. Some animal studies suggest that emu oil is more effective in acute inflammation than in chronic inflammation.

Emu oil is not known to have any adverse side effects, interactions with foods, interactions with drugs, or interactions with disease states. In theory, it could affect anticoagulant drugs, so patients taking anticoagulant drugs should check with their physician before using emu oil. Perhaps the bottom line on emu oil is that large clinical trials are lacking. There have been several small promising clinical trials that suggest its best use is in acute instances of inflammation and injury to joints or muscles.

Capsicum

Capsicum, which is also called cayenne pepper, chili pepper, or red pepper, is a natural product that has been sold in the United States for the last 10–15 years. Applied topically to relieve pain, capsicum is considered unsafe when used orally, as it can cause liver or kidney damage. Topical capsicum is considered effective for the temporary relief of pain from rheumatoid arthritis, osteoarthritis, and neuralgias due to shingles or diabetic neuropathy.[1] Capsicum has been approved by the FDA as a nonprescription drug for treatment of these conditions.

The mechanism of action of capsicum is fairly well understood. There is a chemical called substance P near the surface of the skin in pain nerve endings. This compound is involved in the transmission of painful stimuli from the periphery to the spinal cord.[2] Initially, when a painful stimulus occurs, substance P is released, causing an increase in the sensation of pain. Upon repeated administration of capsicum, substance P is depleted and pain ceases.[1,2] The onset of pain relief is usually 3 days or less.[2] It should be noted that capsicum does not penetrate more than 2.5 cm, or approximately

1 inch, into the body. If a patient is suffering from pain that is particularly deep (greater than 1 inch), this product probably will not work.

Adverse reactions to this product include burning of the skin and possible contact dermatitis and rash. Capsicum comes in 0.025% and 0.075% strengths. The product is normally applied topically three or four times a day. It has several trade names, but patients can buy a lower cost generic form. It is suggested that patients start with the lower strength of 0.025% and then go to the higher strength of 0.075% if the condition warrants. Patients should always wash their hands after applying this product.

St. John's Wort

St. John's Wort, a natural product used widely in the Middle Ages, had fallen out of use until about 10 years ago. St. John's Wort is an aromatic perennial native to Europe but is now found throughout the United States and parts of Canada. Considered an aggressive weed, it grows in the dry ground in roadsides, meadows, woods, and hedges. The plant has oval-shaped leaves and yields golden-yellow flowers that bloom from June to September. Some say that its brightest blooms coincide with the birthday of John the Baptist on June 24, hence the name St. John's Wort.

Hypericum perforatum has gotten a lot of press in recent years because of its antidepressant effect. The active component hypericum creates the anti-depressant effect. In the Middle Ages, St. John's Wort was used for its anti-inflammatory and wound-healing abilities, but these uses have not been readily validated by current scientific research. In more than 19 recent, double-blind clinical trials, however, this product was shown to be safe and effective with fewer side effects than traditional antidepressant therapy. St. John's Wort works by inhibition of serotonin uptake by postsynaptic receptors. In one study, hypericum caused a 50% inhibition of serotonin uptake by rat synapses.

St. John's Wort has several contraindications. It is not recommended for use with concomitant antidepressant medications. Excessive doses may potentiate existing monoamine oxidase inhibitor antidepressant activity. Also, patients can become photosensitized by St. John's Wort, particularly in higher doses and if they are fair skinned. Patients taking other prescription products should be encouraged to talk with a pharmacist, as St. John's Wort has been implicated in more than 100 drug interactions.

SAMe

One of the current darlings of the natural product market is SAMe, S-adenosyl-L-methionine. Like most natural products, SAMe is purported to help a whole slew of medical conditions. Its two best documented uses, as well as the ones that are likely to be effective, are in the treatment of depression and in the treatment of osteoarthritis. This product has been available by prescription only in Europe since the mid-1970s, but in the U.S. market, it is available as a nutritional supplement. In a study with more than 20,000 subjects, the discontinuation rate of SAMe was only about 5%. There have been numerous clinical trials with SAMe in treating osteoarthritis. These studies have shown that SAMe is superior to placebo and comparable to NSAIDs for decreasing osteoarthritis symptoms.[2] These studies have ranged in length from several months up to 2 years.

The second use of SAMe is in the treatment of depression. It can be used either alone or in combination with tricyclic antidepressants. The dose of SAMe varies according to the clinical condition being treated.[2] The dose of SAMe for depression is 400–1600 mg per day. In most clinical trials, the daily dose is 1600 mg. In the treatment of osteoarthritis, an oral dose of 200 mg three times a day is typically used.

Most of the ADRs associated with this drug, such as flatulence, vomiting, diarrhea, and nausea, are related to the GI tract. Headache has also been reported. This product is contraindicated in persons with bipolar disorder (manic depression), as it can exaggerate the manic episodes. SAMe should be used only with the older tricyclic antidepressants. It should not be used with newer antidepressants, that is the serotonin reuptake inhibitors (Prozac®, Zoloft®, Paxil®, and Celexa®), because it can trigger the sometimes fatal serotonin syndrome.

SAMe is a rather pricey natural product and there is no literature stating that it works any better than other prescription products in the treatment of osteoarthritis or depression. It is merely an alternative and can be a fairly expensive one at that.

KEY POINTS

- Most elders do not mention their use of herbal medications; pharmacists and other health care professionals must be proactive in taking drug histories and in observing which products they purchase.

- Although many natural products have ingredients with centuries of use, that does not mean they are all safe and effective.
- Natural medicines are widely used, but their use is influenced by many factors, especially local custom and tradition.
- Few natural products have scientific documentation for their use and effectiveness; most rely on testimonials.
- All elderly patients who use herbal products should be encouraged to let their health care professionals know what they are using, as many have interactions with prescription medications.
- Quality of marketed products varies considerably. Lack of regulation and standardization contribute to the possibility of consumers not getting what they paid for.
- Herbal products are involved in many drug interactions and the list is growing.
- To learn more, try these web sites:
  - The National Center for Complementary and Alternative Medicine
    - This is a division of the National Institutes of Health (NIH); it serves as the federal government's clearing house on matters relating to CAM:
      - www.nccam.nih.gov
  - The American Botanical Council
    - An independent group that promotes the proper use of herbals:
      - www.herbalgram.org
  - University of Washington School of Medicine
    - The Department of Family Medicine at the University of Washington has a web site that contains reviews of popular herbal medicines for use by health professionals:
      - www.fammed.washington.edu/predoctoral/cam/herbsupp.html
  - The Dietary Supplement Education Alliance
    - This joint industry and academic organization promotes the responsible use of herbals, vitamins, and other dietary supplements:
      - www.supplementinfo.org

REFERENCES

1. Eisenberg DM, Davis RB, Ettner SL, et al. Trends in alternative medicine use in the United States, 1990–1997. *JAMA*. 1998;280(18):1569–75.
2. Bauer BA. Herbal therapy: what a clinician needs to know to counsel patients effectively. *Mayo Clin Proc*. 2000;75(8):835–41.

3. Lessard S, DeYoung J, Vazzana, N. Medication discrepancies affecting senior patients at hospital admission. *Am J Health Syst Pharm.* 2006;63(8):740–3.

4. Sleath B, Rubin RH, Campbell W, et al. Physician–patient communication about over-the-counter medications. *Soc Sci Med.* 2001;53(3):357–69.

5. Top 200 OTC/HBC brands in 2004. Available at: http://www.drugtopics.com/drugtopics/article/articleDetail.jsp?id=156502.

6. Lewis JD, Kimmel SE, Localio AR, et al. Risk of serious upper gastrointestinal toxicity with over-the-counter nonaspirin nonsteroidal anti-inflammatory drugs. *Gastroenterology.* 2005;129(6):1865–74.

7. Barnes PM, Powell-Griner E, McFann K, et al. Complementary and alternative medicine use among adults: United States, 2002. Advance Data From Vital and Health Statistics; Number 343. Hyattsville, Maryland: National Center for Health Statistics; 2004. Available at: http://www.mbcrc.med.ucla.edu/PDFs/camsurvey2.pdf.

8. Jellin JM, Gregory PJ, Batz F, et al. *Pharmacist's Letter/Prescriber's Letter Natural Medicines Comprehensive Database.* 7th ed. Stockton, CA: Therapeutic Research Faculty; 2005.

9. DerMarderosian A, Beutler JA, eds. *The Review of Natural Products.* St. Louis, MO: Wolters Kluwer Health; May 2006.

10. Foster S, Tyler VE. *Tyler's Honest Herbal: A Sensible Guide to the Use of Herbs and Related Remedies.* 4th ed. Binghamton, NY: The Haworth Press Inc.; 1999.

11. Blumenthal M. Herb sales down 7.4 percent in mainstream market. *HerbalGram.* 2005; 66:63.

12. Blumenthal M, ed. *The Complete German Commission E Monographs—Therapeutic Guide to Herbal Medicines.* Austin, TX: American Botanical Council; 1998.

13. Clegg DO, Reda DJ, Harris CL, et al. Glucosamine, chondroitin sulfate, and the two in combination for painful knee osteoarthritis. *N Engl J Med.* 2006;354(8):795–808.

14. Poolsup N, Suthisisang C, Channark P, et al. Glucosamine long-term treatment and the progression of knee osteoarthritis: systematic review of randomized controlled trials. *Ann Pharmacother.* 2005;39(6):1080–7.

15. Burr ML, Fehily AM, Gilbert JF, et al. Effects of changes in fat, fish, and fibre intakes on death and myocardial reinfarction: diet and reinfarction trial (DART). *Lancet.* 1989;2(8666):757–61.

16. Calo L, Bianconi L, Colivicchi F, et al. N-3 Fatty acids for the prevention of atrial fibrillation after coronary artery bypass surgery: a randomized, controlled trial. *J Am Coll Cardiol.* 2005;45(10):1723–8.

17. Peet M, Stokes C. Omega-3 fatty acids in the treatment of psychiatric disorders. *Drugs.* 2005;65(8):1051–9.

13

Ethical Prescribing in the Geriatric Patient

KAREN KOVACH AND JOHN M. BOLTRI

I will follow that system or regimen which, according to my ability and judgment I consider for the benefit of my patients, and abstain from whatever is deleterious and mischievous.

—Hippocratic oath, 5th century BC

OVERVIEW

This chapter, which looks at the process of prescribing and how bioethical issues in the contemporary setting can make it difficult for any prescriber, is intended to help health professionals grasp the nuances of clinical decision-making and appreciate why the best decisions are usually made by shared means, especially when the elderly are involved. These shared means are related to doing what is necessary to help the elderly come to terms with their treatment options when there are differences in vulnerability, risks, adherence, skepticism, and other factors deep in the person's value system, health beliefs, and goals for a therapeutic outcome. Following a quick review of adherence and concordance to medical regimens, this chapter provides a nine-step guide to ethical and shared decision-making that is founded on best practices and based on evidence-based medicine.

Mary Anderson, who is 81 years old, comes in for a follow-up appointment. She is remarkably healthy except for a 10-year history of diabetes and a 2-year history of atrial fibrillation. She takes metoprolol for blood pressure and rate control and she takes warfarin to prevent the development of clots secondary to the chronic atrial fibrillation. During the current visit she gives you her self-monitored blood pressure record. Her blood pressures have steadily increased during the past 3 months and are now not controlled. She is also experiencing frequent palpitations but no chest pain or shortness of breath. Of even greater concern, her PT/INR test, performed yesterday, is low (INR is only 1.2). Past results of this test remained in the therapeutic range (INR 2–3). This new low result alerts you that she is most likely not taking her medication as prescribed.

Upon further questioning you discover that Mary developed a fear of bleeding when a friend was recently admitted to the hospital with rectal bleeding. Due to this fear and being uncertain which medication caused her blood to thin, she stopped taking both the metoprolol and the warfarin. You perform a focused physical exam and find her blood pressure to be very elevated and her pulse rate at the upper limit of normal. You perform an electrocardiogram; except for the increased rate there are no new findings. You then review Mary's goals for her care as well as the risks and benefits of each medication. You answer her questions, discuss alternative medications and treatments, and give your recommendations. After careful consideration, Mary chooses to resume the metoprolol but to stop the warfarin and take aspirin once daily instead. She agrees with your request to have a discussion in the future regarding the risks and benefits of resuming warfarin. She also decides to continue monitoring her blood pressure and to follow up with you in 4 weeks to review her progress.

BIOETHICAL PROBLEMS AMONG THE ELDERLY

Bioethical problems typically arise when there are conflicts among the several goals and values of medicine. It may, for instance, be unclear how much risk should be taken to restore a patient's health. The provider's duty to put clinical expertise to the service of the patient's good may, in one way or another, collide with the ethical demands of respect for the individual. Such problems as these are as likely to arise in the context of prescribing as in any other therapeutic context.

However, certain characteristics of drug therapy create additional ethical concerns. Patients request medical procedures infrequently, but they routinely request medications. Drug therapy necessarily involves the active participation of patients in the management of their own medical problems, but many patients do not adhere to their medication regimens. Pharmaceutical companies employ sophisticated marketing techniques and vast economic resources to influence the prescribing habits of patients and health care providers. Some patients request prescriptions for the purpose of ending their own lives or seek advice about how medications can be used to achieve this end.

Because the elderly are more likely to have chronic illnesses, they are more likely to take both prescription and nonprescription medications. The elderly are more likely to have multiple medical problems and are, therefore, more likely to take multiple medications simultaneously. Older patients are more vulnerable to some of the side effects of drugs, to the risks of polypharmacy, and to the potential harms of nonadherence. Having a complex drug regimen is one risk factor for nonadherence, and older patients frequently have other characteristics that can make adherence to drug therapy difficult.[1]

- The elderly patient may not be able to read standard medication labels or open a medication package.[2]
- Older patients are also more likely to have characteristics that complicate the communication necessary for shared decision-making and genuine informed consent to a drug treatment plan.
- They are more likely to suffer from diseases that involve impairment of cognition, more likely to suffer impaired cognition from depression, and more likely to suffer impaired cognition as a side effect of medication.
- The elderly are more likely to be economically, functionally, or socially dependent.
- They are more likely to lack strong familial or social support.
- The elderly experience pain more frequently.
- By definition, the elderly patient is more likely to be nearing the end of life.

These facts all contribute to the complex ethical issues inherent in prescribing for the elderly. This chapter is a discussion of the ethics of prescribing, with special attention to the peculiar needs of the elderly.

Shared Decision-Making, Consent, and Adherence

Patients have the right to participate in decision-making about the care they will receive and to refuse particular treatments. It follows that they have the right to understandable information about diagnosis, prognosis, treatment options, and the consequences of not treating. The ethical requirement of obtaining patient consent for treatment applies as fully in the context of prescribing as in that of performing surgery or other procedures. Especially in the context of prescribing, engaging in a process of shared decision-making may be therapeutically advantageous as well as morally sound.

Unlike the performance of a procedure, which may be a discrete event, the act of prescribing begins a treatment that will typically be ongoing for substantial periods of time and require for its success the sustained active involvement of the patient. Patients have daily opportunities to alter or opt out of drug therapy and to do so without the agreement of the prescribing physician. This fact has implications for the ethics of obtaining consent to drug therapy and for the responsible monitoring of treatment.

When the patient has authorized the start of a course of drug therapy, the provider writes a prescription. It is, however, the patient who must fill the prescription and take the medication in the correct dose, at the appropriate time intervals, and for the prescribed period of time. Patients not infrequently leave the health care provider's offices with prescriptions that they will never fill or will not take "as directed." This is the problem of nonadherence or what used to be called noncompliance. Roughly 50% of patients in countries in the developed world are nonadherent to drug therapies for chronic illnesses, including hypertension, heart disease, diabetes, cancer, osteoarthritis, and depression, all illnesses common in the geriatric population. The prevalence of nonadherence in the geriatric population is roughly the same as in the general population.[1]

A patient is nonadherent with drug therapy when she displays an intention to follow a particular treatment plan—by explicitly expressing that intention or simply by accepting a prescription from her provider—but then fails to follow through by taking the prescribed medication in accordance with the plan. Whenever a person fails to perform an action that she had exhibited an intention to perform, at least one of three sorts of explanations would seem to be at play:

1. A person may unintentionally fail to do what she had intended to do. In this case, the patient is unintentionally nonadherent to a treatment plan.

2. He may fail to take his medication appropriately because he has misunderstood how it is to be taken or forgets either how or, on occasion, that it is to be taken. Alternatively, a person may intentionally choose not to perform an action that she had previously expressed an intention to perform. She may change her mind, or she may never actually have intended to perform the act she expressed an intention to perform.
3. A patient is intentionally nonadherent if she fails to take her medication as directed because she chooses not to do so, whether she has changed her mind or never fully committed to doing so in the first place.

Willing and unwilling intentional nonadherence can be distinguished further. A patient is intentionally but unwillingly nonadherent if she would choose to adhere to the treatment plan but cannot; it may, for example, be financially impossible for her to do so. Given this obstacle, she chooses not to take her medication as prescribed. A patient is willingly intentionally nonadherent to a particular therapeutic plan when she decides not to take the medication that has been prescribed for her or to take it in doses other than those recommended, not because it would be, as a practical matter, difficult for her to follow the direction she has been given, but because she does not believe doing so would be the best choice.

There is some evidence that physicians tend to underestimate the prevalence of nonadherence among their own patients.[3] Providers should be knowledgeable about the prevalence of nonadherence in their own therapeutic areas and about ways to simplify drug therapy. They should be willing to address the practical difficulties patients have in adhering to therapy and should be skilled in communicating with patients about all of the complex issues associated with medicinal therapy.[4]

A great deal of work has been done to improve support for patients with functional or cognitive impairments that interfere with medication self-management. Large print can be used for both medication labels and information sheets for elderly patients with poor eyesight. Information formats can be simplified, although this typically involves providing less information, a change not welcomed by all patients. Some researchers have investigated the question of how information is most effectively organized and presented to older patients.[5-8] Here are some suggestions:

- In this population, lists are more effective than prose.
- Adding readily decipherable icons to written instructions may aid understanding and recall.

- Support that addresses memory problems will be especially important for many older patients.[9,10]
- Patients may benefit from medication packaging that incorporates the timing of doses or from pillboxes with compartments that can be filled so that each contains all and only those medications that are to be taken at a particular time.[11]
- Memory aids that help patients know when to reach for the next dose are also available.[12]

In addition, inpatient self-medication programs seem to improve adherence following hospital discharge, a particularly challenging time for older patients, whose medication regimens are often radically revised during hospitalization.[1,13] Educating a patient's family about the illness and its treatment can improve adherence by helping family members support the patient's efforts to adhere. Both intentional and unintentional failures to do so should be addressed.[14] Some evidence suggests that improving shared decision-making in the context of prescribing might improve patient understanding of both how to take medications appropriately and why the patient has good reason to do so, thereby reducing both unintentional and intentional nonadherence.[15–19]

Shared decision-making and the problem of nonadherence to drug therapy for chronic illness were brought together in a much-cited report of a task force of the Royal Pharmaceutical Society of Great Britain.[20] The report recommended that the concept of compliance be replaced with that of concordance—a state of affairs that is achieved when provider and patient reach agreement on a treatment plan by engaging in a process of shared decision-making that is fully responsive to the beliefs and values of the patient.[21,22]

There is reason to think that decision-making processes that lead to concordance will also improve adherence and outcomes.[23] Whether or not they do, shared decision-making in the context of prescribing would seem to be the best approach to satisfying the moral requirement that providers obtain genuine informed consent for treatment. The central idea of concordance is that there should be a partnership, rather than an authoritarian relationship, between prescriber and patient. In partnership, prescriber and patient should work out the drug therapy that will work best for the patient, taking into account the fact that no proposed therapy can be best if it is not one to which the patient will adhere. This effort to reach agreement between provider and patient should lead to further efforts to maintain agreement throughout the course of treatment. The patient remains engaged in the decision-making process after he has gained experience with the costs—financial, physical, and personal—of taking the drug.

One study suggests that provider efforts to achieve concordance improve adherence by significantly improving patient understanding of the drug regimen.[24] This is not terribly surprising. When conversation with others is guided by the aim of reaching agreement with them, speakers work harder at making themselves clear, as they have something at stake. Providers can provide patients with decision aids or other written information in anticipation of decision-making discussions or medication reviews. During shared reviews, the provider has opportunities to assess not only how adherent the patient has been but also potential barriers to future adherence. She can tailor her support of the patient to the patient's specific needs.

Patients frequently attribute their own nonadherence to skepticism concerning the necessity of the drug at issue for them or its value or safety if taken in the amounts for which the prescription was written. Patient skepticism is not necessarily entirely unreasonable. It is useful to remember—and it may be useful for providers to acknowledge to patients—that drugs are sometimes inappropriately prescribed or inadequately monitored. Mistakes are not uncommon in medicine nor, in particular, are they uncommon in prescribing.[25] Studies conducted in a variety of care settings show a substantial amount of inappropriate prescribing and monitoring in the geriatric population.[26-29] According to one study in 1999, roughly 7 million elderly patients (65 years of age and older) in the United States received "potentially inappropriate" drugs.[30]

Some patients believe that they should use medications as little as possible. Some have a substantial degree of confidence in alternative therapies and may get advice from both a traditional and an alternative practitioner before deciding how they will treat their illness, relying on one or the other or, frequently, both. Very few of those patients who use complementary medicine reveal this fact to their physicians.[31] Ideally, the provider is interested in and respectful of the considered opinions of his patients and is open to the possibility that there is or could be value in a particular patient's use of a particular complementary therapy.

Especially when prescribing for elderly patients, for whom polypharmacy is a significant problem, alternatives to pharmacotherapy should be explored and, where possible, encouraged. At the least, it should be acknowledged that the patient is the most promising source of information about what he is actually willing to do. Engaging the patient in an open, mutually respectful conversation about the value of a particular drug therapy in managing his illness will provide the patient with an opportunity to describe his perceptions of his illness, his views of medicine, and his goals for treatment. At the same time, open discussion of complementary medicine provides important opportunities for the provider to communicate her reasons for accepting or rejecting particular alternative treatments and to help the patient evaluate the competence of the particular alternative practitioner she consults.

It is, of course, impossible to predict all of the many ways in which the beliefs and values of patients may complicate medical decision-making, and it is not necessary to do so. Patients will bring their particular beliefs and values to their consultations with physicians. Providers should, however, bring some understanding of where the contributions of patients belong in the decision-making processes and possess the communication skills necessary for shared decision-making. Despite growing acceptance of the importance of shared decision-making in health care, there is no consensus on precisely when it should be engaged or what it should entail.[32]

Entwistle and O'Donnell have offered one model of patient involvement in clinical decision-making.[33] Of course, breaking decision-making down into its components has an air of artificiality, because providers do not start from scratch in their thinking about how to treat the particular medical problems addressed in a particular patient encounter. Doing so, however, helps to clarify at which points in the decision-making process the patient's point of view is appropriately taken into account. A model of shared medical decision-making presupposes a model of clinical decision-making in general, and Entwistle and O'Donnell's discussion presupposes an evidence-based medicine model.

This model is loosely understood as clinical practice that makes use of "best current evidence to provide the most appropriate health care for individual patients." Evidence-based decision-making involves:

- Formulating a clinical question.
- Seeking out relevant research evidence.
- Evaluating the evidence found.
- Making a decision based on the best available evidence.

With this model, patients may be involved at all stages, but patient involvement is most important in the first and last stages, when questions are formulated and decisions are made.

Entwistle and O'Donnell do not restrict the application of their model. It is intended to apply to clinical decision-making in general. There are those who believe that shared decision-making is appropriate only in situations in which the provider sees more than one treatment choice as legitimate.[34,35] It may be that patient involvement is especially important in that context, but it is also especially important in prescribing, because of the role that patients play in successful drug therapy. Involving the patient in decision-making is generally valuable as a means to improved mutual understanding and trust between patient and provider.[36]

A Guide to Patient–Provider Discussions

A model of shared decision-making in medicine should provide guidance for provider–patient conversations in which treatment decisions are to be made. It is difficult to specify the steps of a successful conversation, because actual conversations have a life of their own and are often only pieces of larger relationships. The provider may come to a particular meeting with a patient with some knowledge of that patient, the decision may concern issues they have discussed before, and the patient may come with questions or discussion points of his own. The following, then, should be seen as a rough guide to discussions that are more likely to eventuate in shared decisions.

1. **Assess the patient's decision-making capacity.** The patient must be able to make the treatment decision at issue, based on relevant information and out of a reasonably constant set of values. While decision-making ability is a spectrum concept—admitting of all degrees of variation—decision-making capacity, in the technical sense in which it is used in the context of health care, is a status concept. One either possesses the capacity to make a particular decision or one does not, and in the balance hangs whether one will be permitted to make that decision for oneself or a surrogate decision-maker will be consulted. It is possible, then, and common for a patient with decision-making capacity to have all the same a great deal of difficulty comprehending complex information or making reasoned decisions. Such patients may need more assistance. If the patient does not have decision-making capacity, treatment decisions will be made with a surrogate. Surrogates also have the right to be adequately informed of treatment options and to participate in the decision-making process, with an eye to making choices consistent with the patient's beliefs and values. Steps 2–9 are as appropriate in the context of shared decision-making with surrogates as in the context of deciding with patients.

2. **Discuss the patient's involvement in decision-making with the patient (optional).** Explicitly forming a "partnership" with the patient has been recommended by some researchers on shared decision-making and rejected by others.[4,34] It will be necessary to explore in some way the patient's preferences for receiving information, sharing concerns, and contributing ideas:

   - Would she like others to be involved?
   - Would she like guidance in researching her illness?
   - Does she need time to formulate questions?

3. **Listen to the patient.** Patient encounters will vary in their origin. Some are initiated by patients, others by providers for routine checks and reviews of treatment. In either case, it is appropriate to begin by listening to the patient's perception of her health, her medical problems, her treatment, and her needs.

4. **Present treatment options to the patient, taking into account the patient's perceptions.** The provider presents what he takes to be clinically responsible responses to the patient's medical problems, with the risks and benefits of each treatment option, including the option of not treating. It may be insufficient to say that "medication" is an option. The patient should be informed of the availability of alternative medications when there are differences among them that either a reasonable person may be expected to think relevant or the provider has reason to believe the particular patient would wish to take into account. Special care should be taken to convey risk information as clearly and objectively as possible.[37] Decision aids for patients have been developed for some diseases.[38,39] The provider should offer his advice and make clear his reasons for preferring one course to the others. He should also describe any life-style changes that will be caused or required by a particular medication.

5. **Consider the options together.** Listen to the patient's view of how the plan would work for her.

   - Does she understand the information she has been given?
   - Does she expect to follow self-management aspects of the proposed plan?
   - Does she believe she will be able to?
   - Does she believe it is appropriate care for her condition?
   - Does she plan to follow the plan while simultaneously addressing her health problems in alternative ways?
   - Can she afford the proposed treatment? Is she willing to pay for it?
   - Does she have reservations about any aspect of treatment?

6. **If necessary, negotiate with the patient.**
   - Can her concerns be addressed?
   - Can perceived difficulties be avoided?
   - Would complementary therapies help?
   - Will they cause harm?
   - Would she like family members to be educated about her medical problem and the proposed treatment?
7. **Agree on a plan.** Is the patient clear about her responsibilities in carrying out the plan? When will treatment be reviewed? It should be made clear to the patient that the conversation can resume if necessary, and that the provider should be contacted if she has any trouble with the medication regimen or changes her mind about it. The patient should be reminded of potential risks and how to avoid injury. She should be advised of signs and symptoms that would warrant timely reporting.[40]
8. **Write prescription(s).**
9. **Review prescription drug therapy with the patient at appropriate intervals.**

Although this process may seem arduous, there is some evidence to suggest that conversations aimed at concordance do not take much more time.[4]

Recent discussions of the problem of adherence have also suggested enhancing the role of pharmacists, nurses, and health care administrators in supporting patient adherence.[14,41,42] Primary health care providers should continue to accept full responsibility for working with patients on prescribing decisions, education, monitoring, and addressing practical difficulties in carrying those decisions through, but they should also be open to working across disciplines to improve support for patients. Working well with other professionals is as much a skill as working well with patients. Very broadly, it involves the ability to benefit from the expertise of others and to share one's own expertise with others without losing control over the patient's care. In addition, it is common for older patients to have a number of prescribing providers, and it is necessary for each to remain knowledgeable about and confident in the patient's medication regimen. In this context too, communication and negotiation skills are needed for the responsible sharing of patient care.

THREE AREAS OF ETHICAL ISSUES
IN A MODERN SOCIETY

Patient Requests for Medication

Both prescription and nonprescription medications are advertised to patients, and patients can be led to request drugs that good clinical judgment would not recommend. Providers must educate patients and limit patient choice in this peculiar social context. Frequently, however, providers agree to provide prescriptions for drugs that patients have discovered through direct-to-consumer advertising (DTCA), despite reservations about the drug's appropriateness for that patient.[43] Furthermore, patients who request particular drugs are more likely to receive a prescription for some drug or other.[43,44]

Advertising campaigns for particular drugs often boost sales for all drugs of the same class and may, as a whole, contribute to creating or sustaining cultural norms of overreliance on drugs. If DTCA did not lead to significant increases in the prescribing of particular drugs, the pharmaceutical industry would likely not spend much money on it. In 2001, $2.7 billion was spent on DTCA in the United States.[43]

In a national survey, American physicians judged that 49% of requests from patients originating from DTCA were clinically inappropriate. In response to these requests for inappropriate interventions, 69% of physicians agreed to provide the intervention, fully or in part.[45] It is problematic to see patient choices that have been substantially formed by marketing interests as genuinely autonomous choices.

Many DTCA-originating patient requests are for "lifestyle drugs" or for drugs that treat discomfort, distress, or displeasure: pain, heartburn, anxiety, or the symptom-centered illness of depression. There is no uniform definition of a lifestyle drug, but it is generally understood to be a drug that is, in some sense, not medically necessary for a particular patient. Some drugs are never, strictly speaking, clinically indicated, such as medications to address baldness, for instance. Most of the lifestyle drugs are drugs that are clinically indicated for some patients but are not clinically indicated for many of those who wish to use the drug. A single drug, like an antidepressant or an appetite suppressant, might be a lifestyle drug for one patient but not for another. Providers should discourage the use of drugs when healthier approaches to treating health problems are at least as likely to succeed, but they should remain open to patients' explanations of why alternatives seem inadequate to them.

One major advertiser of lifestyle drugs is the Internet pharmacy industry, a poorly regulated industry that has grown substantially in recent years. Inappropriate patient choices are less likely to be challenged by Internet pharmacies. Of most concern are Internet pharmacies that offer online prescribing as well as traditional pharmacy services or illegally provide prescription drugs with no prescription at all. The AMA has come out strongly against the prescribing of medications for patients whom the physician has not met face-to-face and cannot have examined.[46,47] A doctor–patient relationship cannot develop in the context of fleeting exchanges of information online.[48] Typically, no arrangements are made for medication review. Given the medium, medications are necessarily irresponsibly prescribed when they are prescribed by online pharmacies. In addition to refraining from professional involvement with Internet pharmacies, providers should discuss with patients where they fill prescriptions and whether they purchase medications online.

Drug therapy is the principal treatment for pain, and the prescribing of medications for the relief of pain raises additional ethical concerns. Pain has often been undertreated. Providers have a duty to treat pain adequately to the extent that it is possible to do so, given the patient's goals of care. Some patients prefer to take less pain medication than needed to fully alleviate pain in order to avoid the side effects associated with pain medications. Patient preferences should be respected.

Pharmaceutical companies advertise their products to providers and to patients. While industry promotions contribute to provider and patient awareness of new drugs, the main purpose of advertisement is, of course, to sell as much of the company's products as possible. It has been argued that DTCA empowers patients and enhances the doctor–patient relationship.[49,50] It would, however, be possible to provide information to providers and to the public without employing the tools of marketing, that is without appealing to emotions and putting persuasiveness before accuracy in the advertisement.[51] The principal aim of industry's promotional activity is not the provider's aim of ensuring that each patient gets precisely that drug therapy that would be best for her. It is to increase profit by creating and nurturing a desire or need for particular drugs. It is necessary for providers to resist the enticements of pharmaceutical company salesmanship and to help their patients do so as well.

Although pharmaceutical representatives often provide useful information regarding new medications, new uses for old medications, and new evidence about side effects of medications, the main purpose of marketing by pharmaceutical companies is to increase sales of a particular drug. First, marketers try to persuade providers, through the use of advertisements and informational material, to accept positive claims about their products when those claims may not have been substantiated by independent, high-quality research. They mislead by presenting positive research evidence and withholding negative research evidence.[44,52,53] Marketing campaigns often appeal to the emotions, and considerable sums of money are spent to shape provider attitudes about particular pharmaceutical companies and about the industry as a whole.

Pharmaceutical companies manipulate provider attitudes through advertisements, of course, but also by providing gifts, grants, and educational support to providers and to their professional organizations. The AMA has issued guidelines concerning "gifts to physicians from industry," which lay out the conditions under which it is ethically permissible for physicians to accept gifts from pharmaceutical companies.[54] According to the AMA guidelines, acceptable gifts "primarily entail a benefit to patients and should not be of substantial value." Examples of acceptable gifts include:

- Books.
- Modest meals.
- Drug samples for patient or personal use.
- Financial support of professional meetings (with disclosure, and with monies going to the sponsor to support the meeting itself rather than for the travel expenses of participants).

The guidelines also require that there be no strings attached to the acceptance of a gift; i.e., it would be unacceptable for physicians to agree to alter their prescribing practices in exchange for a gift.

While not all providers have been following the AMA guidelines, a good many have and yet the pharmaceutical industry continues to spend many billions of dollars on marketing.[44,55] It is plausible to suppose that the industry believes that it can strongly influence provider prescription practices even when these guidelines are followed.

Gifts as a Form of Marketing

The AMA guidelines have been criticized in a number of ways for not being strict enough. First, it has been noted that a gift of minimal value (which the AMA has specified as less than $100) may be influential and that, while the AMA has put a limit on the value of any one gift, it has put no limit on the number of gifts a physician might accept.[44] Second, the point of the condition that gifts "primarily entail a benefit to patients" is unclear. From the fact that a gift will be used in the service of patients, it surely does not follow that it is the patients who benefit from the gift. Suppose a physician is offered a free medical instrument. It would, of course, be used in the care of patients. But had he not been given this instrument, he would presumably either have bought one or have been able to provide satisfactory patient care without it.

Perhaps most importantly, the AMA approach to the ethics of accepting gifts from pharmaceutical companies presupposes that when physicians are influenced by gifts, they are consciously influenced by gifts, intentionally favoring the gift-giver over other companies or favoring pharmacotherapy over other treatments. The evidence suggests, however, that physicians are not aware of the effect of pharmaceutical industry marketing on their own clinical judgment and that gifts of very minimal value are effective marketing tools.[56-58]

The American College of Physicians has offered its own "general" and "specific" guidelines for the permissibility of accepting gifts from industry.[59] Its specific guidelines mirror the AMA's: "low-cost gifts of an educational or patient-care nature (such as medical books) and modest hospitality."

There are two components to the discussion that precedes these specific guidelines, however, and it is not clear how they fit together. First, the ACP acknowledges the research showing both the insignificance of gift value in determining whether the behavior of the recipient will be influenced and the lack of self-awareness among physicians regarding the influence of pharmaceutical companies on their own clinical judgment. Second, it recommends, as general guidelines, that physicians ask themselves two questions. (Question 1) What would my patients/colleagues/the public think of my accepting this gift? (Question 2) What is the purpose of the industry offer? It is clear that Question 1 would lead to the conclusion that modest educational or patient-care gifts are acceptable. What is not clear is how acknowledging the research evidence on gift-giving could lead to the claim that answering Question 1 will help root out conflicts of interest in prescribing. Since most patients do not have access to the evidence that untutored physician intuitions about the effects of gifts on clinical judgment are deeply flawed, responding to that evidence by suggesting a reliance instead on untutored patient intuitions is remarkably ill conceived. Question 2, on the other hand, is a perfectly sensible question to ask about the offer of any gift. What is unclear is how answering Question 2 could lead to the claim that it is permissible to accept the kinds of gifts from pharmaceutical companies that are mentioned in the specific guidelines. Surely the point of any of these offers is to promote the company and its products.

Patient Requests for Physician-Assisted Suicide

Physician-assisted suicide (PAS) is illegal in every state but Oregon. The question of whether it should be legalized (as it was in Oregon when the Oregon Death with Dignity Act was passed) or decriminalized is highly controversial in this country, no less among physicians and medical ethicists than in the general population.[60] Physicians in all states are asked for assistance in dying and some physicians outside of the state of Oregon are willing to provide it.[61,62]

Whatever their position on this question of political morality, physicians have reason to consider how to respond in a morally responsible way when a patient expresses interest in obtaining information about the use of medications to bring about his or her own death or a prescription for medication to be used for that purpose. Questions about the moral permissibility of PAS, about whether PAS should be legal in some circumstances, and about the moral permissibility of civil disobedience in the context of PAS are questions about which reasonable people can disagree. There may be more than one morally responsible clinical response to a patient's request for PAS.

Arguments for the moral permissibility of PAS are grounded in the principles of beneficence and autonomy. Physicians have a duty to respond to the suffering of their patients, to relieve it if possible, and to aim at the patients' good. One way to respond to the suffering of patients is to make high-quality palliative care available at the end of life, but this will not necessarily relieve a particular patient's suffering. The issue of PAS arises because not all kinds of suffering are treatable and because, not infrequently, suffering that undeniably could be avoided with expert palliative care is not avoided—many patients do not have access to that expertise. Fifty percent of patients studied in the 1995 SUPPORT study suffered substantial pain during the last days of life.[63] Since then, a good deal of attention has been paid to the importance of physician training in palliative care, but there remains a gap between what can be done for dying patients and what is done.

In addition to the duty of beneficence, physicians have a duty to respect patient autonomy. Particularly when it comes to decisions so personal as how one will die and how far one will allow one's body to deteriorate at the end of life, caregivers respect the moral personalities of others by respecting the choices they make.[64] From the fact that palliative care is an important option for patients at the end of life, it does not follow that it is the option of choice for all patients. Some would prefer to die sooner in order:

- To relieve suffering and the fear of future suffering.
- To avoid burdening family or friends with the emotional or practical costs of an extended illness or prolonged death.
- To prevent the "loss of self" that commonly occurs at the end of life.[65,66]

Arguments against the moral permissibility of PAS center on the moral significance of the difference between killing (and, by extension, assisting in the taking of a life) and "letting die." Despite continuing disagreement over details, there is substantial consensus on the claim that it is, in some circumstances, morally permissible to allow a person to die. When, for example, a competent patient who will die without a particular medical intervention refuses that intervention, it is widely accepted that physicians respect that patient's rights, and so act in a way that is not only morally permissible but also morally obligatory when they refrain from providing the intervention.

Very few people believe that killing is never morally permissible—most allow killing in self-defense, for instance, or in the conduct of a just war. The prima facie duty not to kill is, however, taken to be much stronger than the prima facie duty not to allow another person to die. The burden of showing how other moral considerations outweigh this strong prima facie duty would seem to lie with those who would argue for helping seriously ill and suffering patients to die.

In an important philosophical paper published in 1975 in the *New England Journal of Medicine*, James Rachels argued that intuitions about this intrinsic moral difference between killing and letting die are explicable in terms of contingent features of typical acts of killing and the omissions called "letting die"—features such as the motives of the agents and the consequences of their choices.[67] Between cases of physicians' respecting treatment refusals that will eventuate in death and cases of PAS, such contingent factors do not differ as they typically do between cases of letting die and cases of killing. Without those differences, Rachels argued, no moral difference remains.

It has been argued that even if there is nothing intrinsically morally wrong with helping a suffering, dying patient hasten her own death, physician assistance with dying is inconsistent with the traditional goals of medicine, on which depend the integrity of the profession and extensive trust in physicians. The tradition of medicine as a healing profession inherently gives physicians moral reason not to participate in PAS, as does the fact that doing so could endanger public perceptions of the profession. Another troubling possible consequence of helping some patients to die is that doing so might begin a "slippery slope" from careful fulfillment of autonomous patient choices to less careful satisfaction of patient requests. "Slippery slope arguments" have played a significant role in the debate over legalizing or decriminalizing PAS. Allowing assistance in dying in some circumstances could open the door to abuse. Supporters of legalization point out that PAS is practiced now. Abuse may be more likely when it is engaged in secretly and without controls.

Others have argued that members of social groups that are disvalued in today's society—in particular, the elderly, the disabled, and members of minority groups—will be particularly vulnerable to potential abuses of PAS should it become an accepted part of medical practice. It has, for example, been argued that the lives of the disabled are less good than they could be because sufficient care is not taken of those members of society who depend more on assistance. If not enough is done to support disabled individuals, then they may be coerced by avoidable circumstances to end their lives prematurely. This argument would seem to work better as a call for more humane social responses to the fact that some are disabled in one way or another than as an argument against PAS. If the circumstances of one's life are such as to make death seem preferable, it hardly addresses the problem to rule death out as well as the achievement of a decent life. It has, in addition, been argued that efforts to protect disabled persons from the choices they would make for themselves are paternalistic and disrespectful of their equal capacities for autonomous choice.[68]

In Oregon, physicians have the legal right to assist patients in dying. It is, of course, necessary to consider a particular request for PAS very carefully, exploring with the patient the reasons for the request and working with the patient to address those forms of suffering or difficulty that can be addressed. It is necessary to determine that the patient has decision-making capacity and reasonable to hold the bar for capacity to make this particular decision rather high. It is also necessary to make sure that the patient has an accurate understanding of her circumstances—of the prognosis and of all available options for treatment, for refusals of treatment, and for palliative measures. Physicians should be attentive to the differences that may exist between the care that is available in theory and the care that is actually available for this patient. For the physician who either believes that PAS is not morally permissible or is unwilling to participate in it, the same explorations and efforts to assist the patient are appropriate. The physician should share with the patient his beliefs about PAS or about his own involvement, in order to make clear that he is unwilling to assist the patient and his reasons for refusing. He should not, however, discuss his beliefs with a view to changing the patient's mind on these large and controversial moral and political questions.

The American physician outside of the state of Oregon has to consider as well the illegality of the act that is being requested. Clearly, the integrity of the profession is to some extent dependent on the willingness of its members to follow laws designed to limit its powers. More generally, in a reasonably just society, physicians share with other citizens prima facie reasons to obey the law. It might, however, be argued that when physicians write prescriptions for patients who wish to die after careful and caring consideration of the circumstances of that request, they engage in a morally permissible illegal act. A physician might believe that the law regarding PAS is unjust or he might believe that, while the law is as it should be, there ought to be exceptions.[69] It is harder to argue for morally motivated noncompliance with the law in the case of PAS than it is in such clear-cut cases as those taken from the civil rights movement because it is not nearly as clear that people have a right to assistance with dying as that people have a right to enjoy equally the rights of citizenship and of fundamental social acceptance.

KEY POINTS

- The ethics of prescribing has essentially to do with the decision-making processes that lead to the writing of prescriptions.
- The provider should welcome the patient's participation in the choice of a treatment plan and in reassessment of drug therapy.
- Patients should be supported in their efforts to educate themselves about the medical problems they face and the treatments available.
- There are, at the same time, limits to the choices that patients may make, and it is sometimes necessary to refuse patient requests for particular medications or advise against particular plans concerning treatment.
- Providers have a general duty to maintain expertise in the areas in which they practice and to consult with experts when their patients' needs call for knowledge or skills that they do not possess. This duty

applies as fully to the rapid developments in pharmacotherapy as to any other area of medical progress.

- Providers have a duty to avoid conflicts of interest that may interfere with clinical judgment. It may be that potential conflicts are nowhere more pervasive than in the area of prescribing drugs.
- Responses to patient requests for assistance in dying should be guided by reasoned consideration of the ethical requirements of the duties of beneficence and respect for patient autonomy.

REFERENCES

1. Schlenk EA, Dunbar-Jacob J, Engberg S. Medication non-adherence among older adults: a review of strategies and interventions for improvement. *J Gerontol Nurs.* 2004;30(7):33–43.
2. Ruscin JM, Semla TP. Assessment of medication management skills in older outpatients. *Ann Pharmacother.* 1996;30(10):1083–8.
3. Dunbar-Jacob J, Schlenk EA. Patient adherence to treatment regimen. In: Baum A, Revenson TA, Singer JE, eds. *Handbook of Health Psychology.* Mahwah, NJ: Lawrence Erlbaum Associates, Inc.; 2001:571–80.
4. Towle A, Godolphin W. Framework for teaching and learning informed shared decision making. *BMJ.* 1999;319(7212):766–71.
5. Morrow DG, Hier CM, Menard WE, et al. Icons improve older and younger adults' comprehension of medication information. *J Gerontol B Pyschol Sci Soc Sci.* 1998; 53(4):P240–54.
6. Morrow DG, Leirer V, Altieri P. List formats improve medication instructions for older adults. *Educ Gerontol.* 1995;21:151–66.
7. Morrow D, Leirer V, Altieri P, et al. Elders' schema for taking medication: implications for instruction design. *J Gerontol.* 1991;46(6):P378–85.
8. Morrow DG, Leirer VO, Andrassy JM, et al. The influence of list format and category headers on age differences in understanding medication instructions. *Exp Aging Res.* 1998;24(3):231–56.
9. Col N, Fanale JE, Kronholm P. The role of medication noncompliance and adverse drug reactions in hospitalizations of the elderly. *Arch Intern Med.* 1990;150(4):841–5.
10. Pettinger MB, Waclawiw MA, Davis KB, et al. Compliance to multiple interventions in a high risk population. *Ann Epidemiol.* 1999;9(7):408–18.
11. Ware GJ, Holford NH, Davison JG, et al. Unit dose calendar packaging and elderly patient compliance. *N Z Med J.* 1991;104(924):495–7.
12. Miller CA. Teaching older adults medication self-care. *Geriatr Nurs.* 2004;25(5):318–9.
13. Gray SL, Mahoney JE, Blough DK. Medication adherence in elderly patients receiving home health services following hospital discharge. *Ann Pharmacother.* 2001;35(5):539–45.
14. World Health Organization. *Adherence to Long-Term Therapies: Evidence for Action.* Geneva: World Health Organization; 2003.
15. Kerse N, Buetow S, Mainous AG 3rd, et al. Physician–patient relationship and medication compliance: a primary care investigation. *Ann Fam Med.* 2004;2(5):455–61.

16. Maly RC, Leake B, Frank JC, et al. Implementation of consultative geriatric recommendations: the role of patient–primary care physician concordance. *J Am Geriatr Soc.* 2002;50(8):1372–80.

17. Vedsted P, Mainz J, Lauritzen T, et al. Patient and GP agreement on aspects of general practice care. *Fam Pract.* 2002;19(4):339–43.

18. Stewart MA. Effective physician–patient communication and health outcomes: a review. *CMAJ.* 1995;152(9):1423–33.

19. Stewart M, Brown JB, Boon H, et al. Evidence on patient–doctor communication. *Cancer Prev Control.* 1999;3(1):25–30.

20. Royal Pharmaceutical Society of Great Britain. *From Compliance to Concordance: Achieving Shared Goals in Medicine Taking.* London: Royal Pharmaceutical Society of Great Britain; 1997.

21. Marinker M, Shaw J. Not to be taken as directed. *BMJ.* 2003;326(7385):348–9.

22. Medicines-Partnership.org [home page on the Internet]. London: Medicines Partnership of the Department of Health, UK.; c2002 [updated 2005 Jun 13]. Available from: www.concordance.org, www.medicines-partnership.org

23. Stewart M, Brown JB. Patient-centredness in medicine. In: Edwards A, Elwyn G, eds. *Evidence-Based Patient Choice: Inevitable or Impossible?* New York: Oxford University Press; 2001:97–117.

24. Heisler M, Bouknight RR, Hayward RA, et al. The relative importance of physician communication, participatory decision making, and patient understanding in diabetes self-management. *J Gen Intern Med.* 2002;17(4):243–52.

25. Institute of Medicine. *To Err is Human: Building a Safer Health System.* Washington, DC: Institute of Medicine; 1999.

26. Meredith S, Feldman PH, Frey D, et al. Possible medication errors in home healthcare patients. *J Am Geriatr Soc.* 2001;49(6):719–24.

27. Willcox SM, Himmelstein DU, Woolhandler S. Inappropriate drug prescribing for the community-dwelling elderly. *JAMA.* 1994;272(4):292–6.

28. Gurwitz JH, Soumerai SB, Avorn J. Improving medication prescribing and utilization in the nursing home. *J Am Geriatr Soc.* 1990;38(5):542–52.

29. Ray WA, Taylor JA, Meador KG, et al. Reducing antipsychotic drug use in nursing homes. A controlled trial of provider education. *Arch Intern Med.* 1993;153(6):713–21.

30. Stuart B, Kamal-Bahl S, Briesacher B, et al. Trends in the prescription of inappropriate drugs for the elderly between 1995 and 1999. *Am J Geriatr Pharmacother.* 2003;1(2):61–74.

31. Eisenberg DM, Davis RB, Ettner SL, et al. Trends in alternative medicine use in the United States, 1990–1997: results of a follow-up national survey. *JAMA.* 1998;280(18):1569–75.

32. Elwyn G, Charles C. Shared decision making: the principles and the competences. In: Edwards A, Elwyn G, eds. *Evidence-Based Patient Choice: Inevitable or Impossible?* New York: Oxford University Press; 2001:118–43.

33. Entwistle V, O'Donnell M. Evidence-Based Health Care: What Role for Patients? In: Edwards A, Elwyn G, eds. *Evidence-Based Patient Choice: Inevitable or Impossible?* New York: Oxford University Press; 2001:34–49.

34. Elwyn G, Edwards A, Kinnersley P, et al. Shared decision making and the concept of equipoise: the competences of involving patients in healthcare choices. *Br J Gen Pract.* 2000;50(460):892–9.

35. Ashcroft R, Hope T, Parker M. Ethical issues and evidence-based patient choice. In: Edwards A, Elwyn G, eds. *Evidence-Based Patient Choice: Inevitable or Impossible?* New York: Oxford University Press; 2001.

36. Mainous AG 3rd, Baker R, Love MM, et al. Continuity of care and trust in one's physician: evidence from primary care in the United States and the United Kingdom. *Fam Med.* 2001;33(1):22–7.

37. Edwards A, Bastian H. Risk communication—making evidence part of patient choices. In: Edwards A, Elwyn G, eds. *Evidence-Based Patient Choice: Inevitable or Impossible?* New York: Oxford University Press; 2001:144–60.

38. O'Connor A, Edwards A. The role of decision aids in promoting evidence-based patient choice. In: Edwards A, Elwyn G, eds. *Evidence-Based Patient Choice: Inevitable or Impossible?* New York: Oxford University Press; 2001:220–42.

39. Rosenberg W. Evidence-based patient choice in secondary care. In: Edwards A, Elwyn G, eds. *Evidence-Based Patient Choice: Inevitable or Impossible?* New York: Oxford University Press; 2001:191–205.

40. Benjamin DM. Reducing medication errors and increasing patient safety: case studies in clinical pharmacology. *J Clin Pharmacol.* 2003;43(7):768–83.

41. Rich MW, Gray DB, Beckham V, et al. Effect of a multidisciplinary intervention on medication compliance in elderly patients with congestive heart failure. *Am J Med.* 1996;101(3):270–6.

42. Lowe CJ, Raynor DK, Purvis J, et al. Effects of a medicine review and education programme for older people in general practice. *Br J Clin Pharmacol.* 2000;50(2):172–5.

43. Mintzes B, Barer ML, Kravitz RL, et al. How does direct-to-consumer advertising (DTCA) affect prescribing? A survey in primary care environments with and without legal DTCA. *CMAJ.* 2003;169(5):405–12.

44. Angell M. *The Truth about the Drug Companies: How They Deceive Us and What To Do about It.* New York: Random House; 2004.

45. Murray E, Lo B, Pollack L, et al. Direct-to-consumer advertising: physicians' views of its effects on quality of care and the doctor–patient relationship. *J Am Board Fam Pract.* 2003;16(6):513–24.

46. American Medical Association. Internet Prescribing, Board of Trustees Report 35-A-99, 1999, www.ama-assn.org/meetings/public/annual99/reports/onsite/bot/rtf/bot35.rtf.

47. American Medical Association. Guidance for Physicians on Internet Prescribing, Board of Trustees Report 6-A-02, 2002, www.ama-assn.org/ama1/upload/mm/annual03/bot7a03.doc.

48. Hochberg JW. Nailing Jell-O to a wall: regulating Internet pharmacies. *J Health Law.* 2004;37(3):445–71.

49. Holmer AF. Direct-to-consumer prescription drug advertising builds bridges between patients and physicians. *JAMA.* 1999;281(4):380–2.

50. Holmer AF. Direct-to-consumer advertising—strengthening our health care system. *N Engl J Med.* 2002;346(7):526–8.

51. Woloshin S, Schwartz LM, Tremmel J, et al. Direct-to-consumer advertisements for prescription drugs: what are Americans being sold? *Lancet.* 2001;358(9288):1141–6.

52. Liberati A, Magrini N. Information from drug companies and opinion leaders. *BMJ.* 2003;326(7400):1156–7.

53. Lexchin J. What information do physicians receive from pharmaceutical representatives? *Can Fam Physician*. 1997 May;43:941–5.

54. American Medical Association, Council on Ethical and Judicial Affairs. Opinion 8.061: Gifts to Physicians from Industry: Code of Medical Ethics: Current opinions of the Council on Ethical and Judicial Affairs. Chicago: American Medical Association. Updated Nov. 2004.

55. Blumenthal D. Doctors and drug companies. *N Engl J Med*. 2004;351(18):1885–90.

56. Wazana A. Physicians and the pharmaceutical industry: is a gift ever just a gift? *JAMA*. 2000;283(3):373–80.

57. Watkins C, Moore L, Harvey I, et al. Characteristics of general practitioners who frequently see drug industry representatives: national cross sectional study. *BMJ*. 2003;326(7400):1178–9.

58. Chren MM. Interactions between physicians and drug company representatives. *Am J Med*. 1999;107(2):182–3.

59. Coyle SL. Ethics and Human Rights Committee, American College of Physicians-American Society of Internal Medicine. Physician-industry relations. Part 1: individual physicians. *Ann Intern Med*. 2002;136(5):396–402.

60. Stell L. Physician-assisted suicide: to decriminalize or to legalize, that is the question. In: Battin M, Rhodes R, Silvers A, eds. *Physician-Assisted Suicide: Expanding the Debate*. New York: Routledge; 1998:225–51.

61. Meier DE, Emmons CA, Wallenstein S, et al. A national survey of physician-assisted suicide and euthanasia in the United States. *N Engl J Med*. 1998;338(17):1193–201.

62. Emanuel EJ, Fairclough D, Clarridge BC, et al. Attitudes and practices of U.S. oncologists regarding euthanasia and physician-assisted suicide. *Ann Intern Med*. 2000;133(7):527–32.

63. A controlled trial to improve care of seriously ill hospitalized patients. The study to understand prognoses and preferences of outcomes and risks of treatment (SUPPORT). The SUPPORT Principal Investigators. *JAMA*. 1995;274(20):1591–8.

64. Dworkin R, Nagel T, Nozick R, Rawls J, Scanlon T, Thomson JJ. The Philosophers' Brief. State of Washington v. Glucksberg; Vacco v. Quill, nos. 95-1858, 96-110, October term, 1996, December 10, 1996, Brief for Ronald Dworkin, Thomas Nagel, Robert Nozick, John Rawls, Thomas Scanlon, and Judith Jarvis Thompson as amici curiae in support of respondents.

65. Pearlman RA, Starks H. Why do people seek physician-assisted death? In: Quill T, Battin M, eds. *Physician-Assisted Dying: The Case for Palliative Care and Patient Choice*. Baltimore: John Hopkins University Press; 2004:91–101.

66. Lavery JV, Boyle J, Dickens BM, et al. Origins of the desire for euthanasia and assisted suicide in people with HIV-1 or AIDS: a qualitative study. *Lancet*. 2001;358(9279):362–7.

67. Rachels J. Active and passive euthanasia. *N Engl J Med*. 1975;292(2):78–80.

68. Silvers A. Protecting the innocents from physician-assisted suicide: disability discrimination and the duty to protect otherwise vulnerable groups. In: Battin M, Rhodes R, Silvers A, eds. *Physician-Assisted Suicide: Expanding the Debate*. New York: Routledge; 1998:133–48.

69. Childress JF. Civil disobedience, conscientious objection, and evasive noncompliance: a framework for the analysis and assessment of illegal actions in health care. *J Med Philos*. 1985;10(1):63–83.

14

Improving Medication Use in the Elderly: Seven Prescriptions for the H.E.L.P.I.N.G. Professional

WILLIAM N. TINDALL AND CYNTHIA G. OLSEN

Teamwork delivers a better product.

—Dr. Robin A. Harvan, Colorado AHEC

OVERVIEW

A case study is used to present some nuances associated with aging physiology, multiple chronic disorders, polypharmacy, and inappropriate prescribing of medications as well as to illustrate what can happen as a result of nonadherence to a complex medication regimen. This chapter also details seven behaviors or tenets that if followed by caring health professionals would help the elderly achieve the most benefit from their medications. These tenets focus the helping health professional on ways to become an advocate, a protector, a knowledgeable educator, and a friend who is willing to assist the elderly with drug-related problems through a long-term commitment and effective teamwork. The elderly are presented as persons who more often than not should be engaged as capable and willing partners in any activity aimed at managing their health care, especially when they are given appropriate education and support.

When Margot Keys moved to Florida, her motivation was her strong desire to take care of her aging parents, Frank and Carol Forman. That was 10 years ago. Mr. Forman has since died and Margot, rather than moving her mother to an assisted-living facility, now provides total care for her mother in her home. Since moving to Florida, Margot has used the same family medicine clinic and local pharmacy for herself and her family as well as her parents.

Since her father passed away 18 months ago, Margot has noticed a decline in her mother's cognitive abilities. Margot recently requested a change to another family physician. This happened after she met a "lady doctor" at her family medicine clinic who she believes better understands her and better understands her mother's needs. When Margot moved her mother into her home, her husband was supportive because he has a job that requires him to travel a great deal and he thought the two women would be great company for each other. Margot has several citrus fruit trees in her yard and loves to pick her mother a fresh grapefruit every morning. This has quickly become a delightful, shared, experience for the two of them.

One afternoon Margot returned from a short shopping trip to find her mother in a state of anxiety and wandering about the neighborhood. Frantic and worried, she took her mother to their lady doctor—Dr. Lois Wilson— who subsequently placed Mrs. Forman on Risperdal® 1.5 mg BID.

Six weeks later Margot had to rush her mother to the emergency department at the local hospital after she came home to find her mother lying on the floor. Her mother had tripped on a loose rug and was in terrible pain, the result of a broken wrist. Mrs. Forman was rushed to the ER, and within 2 hours a physician had put her wrist in a cast and prescribed Duragesic® 25 mcg/day via a patch for the pain. Two days later Margot takes her mother to Dr. Wilson for follow-up and to check things out. Dr. Wilson then reviews with Margot the status of her mother's hypertension, insomnia, restlessness, and depression and then notices in her chart that Mrs. Forman continues to take medications prescribed by her previous physician. She also notices that a nurse had recorded Mrs. Forman's BP as 148/98 mm Hg during her last visit.

The chart further reveals that Mrs. Forman's current drugs are:

1. Verapamil 40 mg TID
2. Paxil® 20 mg OD
3. Metoprolol CR 50 mg BID
4. Cardizem® 180 mg HS
5. Restoril® 7.5 mg HS

6. Diazepam 2 mg generic 1 at HS
7. Risperdal 1.5 mg BID

Dr. Wilson now picks up her phone and calls the local pharmacist. "Can you help me out here?" she asks. "You know Margot and her mother as well as I do and since Margot thinks so highly of us both I thought we could work on Mrs. Forman's medication issues together." She reads the list of drugs from Mrs. Forman's chart to the pharmacist and asks whether the pharmacy's records indicate that she is on anything other than these drugs. The pharmacist replies, "Yes, I added a new drug, Duragesic, a couple of days ago, but my medication profile lists the same medicines as yours. However, I did make a notation that Margot gives her mother a multivitamin every day and a baby aspirin. I have talked to them both about the large amount of Metamucil® they buy, and I did express my concern over their eating so much grapefruit." Dr. Wilson goes on to ask several other questions: Do you think any of her drugs could have been responsible for the recent fall? If so, which ones? Do you have any recommendation for changing Mrs. Forman's drugs to prevent her from falling again? Do we need to change any of her dosages?

- What is it about Mrs. Forman's drug therapy, her diseases, or Mrs. Forman herself that would indicate why her fall may have had something to do with an adverse drug reaction (ADR)?
- Do you suspect there might be some drug interactions going on? If so, what are they?
- What nondrug measures could Margot initiate to help keep her mother from falling again or wandering off?
- If Mrs. Forman is on only eight medications and a couple of nonprescription medications, does she qualify as a victim of polypharmacy?

In this case, the physiological changes of aging, disease pathology, a complex drug regimen, and polypharmacy are all at play. Mrs. Forman is on a beta-blocker and a calcium channel blocker which together can heighten the risk of bradycardia and heart block. Serotonin syndrome is also a possibility due to Paxil and Duragesic. Enhancement of the sedative effect of diazepam is also possible due to combining Duragesic and Paxil.

After Dr. Wilson and the pharmacist review Mrs. Forman's medications, they could stop the Duragesic and use a less potent analgesic. Stopping the diazepam is also prudent. Stopping or decreasing the dose of metoprolol and considering control of Mrs. Forman's hypertension with a thiazide or loop diuretic and an angiotensin-converting enzyme (ACE) inhibitor is also an option because her BP remains high despite her current therapy. Stopping the verapamil and Cardizem combination may also be prudent. Since the Paxil was prescribed to help Mrs. Forman deal with the death of her husband several years ago, it may be time to discontinue it as well. If she's taking Metamucil at the same time as other medications (likely at bedtime), it may be binding to a prescription drug and causing it to be less bioavailable and hence less effective.

Approximately one-third of all drugs prescribed in the United States are considered unnecessary, and this is likely with Mrs. Forman. Polypharmacy is the unnecessary and excessive use of prescription and nonprescription medications, and it increases the risk for ADRs and drug–drug interactions. The question is what number of medications is considered excessive?

The answer is, it depends. Older, community-dwelling, independent women are at the highest risk for polypharmacy. Mrs. Forman is not living alone, but she likely has age-related changes affecting her pharmacokinetic and pharmacodynamic responses to medications. The effects of these changes are further complicated by the presence of comorbidities that require pharmacologic management. If her rate of unintentional noncompliance with her therapeutic regimen were high, she would really be in trouble. Fortunately, her daughter is trying hard to keep her on the correct medication regimen. In addition, the pharmacist, who knows both women, is monitoring refill rates to make sure they are adhering to the prescribed regimen. Mrs. Forman's previous physician may have contributed to the polypharmacy by prescribing medications considered inappropriate for the elderly (diazepam, Paxil). Dr. Wilson is trying to avoid ADRs and drug interactions with her team approach, which includes family input from both Margot and her mother as well as the assistance of a pharmacist.

A COGNITIVE SHIFT: MAKING PROFESSIONALS BETTER AT HELPING THE ELDERLY

The aging of the U.S. population has raised concerns about the social and economic burdens associated with managing an increasing number of elderly people with chronic diseases. The fact that the elderly are enjoying increased longevity does not imply that they are also seeing an increase in "good health." In fact, the leading causes of death among older people are chronic diseases such as heart disease, cerebrovascular disorders, respiratory disorders, diabetes, and renal and hepatic disorders. What is common among these chronic diseases is their reliance on medications to control them and the patient's need for caring, competent, and gifted health professionals to work as a team to help with medication-related problems.

For example, coronary heart disease is the major cause of death in both elderly men and women. Yet well into the 1980s many physicians did not believe that antihypertensive drugs could improve health outcomes and quality of life for the elderly, so they did not treat coronary heart disease with antihypertensive drugs. This practice of not using antihypertensive drugs was hard to understand considering the abundance of evidence to the contrary.[1,2] In addition, valid evidence showed that antihypertensive therapy reduces blood pressure to below 140/90 mm Hg in up to 70% of elderly patients.[3] Furthermore, not treating hypertension in the elderly became even more disconcerting when published evidence demonstrated that, in most instances, elderly patients adhere to antihypertensive drug therapy at least as well as younger patients and also tolerate these medications just as well if the drugs are administered properly.[4]

Today, the taking of any medication, whether prescription, nonprescription, herbal, nutraceutical, or supplement, is still the number one medical intervention utilized by the elderly, who view taking medications more as looking for relief from symptoms, not necessarily as a cure. However, physiological changes in the elderly, their chronic illnesses, their frailties, and their increased use of drugs contribute to their risk for developing a drug-related problem. The following eight types of "drug-related problems" are potential causes of an undesirable medication use outcome for anyone, including the elderly, although the elderly have a higher percentage of drug swapping, self-administering, and use of nonprescription products and herbals:[5]

1. Untreated indications
2. Improper drug selection
3. Subtherapeutic dosage
4. Failure to obtain the drugs
5. Overdosage
6. ADRs
7. Drug interactions
8. Use of a drug without an indication

Fortunately, these eight drug-related problems are all preventable. A ninth drug-related problem that has been described but is largely unrecognized also is preventable. This phenomenon is known as the "prescribing cascade."

The prescribing cascade occurs when an ADR is misinterpreted as a new medical condition and another new drug is prescribed on top of all the other drugs to treat the "new" condition.[6] The prescribing of an additional new drug brings added risk of an ADR, especially when the added drug is unnecessary. Fortunately, a growing body of literature encourages providers to consider any new signs and symptoms a patient exhibits to be the result of one or more of the drugs already being taken.[7]

Because there is a growing interest in drug-related problems among the elderly, more than ever there are also numerous opportunities for health professionals to assist the elderly with their medication needs. However, such opportunities go wanting unless there is effective teamwork among physicians, pharmacists, physician assistants, nurses, and nurse practitioners. But more important, patients must be given an active role that allows them to help "manage" their chronic disease(s).

Today, many health professionals are initiating what they believe are "disease management programs." In fact, over the past several decades an entire industry has been built using health professionals in chronic disease management interventions. Some of this has been an outgrowth of the four-decade shift in the United States into refinancing its health care system and reformatting the health care system as one based on "managed care."

But how can a health professional or a corporation or an agency "manage" someone else's health care? Furthermore, how can a corporate entity provide "care"? As traditional models of care give way to newer models of care, some health professionals are positioning themselves as "managing" whatever intervention it is that patients are provided. Although pharmacists, physicians, case managers, nurses, and others focus on "managing" drug interactions, ADRs, complex dosing schedules, and polypharmacy through "disease management" or "medication therapy management" or "pharmaceutical care" interventions, the truth is that the person who was given the medication and who has a chronic disease must "manage" them both. This is especially noteworthy in cases of chronic medication use among community-dwelling, ambulatory elderly. Thus, when nonadherence to a medication regimen occurs it is seen not as a failure on the part of any one health professional but rather as a failure on the part of a team of health professionals who did not work effectively and together at helping an elderly person understand what was expected: that he or she could "manage" his/her own medication situation or disease.[8]

To be better at helping the elderly, some health professionals need to undergo a cognitive shift when they become frustrated over their well-intentioned medication management interventions not being as successful as hoped. This

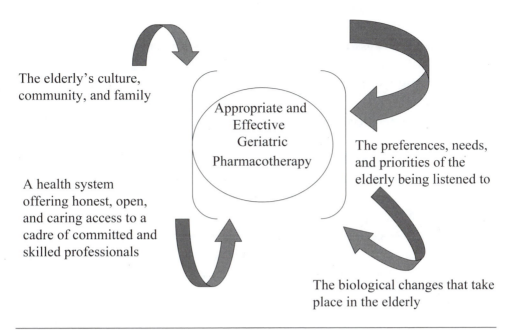

The elderly's culture, community, and family

A health system offering honest, open, and caring access to a cadre of committed and skilled professionals

Appropriate and Effective Geriatric Pharmacotherapy

The preferences, needs, and priorities of the elderly being listened to

The biological changes that take place in the elderly

Figure 1   Forces that affect how the elderly get the best use out of their medications.

cognitive shift involves accepting a viewpoint that medication therapy management must be a partnership in which all health professionals facilitate elderly patients and their caregivers into "management" of their chronic diseases through encouragement, information, and empowerment that results in patients taking responsibility for their own behavior and decisions. After all, if a patient goes into a pharmacy for a 15-minute visit with a pharmacist every 2 months, who is truly "managing" that patient's health the other 59 days, 23 hours, and 45 minutes between visits? Isn't it the patient and those who are the patient's caregivers?

SEVEN TENETS FOR THE H.E.L.P.I.N.G. PROFESSIONAL

There are six foundational "truths" on which the following seven tenets are built. Buffeting these six truths are forces that affect how the elderly may or may not get the best use of their medications, depending on how all these factors interplay (Figure 1). These truths are:

- Treating all of the chronic and multiple conditions that often plague the elderly is a complex issue.
- ADRs to the drugs used to treat chronic and multiple conditions remain the fourth leading cause of death in the elderly, following close behind heart disease, cancer, and stroke.[9]

- Medications and doses of them that are quite appropriate in younger persons can become quite inappropriate in older patients. This is true when drugs are given to the elderly in doses that are considered "normal" in a younger person and when such doses ignore the age-related physiological and pharmacokinetic changes that occur in the elderly.
- Any elderly patient can become nonadherent to a complex medication regimen; this does not make the patient a "bad person."
- All elderly persons can have ADRs, drug–drug interactions, food–drug interactions, and drug–disease interactions, all of which can be complicated by physical, sensory, and cognitive losses as a result of normal aging or disease.
- Appropriate care of the elderly requires a dedicated team of health professionals effectively communicating with each other and with the patient and his or her caregivers. Fortunately, health care professionals, physicians, patients, and their families are learning to rely on the expertise of pharmacists whose recommendations, patient education, intervention, surveillance of medication adherence, and monitoring for ADRs have become highly regarded.

To fulfill the need for a team approach to helping the elderly with their drug-related issues, the following seven prescriptive behaviors are offered. These are suggestions for developing a more coordinated and planned approach to the medication care needs of the elderly. After all, wouldn't every elderly person like to know that a team of health professionals is personally involved in caring for them, especially if they thought/believed they were being cared for as one of the professional's own elderly parents or grandparents?[10]

SEVEN PRESCRIPTIONS FOR BECOMING A BETTER H.E.L.P.I.N.G. PROFESSIONAL

The following are offered in no special order, but rather in a way that may be useful in seeing them as action steps that help someone build a pathway leading toward being a better H.E.L.P.I.N.G. professional (Table 1).

1. ℞ H or <u>Hear</u> and see the elderly as whole persons, most of whom are able to participate in decisions regarding their treatment and medications.

   Some reports indicate that the elderly feel they are not "seen" or "heard" when they are engaged in encounters with health professionals. They refer to being "talked to" and not "talked with." Like other people, health professionals bring their biases and stereotypes to the workplace,

Table 1 Seven prescriptions for the H.E.L.P.I.N.G. professional

R H: Hear and see the elderly as whole persons, most of whom are able to participate in decisions regarding their treatment and medications.

R E: Earn the trust of the elderly through caring communication, cultural competence, and being confident in what you recommend.

R L: Lead your professional colleagues into improving their collaborations with each other, which in turn may result in better treatment of the elderly.

R P: Protect the elderly from inappropriate medications, polypharmacy, and ADRs.

R I: Identify high-risk elderly while improving their adherence to medication regimens.

R N: Never forget the age-related changes that affect drug dynamics of absorption, distribution, metabolism, and excretion.

R G: Generate a complete drug history to document care, follow-up, and the outcomes of any recommendation or intervention.

as much as they try not to. So it is not surprising that some stereotyping and "elder bias" does creep into the health care workplace. Only a small percentage of the elderly are in care homes or institutions, so it is among contributing, community-dwelling elders that age discrimination and unintentional discrimination by well-meaning health professionals give rise to health disparities, causing the elderly to receive different levels of care than younger populations. The elderly do want a say in what happens to them and to do so they need unbiased, direct, and targeted information about what their options are. They can and do make good decisions if given half a chance. More and more the elderly are commenting appreciatively on health professionals who stop, listen, explain, and talk directly and clearly with them. Health professionals who are good listeners with the elderly:

- Make eye contact with the elderly so that they are not perceived as being disinterested or not listening.
- Acknowledge the elderly person as having useful things to say by using nonverbal cues such as leaning forward, touching the person's elbow, nodding their head, and using phrases such as, Umm; Yes, I see . . .; or Yes, that is understandable, etc.
- Paraphrase what the elderly have said by making comments such as, What I hear you saying is (or sound's like) you are feeling _____ about _____ .
- Do not interrupt elderly patients; rather, they let them finish a complete thought.
- Do not change the subject when an older person cannot articulate his or her thoughts fast enough.

Remember, growing old per se is not a disease and the elderly should not be seen as a burden to society. The French call growing old "The Third Age" and view it as a time to remain useful, if only by the grace of some medicine that keeps them in good health.

2. ℞ E or Earn the trust of the elderly through caring communication, cultural competence, and being confident in what you recommend.

Editorials, newspaper stories, and lay literature provide forums in which the elderly regularly express disappointment in the health care services they and their families receive. But what they also are expressing is that there is a need to hold health care professionals responsible for the racial and ethnic disparities in health outcomes because of their failure to recognize the changing demographics of American society and to respond with a workforce able to practice across America's cultural and racial spectrum.[11]

Being old does not mean that a person has become useless. As the elderly demonstrate every day, they have talents, make contributions to society, are able to accept many challenges, and carry through with a strong spirit, wit, humility, and inspiring faith. Sometimes all they want is to be let into someone's life, even if only for a short time.

At one time, nearly every society honored its elders, and respect and dignity were accorded to those who persevered into old age. Now, social patterns are changing not only in America but throughout the world. According to a WHO report, people live longer in developed countries that offer a good quality of life. Thus, the elderly residing in countries with a lower quality of life tend to migrate from their nations of origin to partake in a better quality of life in the United States. They often come to the United States to provide care for grandchildren while parents work. Today, the idea of children staying home to care for aging parents is not the norm, which ultimately creates an elderly population that is growing and becoming medically underserved.[12]

3. ℞ L or Lead your professional colleagues into improving their collaborations with each other, which in turn, may result in better treatment of the elderly.

In 2000, during a Washington, DC, conference of physicians, nurses, and pharmacists, the attendees came to a consensus on several recommendations, centered on the need for all three health professions to conduct collaborative research on medication use, share the results with each other, and, even more important translate the results into the language of the public. The same conference produced their collective thinking on the need to improve interprofessional communications so that the benefits of collaborative practice models, best practice models, shared responsibility, sentinel events, and adequate attention paid to ethnic and cultural issues would accrue to American society. Conference participants believed this could all be done in a manner that "requires mutual respect for and appreciation of the contributions of each health care provider."[13]

In an article written by a pharmacist to physicians, the pharmacist encourages "collaboration and communication between the primary care physician, patient, and other health care professionals as essential in keeping the patient healthy, independent, and free of medication mishaps."[14]

In a different report describing a randomized controlled clinical intervention that was to have a pharmacist review a medication record, interview the patient, conduct a drug regimen review, share recommendations for optimal therapy with the patient's physician, and provide medication counseling to the patient or caregiver, it was found that physicians accepted 76% of the pharmacist's recommendations, which in turn resulted in a direct cost avoidance of $250 per patient.[15] Although this study was done in another country, it did indicate a role for pharmacists in positively affecting medication use by the elderly.

4. ℞ P or <u>Protect</u> the elderly from inappropriate medications, polypharmacy, and ADRs.

Inappropriate medication use among the elderly is a serious patient safety issue and a serious health issue.[16,17] But what makes a prescribed medication "inappropriate"? One widely used and accepted criterion for "inappropriate medication use in the elderly" is that of Mark Beers, MD (see Foreword), and his panel of experts. Beers and his experts not only defined the criteria for inappropriate medications but also identified drugs that meet their criteria.[18-20] Others have done follow-up studies to ascertain the prevalence of inappropriate drugs prescribed for the elderly and have found that 12% to 40% of the drugs used by the elderly are indeed inappropriate for their care.[21,22]

In addition, other studies have shown that 2.6% of community-dwelling elderly are taking at least 1 of 11 medications (Table 2) that should be avoided and that 21.3% of Americans over the age of 65 are taking at least one medication included on the Beers' list of inappropriate medications used in the elderly.[23] Health professionals would do well

Table 2   Beers' list of inappropriate medications used in the elderly

Drugs to Always Avoid in the Elderly

Barbiturates	GI antispasmodics
Flurazepam	Belladonna alkaloids
Meprobamate (Equanil®)	Clindinium and chlordiazepoxide (Librium®)
Meperidine (Demerol®)	Dicyclomine (Bentyl®)
Dicyclomine	Hyoscyamine (Levsin®)
Pentazocine (Talwin®)	Propantheline
Trimethobenzamide	

Drugs That Are Rarely Appropriate in the Elderly

Chlordiazepoxide	Propoxyphene
Benzodiazepines, long acting	Carisoprodol
Diazepam	Chlorzoxazone
Chlordiazepoxide	Cyclobenzaprine
Clonazepam	Indomethacin (Indocin®)
Halazepam	Metaxalone
Quazepam	Methocarbamol
Digoxin (Lanoxin)	

Drugs with Some Indications in the Elderly

Amitriptyline (Elavil®)	Hydroxyzine
Chlorpheniramine	Methyldopa (Aldomet®)
Cyproheptadine	Promethazine
Disopyramide (Norpace®)	Reserpine
Doxepin (Sinequan®)	Oxybutynin
Dipyridamole	Ticlopidine (Ticlid®)
Diphenhydramine	

For the complete version of the Beers' list of inappropriate and potentially dangerous medications for the elderly, go to: http://www.tahsa.org/files%2Fmedbeer1.pdf.

to remember that patients over the age of 65 do not need to stop taking all drugs on the Beers' list; however, psychotropics, antidepressants, and muscle relaxants can be hard on aging kidneys, and the "risky drugs" placed on the Beers' list need to be monitored for their potential to induce accidents and hospitalizations. Prospective studies have yet to prove conclusively that the drugs on the Beers' list are associated with "bad outcomes." Although much work is being done to reduce the inappropriate prescribing of these drugs to the elderly,[24] the use of these drugs has remained fairly constant since the revelation of problems.[25] A cross-sectional study of 157,517 elderly subjects enrolled in 10 HMOs demonstrated that at least 28.8% were taking one potentially inappropriate medication[26] from the Beers' list. Since these rates are as high as they were 10 years ago, it behooves all health professionals to understand more fully the significance of the problem and why it occurs and to be vigilant and vigorous in helping get these rates down or at least in making sure that suspect drugs are used within specified doses and duration in the elderly.

Polypharmacy has many definitions. But for practical purposes it is the unwanted duplication of drugs that often results when patients go to multiple pharmacies and physicians. It is implicated in the ADRs that occur whenever five to ten drugs are taken by the same person."[27] Concerns over the existence of polypharmacy are well documented. For example, complications of heart failure are likely to rise because there is an unusually large number of drugs prescribed for someone with heart failure. Furthermore, polypharmacy is a "disease simulator" in that patients may exhibit conditions induced by medications rather than by pathological processes.[28] These are reasons why reducing the frequency of polypharmacy has become a goal of the Healthy People 2010 initiative.[29]

Polypharmacy may be necessary in special need cases when it is supported by expert consensus panels, treatment algorithms, or national guidelines. Examples of "legitimate polypharmacy" are found in some treatment regimens advocated for mental illnesses, hypertension, and cancer. However, the experts generally agree that when polypharmacy does exist, it is dangerous and costly. But when polypharmacy can be reduced, it normally creates a better outcome for the patient. Since the number of medications is reduced, the potential for drug interactions and other harmful events is reduced. For example, it was found that when the average number of medications was reduced from 13.1 to 8.2 in an elderly population receiving more than 10 medications, their hospitalization rates and deaths were reduced by about one-third. Interestingly, the medications removed/reduced the most in this study were the patients' vitamins. As it turned out, the elderly in this study found it easier to take vitamins rather than their prescribed drugs, such as angiotensin-converting enzyme (ACE) inhibitors for treating heart failure.[30]

No matter how many medications the elderly may be taking, fewer is always better than more. The general rule from experts is to classify the elderly at high risk from polypharmacy if they are taking more than 9 medications per day or if they must adhere to a regimen that involves 12 or more doses per day.[31]

One way for a pharmacist to help an elderly patient reduce the risk of polypharmacy and find a safer level of medication use is to maintain a complete medication history. Such a drug history can be of great benefit when it contains all prescribed medicines and also includes topical medications; eye, ear, and nose drops; vitamins; other dietary supplements; herbals; nonprescription medications; and home remedies. While patients may have several sources for obtaining prescriptions and advice on nonprescription medications and other products, there is a trend for most to patronize only one pharmacy.

5. **℞ I or <u>Identify</u> high-risk elderly while improving their adherence to medication regimens.**

The U.S. Chamber of Commerce estimates that about one-half of all prescriptions in the United States are taken incorrectly, which in turn has led to a therapeutic failure rate of 30%–50%.[32] The elderly are often at high risk for nonadherent behavior due to a combination of factors ranging from age-related memory loss to economic issues to complex medication regimens. Medication nonadherence can be intentional or unintentional. Medication nonadherence most often appears as failure to have the prescription filled, underdosing, overdosing, improper timing of medication, missing a dose, or prematurely terminating the therapy. Identifying the elderly at risk for these behaviors takes work, and that work is further complicated when patients see more than one physician. However, if a pharmacist or health professional asks the elderly patient how he or she takes each medication at the time when refills are requested, this simple question could engage the patient in dialogue that could help reverse nonadherence.

The five most common reasons cited for nonadherent medication behavior are:

- Fear of side effects.
- Disbelief in the medication's benefits.
- Difficulty in incorporating the regimen into a daily schedule.
- Fear of becoming dependent on the medication.
- Cost of the medication.

In fact, nonadherence is higher among patients who believe their medicines are expensive.[33] Failing vision, poor packaging of medications, and impaired manual dexterity to open medication containers also play a role in medication nonadherence. Being vigilant to non-adherence is something health professionals should adopt and with it the perspective that medication nonadherence is costly and trouble-some for society and the elderly. For example, 11.4% of patients admit-ted to an acute care hospital were admitted because of nonadherent behavior.[34]

6. R N or <u>Never</u> forget the age-related changes that affect drug dynamics of absorption, distribution, metabolism, and excretion.

Any health professional who wants to help with medication use in the elderly should begin by learning how physiological, pharmacokinetic, and pharmacodynamic changes that occur in this population affect drug responses. Understanding and appreciating the wide variations in drug responses that occur in the elderly, be they a "very fit old person" or a "very frail old person," go a long way toward designing and suggesting an appropriate intervention. The involved health pro-fessional also knows his/her role is to serve as the patient's advocate by keeping a watchful eye over medications that have a very narrow therapeutic index. For example, the patient's altered pharmacokinetics often lead to an altered sensitivity to medications such as anticonvul-sants or Lanoxin®.

Examples of altered pharmacokinetics affecting drug responses are numerous. While drug absorption may be relatively unchanged in the elderly, drug distribution is very much changed. Distribution of a drug throughout the body of an elderly person is affected by decreases in lean body mass and total body water and by increases in total body fat and a small decrease in plasma albumin.

These changes all affect distribution of lipid-soluble drugs and water-soluble drugs. Drug metabolism is affected by enzyme-induc-ing agents or environmental factors, and drug excretion is profoundly affected by age-related changes in the renal system. For example, drug interactions in the elderly become of particular concern when two or more drugs are competing for the same renal or hepatic elimination sites.

7. R G or <u>Generate</u> a complete drug history to document care, to follow-up, and to track outcomes of any recommendation or intervention.

There is an old caveat in health care: if something is not written down, it did not happen. Physicians, nurses, physician assistants, and almost all other care providers are taught to generate records of the care they provide. Only recently has this type of training become popular to document what pharmacists do in helping with drug therapy beyond the dispensing function. Throughout the United States, the need for accurate, accessible, and shareable health information is great, yet illegible handwriting and other documentation practices that diminish the quality of health care continue unabated. The lack of standardization and transferability of health information is being addressed, but it still influences:

- **Patient safety:** inadequate information, illegible entries, misinterpretations, and insufficient information cause teamwork to falter and a noncaring work atmosphere to prevail.
- **Continuity of patient care:** there is a diminished amount of sharing of information among care providers.
- **Health system policies and procedures:** those in the health care system who make policy decisions or conduct research to improve practice behaviors are hampered in doing so because information capture and report generation have become costly and prohibitive due to lack of standardization.

Health care documentation is considered to have two parts: information capture and report generation. Information capture is the process of recording representations of human thought, perceptions, or actions in documenting patient care, as well as device-generated information that is gathered and/or computed about a patient as part of health care. Typical means for information capture are handwriting, speaking, typing, touching a screen, or pointing and clicking on words, phrases, etc. Report generation, or the construction of a health care document (paper or digital), consists of the formatting and/or structuring of captured information. It is the process of analyzing, organizing, and presenting recorded patient information for authentication and inclusion in the patient's health care record. Thus, the documentation challenge for those involved in medication interventions affecting the elderly is to find a means to standardize information capture. This remains a daunting task given the variation in today's proprietary software, yet the need is great for sharing health information among a few types of health practitioners who could use common formats to do so. This need is especially thwarted by inadequate documentation, illegible handwriting, and the use of technical jargon. Thus, it would behoove all practitioners involved in care of the elderly to at least talk with each other and come to some agreement as to what uniform documentation they would accept, even if it is only on a local level, and especially if they want to get paid for the service.

THE ELDERLY, THEIR MEDICATION COSTS, AND MEDICARE PART D

Few options are available to those health professionals who try to help their elderly patients with medication costs. Available options include:

- Obtain samples from a manufacturer's representative.
- Enroll the elderly person in a Patient Assistance Program (PAP); PAPs are offered directly by most major manufacturers.
- Send the patient to a web site that may prove helpful.
- Enroll the patient in a clinical trial.
- Help the patient enroll in the Medicare Part D program, assuming the elderly patient has no pharmacy benefit as a carryover from an employer's group health plan.

Medicare was brought into existence in the mid-1960s to help the elderly with the cost of, and access to, health care. Little about it has changed over 40 years except that the politicians who have responsibility for it have increased entitlements and benefits, and they have allowed an increase in payouts that has left Medicare on a shaky financial footing. The Medicare program did not include an outpatient prescription benefit until December 2003. At that time, President George W. Bush signed into law the Medicare Modernization and Improvement Act. This legislation added an elective prescription benefit for seniors called Medicare Part D (i.e., D for drugs) to the Medicare benefit package.

The law went into effect in January 2006 amid much controversy about its complexity, and a poor understanding of what its costs might be—although the government did estimate its costs over the first 10 years at $720 billion[35]—and with 43 million Medicare beneficiaries having access to new coverage for outpatient prescription drugs.[36]

In January 2006, private organizations began contracting with the Centers for Medicare and Medicaid Services (CMS) to offer Medicare beneficiaries a number of prescription drug plans. Some plans are a "stand-alone" prescription-drug-only program and some are Medicare Advantage combinations (i.e., Medicare Part A, Medicare Part B, or Medicare Part D).

Of interest to all health professionals is the result of a recent poll in which seniors were asked, "Where would you turn for help with understanding Medicare's Part D prescription plan?" Respondents cited their physician as their number one choice[37] despite the many dollars that were spent for TV and newspaper ads asking people to come into a pharmacy for such advice. In 2006, if an elderly individual has an existing drug benefit plan offered by an employer (past or present), they are able to opt out of the Medicare Part D program. However, if that plan is not "creditable" by Medicare standards, they must enroll in Medicare Part D or risk paying a penalty sum that will forever be added to their monthly premiums. (For details on how a privately insured patient will be affected, the patient should obtain a notice from their current private insurance company that informs them if their policy covers as much or more than a Medicare prescription drug plan.) Persons eligible for full benefits, including prescription drugs, under a state Medicaid program, will automatically be switched to the Medicare Part D plan as Medicaid drug coverage is eliminated and the beneficiaries are randomly assigned to a local prescription drug plan (PDP).

Once Medicare enrollees are in a plan, many likely will need assistance. To stay with the plan and its formulary, they may have to switch medications and/or brands. Until Medicare Part D has been in existence for a few years, they will need help understanding the operational details of these prescription plans. By 2009, the legislation that brought forth Medicare Part D is also expected to mandate electronic prescribing to reduce the cost and burden of medication errors. Medicare Part D is destined to be a topic of discussion among the elderly, their caregivers, and their health care providers until the plan is simplified and well woven into the fabric of American health care.

Of special interest to pharmacists is that their involvement in helping the elderly enrolled in a Medicare Part D plan has the potential for payment under a provision in the Plan D legislation. Beginning in 2006, the law defines medication therapy management (MTM) services and states that such services are designed to ensure that medications covered by Medicare are appropriately used to optimize therapeutic outcomes through improved medication use and to reduce the risk of adverse events, including drug interactions. The Medicare beneficiaries targeted by the MTM program are those with multiple chronic conditions, multiple medications, and high costs, about 80% of Medicare beneficaries.[38,39]

The law further states that each of the individual drug plans may determine fees and contracts associated with a range of such services designed to improve the safety and efficacy of drug therapy and which may include pharmacists and other providers delivering them. MTM services are a "distinct service or group of services that optimize therapeutic outcomes for individual patients and that are independent, but they can occur in conjunction with the provision of a medication product."[40]

To maximize or optimize the challenges associated with providing these new services to the elderly, a number of barriers have to be overcome:

- The physical barriers that exist in a pharmacy that hinder private consultation with the elderly.
- The lack of training many pharmacists have in geriatrics.
- The myriad of barriers that keep a team of health professionals from working collaboratively.

The Medicare Part D option to pay for medication therapy management for the elderly does not exclude any professional from becoming a part of that system.[41] While pharmacists could benefit greatly from how Medicare Part D could redefine their profession, their compensation, and their professional standing, there are no assurances they will seize this opportunity or leave it to others. However, the success of the Medicare Part D program will be critically dependent upon them.

KEY POINTS

- Medication therapy management or interventions in the therapy of the elderly are not simple, but simple interventions work better than none.
- Most interventions will take initiative and patience and will involve not only the elderly, but also their caregivers and families, and especially other health professionals.
- One health professional cannot possibly do all that is needed, but one health professional can make a huge difference by trying.
- Figure 1 illustrates the various forces at work; each is distinct and each must be working optimally if the elderly are ever to get the best use of their medications.

REFERENCES

1. Moser M. Hypertension treatment and the prevention of coronary heart disease in the elderly. *Am. Fam Physician.* March 1 1999;59(5): http://www.aafp.org/afp/1990301 ap/1248.html (accessed February 7, 2006).

2. Amery A, Birkenhager W, Brixko P, et al. Mortality and morbidity results from the European Working Party on High Blood Pressure in the Elderly trial. *Lancet.* 1985;1 (8442):1348–54.

3. Moser M, Grellet C, Okin P, et al. Long-term management of hypertension; II. Private practice experience. *NY State J Med.* 1980;80(7 Pt 1):1102–6.

4. Phillips RA, Kostis JB. Treatment of octogenarians: should we and how? *J Clin Hypertens.* 2004;6(5):267–73.

5. Strand LM, Morley PC, Cipolle RJ, et al. Drug related problems: their structure and function. *DICP.* 1990;24(11):1093–7.

6. Rochon PA, Gurwitz JH. Drug therapy. *Lancet.* 1995;346:32–6.

7. Rochon PA, Gurwitz JH. Optimising drug treatment for elderly people: the prescribing cascade. *BMJ.* 1997;315(7115):1096–9.

8. Anderson RM. Is the problem of noncompliance all in our heads? *Diabetes Educ.* 1985;11:31–4.

9. Pratt CC, Simonson W, Lloyd S. Pharmacists' perceptions of major difficulties in geriatric pharmacy practice. *Gerontologist.* 1982;22(3):288–92.

10. Greenland P. What if the patient were your mother? *Arch Intern Med.* 2005;165(6): 607–8.

11. Smedley BD, Stith AY, Nelson AR. *Unequal Treatment: Confronting Racial and Ethnic Disparities in Healthcare.* Washington, DC: National Academy Press; 2003.

12. Healthy Life Expectancy 2002. World Health Organization. http://www3.who.int/whosis/hale/hale/cfm?path=whosis,burden_statistics,hale&language=english (accessed January 5, 2006).

13. Proceedings, medication use systems—recommendations. *Am J Health Syst Pharm.* 2000;57:582–3.

14. Williams BR. Avoiding medication mishaps, a pharmacist's perspective. *Geriatric Times* (1) 1, May/June 2000: http://wwwgeriatrictimes.com/g000634.html (accessed on January 7, 2006).

15. Lim WS, Low HN, Chan SP, et al. Impact of a pharmacist consult clinic on a hospital-based geriatric outpatient clinic in Singapore. *Ann Acad Med Singapore.* 2004; 33(2):220–7.

16. Kohn LT, Corrigan JM, Donaldson MS. *To Err is Human, Building a Safer Health System.* Washington, DC: National Academy Press, 2000.

17. Simon SR, Gurwitz JH. Drug therapy in the elderly: improving quality and access. *Clin Pharmacol Ther.* 2003;73(5):387–93.

18. Beers MH. Explicit criteria for determining potentially inappropriate medication use by the elderly. *Arch Intern Med.* 1997;157(4):1531–6.

19. Beers MH, Ouslander JG, Fingold SF, et al. Inappropriate medication prescribing in skilled-nursing facilities. *Arch Intern Med.* 1992;117(8):684–9.

20. Beers MH, Ouslander JG, Rollingher I, et al. Explicit criteria for determining inappropriate medication use in nursing home residents. *Arch Intern Med.* 1991;151(9): 1825–32.

21. Fick DM, Cooper JW, Wade WE, et al. Updating the Beers criteria for potentially inappropriate medication use in older adults: results of a U.S. consensus panel of experts. *Arch Intern Med.* 2003;163(22):2716–24.

22. Aparasu RR, Sitzman S. Inappropriate prescribing for elderly outpatients. *Am J Health Syst Pharm.* 1999;56(5):433–9.

23. Zahn C, Sangl J, Bierman AS, et al. Potentially inappropriate medication use in the community-dwelling elderly: findings from the 1996 Medical Expenditure Panel survey. *JAMA.* 2001;286(22):2823–9.

24. Leipzig RM, Cumming RG, Tinetti ME. Drugs and falls in older people: a systematic review and meta-analysis: I. psychotropic drugs. *J Am Geriatr Soc.* 1999; 47:30–9.

25. Goulding MR. Inappropriate medication prescribing for elderly ambulatory care patients. *Arch Intern Med.* 2004;164(3):305–12.

26. Simon SR, Chan KA, Soumerai SB, et al. Potentially inappropriate medication use by elderly persons in U.S. Health Maintenance Organizations, 2000-2001. *J Am Geriatr Soc.* 2005;53(2):227–32.

27. Wick JY. Avoiding polypharmacy pitfalls: it's all in your approach. *Pharm Times.* 2006;72(1):40–2.

28. LeSage J. Polypharmacy in geriatric patients. *Nurs Clin North Am.* 1991; 26(2):273–90.

29. *Healthy People 2000: National Health Promotion and Disease Prevention Objectives.* Washington, DC: U.S. Public Health Service; 2000.

30. Farrell VM, Hill VL, Hawkins JB, et al. Clinic for identifying and addressing polypharmacy. *Am J Health Syst Pharm.* 2003;60(18):1830–5.

31. Morley JE. Conundrums of polypharmacy. *Aging Successfully.* (summer 2003);13(2):1–7.

32. Berg JS, Dischler J, Wagner DJ, et al. Medication compliance: a healthcare problem. *Ann Pharmacother.* 1993;27(9 suppl):S1–24.

33. Smith DL. The effect of patient noncompliance on healthcare costs. *Med Interface.* 1993;6(4):74–84.

34. Col N, Fanale JE, Kronholm P. The role of medication noncompliance and adverse drug reactions in hospitalizations of the elderly. *Arch Intern Med.* 1990;150(4):841–5.

35. Lueck S. Drug benefit cost put at $720 billion for first ten years. *Wall Street Journal.* 2005 February 9;Sect D:5.

36. Kostick J. Counseling patients on the new medicare drug plan, *Medscape Pharmacists.* 2005; 6(2): http://www.medscape.com/viewarticle/513887 (accessed December 15, 2005).

37. Kaiser Family Foundation. March/April 2005 Health Poll Report Survey. Henry J. Kaiser Family Foundation; Menlo Park, CA; April 2005: http://www.kff.org/kaiserpolls/upload/march-april-2005-kaiser-health-poll-report-toplines.pdf (accessed December 15, 2005).

38. ASHP Medicare Modernization Act Resource Center: http://www.ashp.org/medicare/mtm.cfm (accessed March 15, 2006).

39. Center for Medicare and Medicaid Services, Public Law 108-73: http://www.cms.hhs.gov/MMA Update/01overview.asp (accessed March 15, 2006).

40. CMS Finalizes Part D Regulations. American Society of Health-System Pharmacists: http://www.ashp.org/news/ShowArticle.cfm?id=9534 (accessed February 15, 2006).

41. Medication Therapy Management Services Definition and Program Criteria. American Association of Colleges of Pharmacy. http://www.aacp.org/Docs/MainNavigation/Resources/6308_MTMServicesDefinitionandProgramCriteria27-Jul-04.pdf (accessed February 15, 2006).

Index

Page numbers followed by the letter "t" designate tables; page numbers in *italics* designate figures.